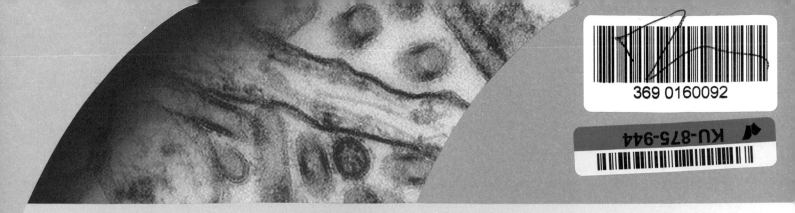

Essentials of Infectious Disease Epidemiology

Manya Magnus, PhD, MPH

George Washington University
School of Public Health and Health Services
Department of Epidemiology and Biostatistics
Washington, D.C.

JONES AND BARTLETT PUBLISHERS
Sudbury, Massachusetts
BOSTON   TORONTO   LONDON   SINGAPORE

World Headquarters

Jones and Bartlett Publishers
40 Tall Pine Drive
Sudbury, MA 01776
978-443-5000
info@jbpub.com
www.jbpub.com

Jones and Bartlett Publishers
Canada
6339 Ormindale Way
Mississauga, Ontario
L5V 1J2
CANADA

Jones and Bartlett Publishers
International
Barb House, Barb Mews
London W6 7PA
United Kingdom

Jones and Bartlett's books and products are available through most bookstores and online booksellers. To contact Jones and Bartlett Publishers directly, call 800-832-0034, fax 978-443-8000, or visit our website www.jbpub.com.

Substantial discounts on bulk quantities of Jones and Bartlett's publications are available to corporations, professional associations, and other qualified organizations. For details and specific discount information, contact the special sales department at Jones and Bartlett via the above contact information or send an email to specialsales@jbpub.com.

This publication is designed to provide accurate and authoritative information in regard to the subject matter covered. It is sold with the understanding that the publisher is not engaged in rendering legal, accounting, or other professional service. If legal advice or other expert assistance is required, the service of a competent professional person should be sought.

Production Credits
Publisher: Michael Brown
Associate Editor: Katey Birtcher
Production Director: Amy Rose
Production Editor: Tracey Chapman
Marketing Manager: Sophie Fleck
Manufacturing Buyer: Therese Connell
Composition: Auburn Associates, Inc.
Cover Design: Kristin E. Ohlin
Cover Image: © CDC/Courtesy of Cynthia Goldsmith, Jacqueline Katz, and Sherif R. Zaki
Printing and Binding: Malloy, Inc.
Cover Printing: John Pow Company

Library of Congress Cataloging-in-Publication Data
Magnus, Manya.
  Essentials of infectious disease epidemiology / Manya Magnus.
     p. ; cm.
  Includes bibliographical references and index.
  ISBN-13: 978-0-7637-3444-2 (pbk.)
  ISBN-10: 0-7637-3444-6 (pbk.)
  1. Communicable diseases—Epidemiology. I. Title.
  [DNLM: 1. Communicable Diseases—epidemiology. 2. Epidemiologic Methods. WC 100 M212e 2007]
  RA643.M33 2007
  362.196'9—dc22
                          2007010527
  6048

Printed in the United States of America
11 10 09 08 07   10 9 8 7 6 5 4 3 2 1

Dedication

For Magus, Hero, & Gryphon Magnus
with love and with gratitude

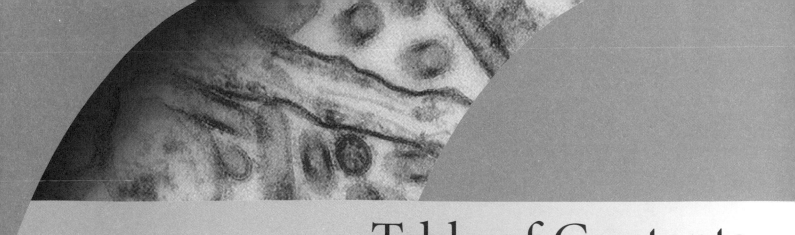

Table of Contents

Acknowledgments

The chance to write a textbook does not present itself every day, and it is a rare honor to develop a work that will go into the hands and minds of students of public health and epidemiology. For this I thank Mike Brown at Jones and Bartlett, Inc., as well as Katey Birtcher, Tracey Chapman, and the wonderful production crew at Jones and Bartlett. I appreciate their giving me the opportunity to write this text, and for believing in the importance of public health education. I also thank Dr. Richard Riegelman, the series editor, who provided me with the opportunity to share in his passion for educating undergraduate and introductory students in public health; without his ongoing encouragement and input, this book would not be a reality. To my students, colleagues, and friends who were supportive and helpful in reviewing and commenting upon the text, a heartfelt thanks to you for helping this to be a better book. I am indebted to the authors of books, research, and articles who have taught me so much, especially to those who created the vast number of resources available through the Centers for Disease Control and Prevention, Health Resources Services Administration, and the National Institutes of Health, without which many of the vivid examples would not be accessible.

To my family, never-ending are my thanks for your love and support.

To you, kind reader, I am hopeful that when you use this text, you feel the thrill of methods in infectious disease epidemiology—and see the vast potential to improve the public health through creative application of the epidemiologic toolkit.

In loving memory of my grandmother, Dr. Ida Russakoff Hoos, 1912–2007.

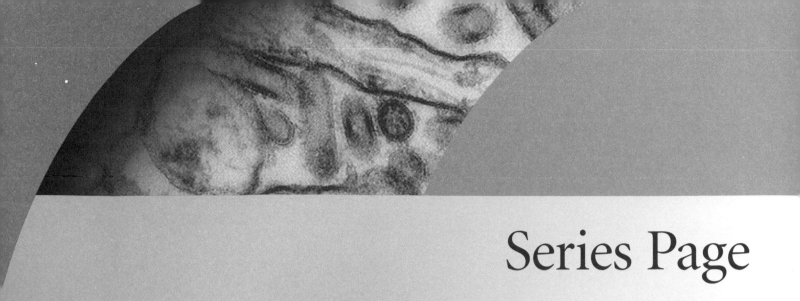

Series Page

See **www.jbpub.com/essentialpublichealth** for the latest information on the series.

ABOUT THE EDITOR:

Richard Riegalman, MD, MPH, PhD, is professor of Epidemiology-Biostatistics, Medicine, and Health Policy and founding dean at George Washington University School of Public Health and Health Services in Washington, DC.

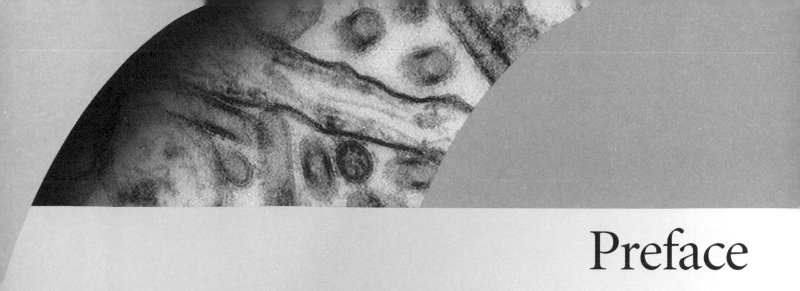

Preface

I hope to have written the book I always wanted to study, but could never find:

One that provides methodologic training going beyond jargon, beyond complexity, to find the simple utility that epidemiology offers. The toolkit that epidemiology provides is powerful, yet sometimes can be lost in its detail. The goal of this text is to find the essential core of the methods, and then see them applied to examples from real-life public health and research.

The layout of this book is designed to mimic your own notebooks: lecture notes in the middle, applied notes in the boxes. This format will enable you to know where to look for the information you need at all times, and simplify assimilation of this powerful methodology.

Epidemiologic methods offer a unique approach to answering questions and dissecting relationships between exposures and outcomes. This text applies these methods to infectious disease, one of the most important public health issues we face today.

I hope that this book excites you and serves as an impetus for future learning. As we evolve, we need epidemiologists who can address emerging and re-emerging infections with creativity and enthusiasm more than ever before.

—Manya Magnus, PhD, MPH

About the Author

Manya Magnus, PhD, MPH, is an Associate Professor in the Department of Epidemiology and Biostatistics, with a secondary appointment in the Department of Health Policy, at the George Washington University School of Public Health and Health Services. Dr. Magnus is co-director of the School's MPH Epidemiology Program and co-director of the Graduate Certificate in HIV/AIDS Studies. Dr. Magnus received her BA from the University of California, San Diego, and her MPH and PhD from Tulane University. Always interested in integrating research with clinical care, Dr. Magnus has collaborated on a variety of epidemiologic studies, including randomized controlled clinical trials, cohort studies, and case-control studies. She now applies epidemiologic methodology to evaluate programs on the local, state, and national level, including CDC-sponsored behavioral surveillance, and Special Projects of National Significance funded by the HIV/AIDS Bureau of the Health Services Resources Administration. Dr. Magnus also participates in a variety of other HIV- and STD-related research activities. The primary focus of her research is HIV/AIDS among women, children, adolescents, and other vulnerable populations, and includes clinical trials, observational studies, and innovative approaches to evaluation research. She also has a side interest in maternal-child health, specifically infertility and decision-making behavior among pregnant women.

Prologue: Essentials of Infectious Disease Epidemiology

If you want to learn to think like an epidemiologist, *Essentials of Infectious Disease Epidemiology* opens the door, turns on the lights, and leads you on the journey. It teaches you to read the scientific literature as well as the daily news. It provides an introduction to the key methods and the essential questions addressed by epidemiology.

To understand the uniqueness of *Essentials of Infectious Disease Epidemiology* you need to appreciate what it is not. It is not a textbook of infectious disease. It is not a textbook of statistical methods. It is not another textbook of epidemiology. Rather, it is as Dr. Magnus writes, the book "I always wanted to study but could never find."

Infectious diseases, for better or worse, represent much of the history as well as the future of public health. Understanding the methods used to investigate their cause and their impact provides an important window on issues of health and disease. *Essentials of Infectious Disease Epidemiology* emphases what is sometimes called "shoe leather" epidemiology. These are basic methods used by epidemiologists who roll up their sleeves, collect the data directly from the affected community, and analyze the data without the need for the latest high-powered computer or statistical technique.

In exploring infectious disease epidemiology, you will ask the basic question such as the *who, when,* and *where* of an outbreak or epidemic. You will come to appreciate what we mean when we say a particular bug or pathogen is the *cause* of a disease. You will understand what is implied when we say that a vaccine or treatment *works*. You will learn to ask the basic questions, think about the methods for answering the questions, and appreciate the meaning of the results.

As editor of the Essential Public Health series, I am delighted to have *Essentials of Infectious Disease Epidemiology* included in our series. It captures the spirit of the series by providing an approachable and engaging introduction. It provides a solid grounding and important insights plus the motivation and resources to continue the journey. The Reader to accompany *Essentials of Infectious Disease Epidemiology* will provide the types of resources needed to help you continue on your way to applying what you have learned.

And now to quote Dr. Magnus: "Let the fun begin."

Richard Riegelman, MD, MPH, PhD
Series Editor—Essential Public Health

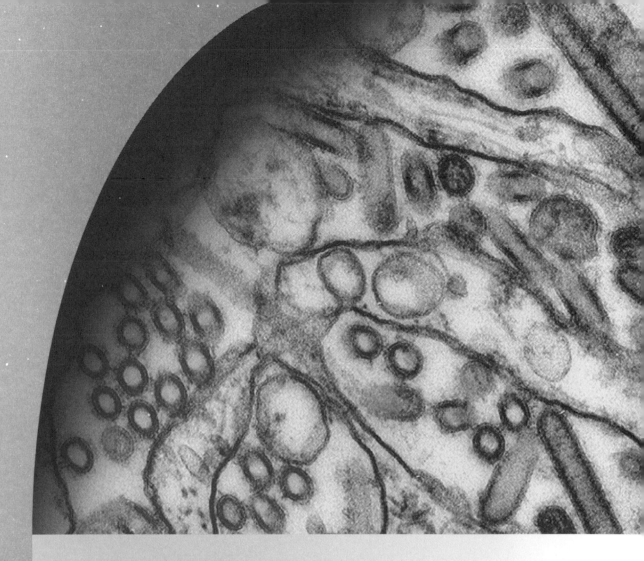

PART I

Background of the Field

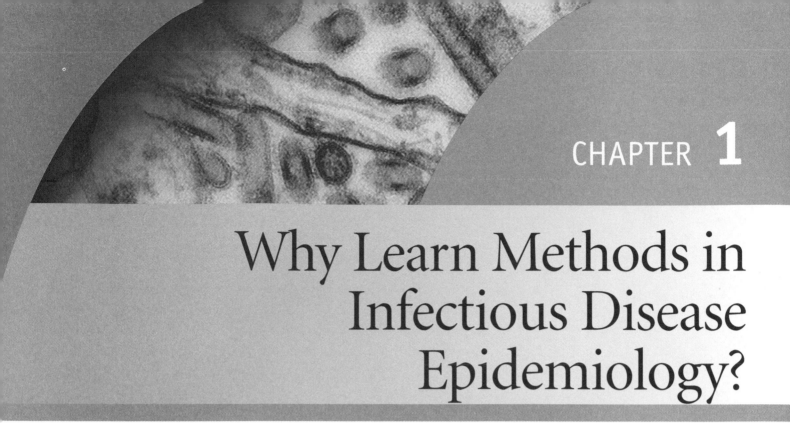

CHAPTER 1

Why Learn Methods in Infectious Disease Epidemiology?

"It is time to close the book on infectious diseases, declare the war against pestilence won, and shift national resources to such chronic problems as cancer and heart disease."

—U.S. Surgeon General William H. Stewart, 1967[1]

"We are standing on the brink of a global crisis in infectious diseases. No country is safe from them. No country can any longer afford to ignore their threat."

—Hiroshi Nakajima, Director-General of the World Health Organization (WHO), 1996[2]

In the four decades since U.S. Surgeon General Stewart declared the book closed on them, we have seen a dramatic and serious increase in infectious diseases, following a period of steep decline (Figure 1-1). In addition to emerging diseases, such as human immunodeficiency virus/acquired immunodeficiency syndrome (HIV/AIDS), severe acute respiratory syndrome (SARS), Lyme disease, Hantavirus, and Ebola hemorrhagic fever,[3–9] we have diseases once cured that have become resistant to our treatments. These include those that we felt confident in our ability to cure, such as bacterial infections.[1,10–17] We have increasingly harmful foodborne conta-

gions occurring in outbreaks that occur with alarming frequency, such as *Escherichia coli* O157:H7.[4,10,11,18] And we have sexually transmitted diseases such as *Chlamydia trachomatis*[9] in epidemic proportions worldwide. Waiting in the wings we have diseases such as Avian flu (H5N1),[19–26] which are on the brink of causing a threat to global health even as we seek methods for their control and risk reduction. Following decades of decline in mortality from infectious diseases, marking significant public health achievement, some of our accomplishments are becoming eroded (Figure 1-2). As WHO Director-General Nakajima says of infectious disease, "No country is safe from them."[2]

For many people, infectious disease is the primary impetus for joining a public health program. There is wide interest in the field—as well as increasing awareness of infectious disease that has accompanied increase awareness of bioterrorism. The importance of and visceral attention to these worldwide changes have created substantial interest in infectious disease epidemiology. Infectious disease epidemiology is engaging and exciting, carrying with it a unique importance. It provides multiple pathways to make an impact on public health. The infectious disease epidemiologist can contribute to the health of populations through work in the field, with local departments of health, health-related industries, research, and government. As undergraduate and introductory public health programs proliferate to meet the needs of the public health workforce,[27–29] so, too, does the need for methodological skills in infectious disease epidemiology. Without these crucial skills, there will be insufficient resources to improve the health of the public, both domestically and globally.

FIGURE 1-1 Crude death rate for infectious diseases—United States, 1900–1996

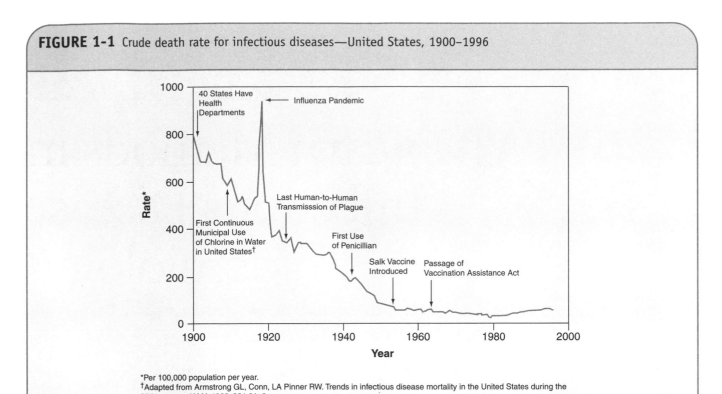

*Per 100,000 population per year.
†Adapted from Armstrong GL, Conn, LA Pinner RW. Trends in infectious disease mortality in the United States during the 20th century. JAMA 1999: 281:61–6.

Tremendous public health strides were made during the last century, most of them in the realm of infectious diseases. In addition to increased awareness and education, access to clean water, improved hygiene, and vaccines to prevent illness, the last century saw the advent of penicillin, marking a new era in public health.

Source: Adapted from Armstrong GL, Conn LA, Pinner RW. Trends in infectious disease mortality in the United States during the 20th century. *JAMA* 1999;281:61–6.

There are several very good books on infectious disease epidemiology aimed at clinicians and advanced students[30–32]; these books have been my teachers, along with the wealth of articles in the peer-reviewed literature. However, there are few texts devoted specifically to the foundational methods required to study infectious disease—those that marry traditional epidemiologic core methods with an infectious disease area of emphasis on a basic level. This book is intended for undergraduate public health students, introductory masters-level public health students, and readers with an interest in infectious disease epidemiology. The goal is to provide you with a methodological scaffolding on which you may later overlay in-depth content area study.

The purpose of this text is to provide readers with a solid foundation in the epidemiologic methods necessary for studying infectious disease. Like all areas of concentration within epidemiology, infectious disease has a unique set of methods for its study, as well as special considerations in the application of standard epidemiologic methods to it. Upon studying *Essentials of Infectious Disease Epidemiology,* readers will be able to:

- Apply epidemiologic methods to the context of infectious disease.
- Critically evaluate the infectious disease literature.
- Understand basic study designs and procedures for evaluating infectious diseases in a variety of settings.
- Conduct introductory-level data analysis of infectious disease data.
- Comfortably enter a masters-level course in infectious disease epidemiology.
- Confidently work in a public health or research setting focused on infectious disease.

This is a methods based text, ideally paired with a more advanced and/or context-based text such as *Infectious Disease Epidemiology*[30] or other available resources that focus on clinical and biological facets of infectious disease. With the many

FIGURE 1-2 Rate of infectious disease mortality, by year—United States, 1900–1996

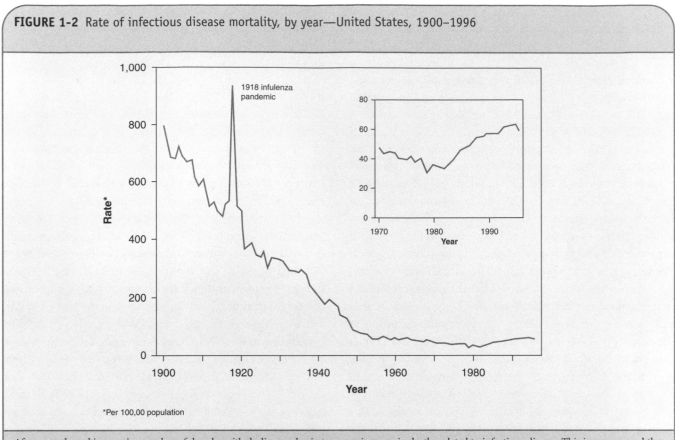

*Per 100,00 population

After a steady and impressive number of decades with decline, we begin to see an increase in deaths related to infectious disease. This increase—and the changes we are currently experiencing in known and unknown pathogens increases the need for skilled epidemiologists who have the skills to rapidly address community needs.

Source: Adapted from Armstrong GL, Conn LA, Pinner RW. Trends in infectious disease mortality in the United States during the 20th century. *JAMA* 1999;281:61–6.

changing diseases and environmental impacts on infectious disease, we cannot possibly know the future of every infectious disease. Most readers do not need an exhaustive knowledge of diseases known to date. Rather, they need to have the skills required to study them and to develop and evaluate public health interventions to address current and yet-to-be-discovered diseases. This book's approach provides the reader with methodological skills that can be readily applied in their professional settings or while pursuing more advanced coursework. Instead of provision of facts and figures to memorize that one later forgets or that become outdated given the rapidly changing times and dynamic public health environment, the goal of this text is to impress upon the reader the methodological skill set unique to studying infectious diseases. Alongside the methods, real-life research and public health examples help integrate the skills.

WHY IS INFECTIOUS DISEASE EPIDEMIOLOGY DIFFERENT FROM OTHER APPLICATIONS OF EPIDEMIOLOGY?

Epidemiology is a toolkit of methods used to answer questions and relate exposures to outcomes. As many conditions and problems as there are in public health—cancer, infectious diseases, environmental exposures, chronic diseases, cardiovascular diseases, promotion of maternal-child health, global and domestic public health issues, and more—epidemiologic tools are an effective way of identifying the problems and assessing the efficacy of solutions. Familiarity with the basic epidemiologic designs is the foundation. Each disease condition or category of exposure has its own "culture" of application of tools, grown out of its unique challenges. For example, within the area of environmental epidemiology, exposure assessment is a key concern. In cardiovascular disease, the long-term, often-subtle, and asymptomatic nature of hypertension (high blood pressure), for example, brings particular methods into focus by making different techniques necessary. For example, identifying and measuring often asymptomatic conditions offers challenges. In epidemiology implemented through applied studies, identification of the appropriate conceptual framework and understanding of the social mores of the target population are essential.

In infectious disease epidemiology, we wrestle with countless heterogeneous organisms. Some cause acute disease, some chronic. Some begin acute and become chronic. Some infectious organisms have little effect in and of themselves, but later cause cancer. There is enormous variety of biologic characteristics that our designs must not only understand, but also know how to study correctly: these include a range of times between exposure and illness, symptomatic and asymptomatic conditions, diseases that require immediate control and those that we are unable to control, and those that we know about and those we do not. Infectious diseases may be contracted in multiple fashions: person-to-person, through needles, exposure to droplets, through sex, from water, from food, and from animals or insects. To handle this variety, epidemiologists generally specialize not only in the field of infectious disease, but also in a specific disease itself—or even a specific disease within a specific population within a specific geographical location. This book on methodological applications in infectious disease epidemiology is intended to assist the reader in learning how to approach infectious diseases, be the detective that one needs to be in order to successfully identify a causal agent and control it, and know how to handle new infectious diseases that will inevitably emerge. Infectious disease is not something that will go away or that we will ever be able to completely eradicate. The more people—in academia, public health, scientists as well as non-scientists—who know about and understand the issues at hand and how to study them, the more people will be capable of noticing and hopefully stopping epidemics before they start.

HOW TO USE THIS BOOK

Readers do not need prior experience with epidemiology in order to learn from this book. The focus is on methods peculiar to infectious disease research, so students who have taken introductory and/or intermediate epidemiology will find the material echoes their methods courses with specific application to disease. Those who have taken clinically-oriented infectious disease courses will find that this book echoes the concepts and content found there, as well as builds a foundation in the methods necessary to study infectious diseases in public health practice. Alongside the narrative, the examples are designed to engage readers as they learn about key issues in infectious disease epidemiology, with an emphasis on methods. The narrative covers methods and core skills (Figure 1-3). The boxes contain examples to help readers integrate the methodological concepts through use. The narrative can be read straight through, in order to focus on the ideas or read alternately with the examples. Those with previous experience in epidemiology may prefer to read through the examples, instead of applying existing knowledge to the real-life examples. The goal of this approach is to facilitate learning by reinforcing the tougher, denser methods with the more lively research and real-life examples. Like your own notebooks, the boxed examples are kept separate from the insides, to maintain clarity throughout the text.

This book distills the vast amount of epidemiologic terms and methods into manageable blocks of information that are

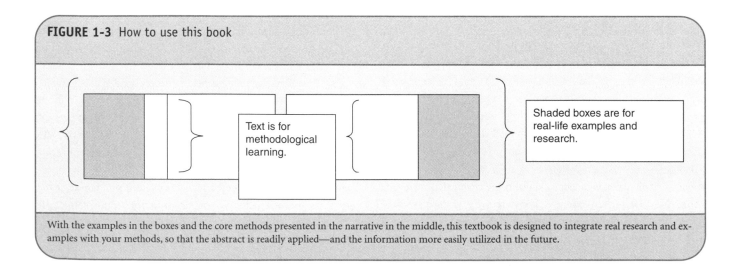

FIGURE 1-3 How to use this book

Text is for methodological learning.

Shaded boxes are for real-life examples and research.

With the examples in the boxes and the core methods presented in the narrative in the middle, this textbook is designed to integrate real research and examples with your methods, so that the abstract is readily applied—and the information more easily utilized in the future.

relatively easy to understand. Through a reduction in jargon (though it is presented so that readers have exposure to it, and can integrate it into their future studies) and technical terms, this textbook will give readers the essence of the methodological skills needed to begin working in the field as well as while reading the scientific literature. Readers should note that this is not a comprehensive text on the biology of infectious disease in general or of the given infections covered in examples throughout the text. It is a methods text, and not a detailed course in study implementation. As such, you will become familiar with the fundamental ways to study infectious diseases epidemiologically, and apply them to your own work. Key concepts that an entry-level epidemiologist needs to have under his or her belt to understand this book are provided, making it useful in tandem with other texts and resources. Chapters in Part I of the text are organized based on a particular study design or topic in infectious disease epidemiology. For chapters on design, the study design is introduced, examples of infectious diseases are provided to illustrate the method and its application, and advantages and limitations of the method are discussed. Additional context-based applications of the method are provided as exercises or datasets available on the website;

discussion questions are provided at the end of each chapter.

In Part II, Special Applications, we explore surveillance, the interface between infectious disease epidemiology and public health and evaluation of public health interventions. Armed with the methods provided in Part I, this section will give the reader familiarity with the more subtle ways in which infectious disease epidemiology methods are encountered in the field.

As with all learning, practice makes the experience richer and more expansive, and the future recall greater. Readers: Do not stop with this book! Extra exercises, reading of the infectious disease literature, and signing up for the publicly available listservs and publications will enrich the reader and expand upon the topics covered in this book. Volunteer, keep apprised of the news, and become involved in the public health settings in your city, state, county, or country. Globally, there is a drastic shortage of public health personnel, in a world filled with emerging, re-emerging, known, and as-yet-unknown diseases. Please take your interest and excitement—which you must have if you have picked up this book—and translate it into activity. Not only might you find a career path where you did not know one existed, you might help—with your infectious disease epidemiologic skills—in ways you never knew you could.

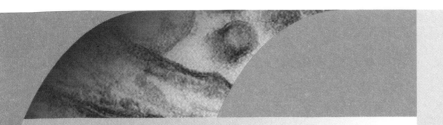

Discussion Questions

1. What emerging or re-emerging infectious diseases have you been aware of in your lifetime? Were you aware of any of the following when first identified:
   a. The first AIDS cases
   b. Toxic shock syndrome related to tampon usage
   c. West Nile Virus
   d. Anthrax
   e. SARS
   f. Avian flu cases in humans
   g. Others

2. What were your first reactions to hearing about these infectious disease situations and outbreaks? How did you first hear of them? Conduct a mini-literature search on one of the outbreaks above that you do not remember. See if you can find information about the first cases, where they were, the characteristics of the first cases, how they were discovered, and what was done to stop the spread of the disease.

REFERENCES

1. Nelson R. Antibiotic development pipeline runs dry. *Lancet.* 2003;362: 1726–1727.

2. Nakajima D-GH. Infectious diseases kill over 17 million people a year: WHO warns of global crisis. 1996. Available at: http://www.who.int/whr/ 1996/media_centre/press_release/en/print.html. Accessed December 20, 2006.

3. Centers for Disease Control. Lyme disease. *MMWR.* 1982;31(27): 367–368.

4. Centers for Disease Control. Preliminary report: foodborne outbreak of *Escherichia coli* O157:H7 infections from hamburgers—western United States, 1993. *MMWR.* 1993;42:85–86.

5. Bwaka M, Bonnet MJ, Calain P, et al. Ebola hemorrhagic fever in Kikwit, Democratic Republic of the Congo: clinical observations in 103 patients. *J Infect Dis.* 1999;179(Suppl.):S1–S7.

6. Centers for Disease Control. Outbreak of severe acute respiratory syndrome—worldwide, 2003. *MMWR.* 2003;52(11):226–228.

7. Centers for Disease Control. Notice to readers: caution regarding testing for Lyme disease. *MMWR.* 2005;54(5):125.

8. Chapman AS. Diagnosis and management of tickborne rickettsial diseases: Rocky Mountain spotted fever, ehrlichioses, and anaplasmosis—United States. *MMWR.* 2006;55(RR-04):1–27.

9. Joesoef MR, Mosure DJ. Prevalence trends in chlamydial infections among young women entering the national job training program, 1998–2004. *Sex Transm Dis.* 2006;33(9):571–575.

10. Centers for Disease Control. Update: multistate outbreak of *Escherichia coli* O157:H7 infections from hamburgers—Western United States, 1992–1993. *MMWR.* 1993;42(13):258–263.

11. Walford D, Noah N. Emerging infectious diseases—United Kingdom. *Emerg Infect Dis.* 1999;5(2):189–194.

12. Brook I. Antimicrobial management of acute sinusitis: a review of therapeutic recommendations. *Infect Med.* 2002;19:231–237.

13. Bukholm G, Tannæs T, Kjelsberg ABB, Smith-Erichsen N. An outbreak of multidrug-resistant *Pseudomonas aeruginosa* associated with increased risk of patient death in an intensive care unit. *Infect Control Hosp Epidemiol.* 2002;23:441–446.

14. Centers for Disease Control. Pertussis—United States, 1997–2000. *MMWR.* 2002;51:73–76.

15. Centers for Disease Control. Summary of notifiable diseases—United States, 2004. *MMWR.* 2004;53:1–80.

16. Murray JJ, Emparanza P, Lesinskas E, Tawadrous M, Breen JD. Efficacy and safety of a novel, single-dose azitrhomycin microsphere formulation vs. 10 days of levofloxacin for the treatment of acute bacterial sinusitis in adults. *Otolaryngol Head Neck Surg.* 2005;133:194–201.

17. Carnicer-Pont D, Bailey KA, Mason BW, et al. Risk factors for hospital-acquired methicillin-resistant *Staphylococcus aureus* bacteraemia: a case-control study. *Epidemiol Infect.* 2006;134:1167–1173.

18. Devasia RA, Jones TF, Ward J, et al. Endemically acquired foodborne outbreak of enterotoxin-producing *Escherichia coli* serotype O169:H41. *Am J Med.* 2006;119:168.e7–168.e10.

19. Centers for Disease Control. Avian influenza infection in humans (bird flu). Available at: www.pandemicflu.gov. Accessed December 25, 2006.

20. Centers for Disease Control. Pandemics and pandemic threats since 1900. Available at: www.pandemicflu.gov/general/historicaloverview.html. Accessed December 25, 2006.

21. Centers for Disease Control. Update: influenza activity—United States, October 1–December 9, 2006. *MMWR.* 2006;55(50):1359–1362.

22. National Institute of Allergy and Infectious Diseases, National Institutes of Health. Focus on the flu: timeline of human flu pandemics. Available at: www3.niaid.nih.gov/news/focuson/flu/illustrations/timeline/timeline.htm. Accessed December 25, 2006.

23. Kilbourne ED. Influenza pandemics of the 20th century. *Emerg Infect Dis.* 2006;12(1):9–14.

24. Krause R. The swine flu episode and the fog of epidemics. *Emerg Infect Dis.* 2006;12(1):40–43.

25. World Health Organization. Cumulative number of confirmed human cases of avian influenza A/(H5N1) reported to WHO. Available at: www.who.int/csr/disease/avian_influenza/country/cases_table_2006_12_27/en. Accessed December 25, 2006.

26. Taubenberger J. 1918 influenza: the mother of all pandemics. *Emerg Infect Dis.* 2006;12(1):15–22.

27. Institute of Medicine. *The Future of the Public's Health in the 21st Century*—Workshop Summary. Washington, DC: National Academies of Sciences Press; 2002.

28. Institute of Medicine. *The Future of the Public's Health in the 21st Century.* Washington, DC: National Academies of Sciences Press; 2003.

29. Association of State and Territorial Health Officials. *State Public Health Worker Shortage Report.* Washington, DC: Association of State and Territorial Health Officials; 2006.

30. Nelson K. *Infectious Disease Epidemiology.* Gaithersburg, MD: Aspen; 2001.

31. Giesecke J. *Modern Infectious Disease Epidemiology.* London: Arnold Publishers/Oxford University Press; 2002.

32. Heymann DL. *Control of Communicable Diseases.* 18th ed. Washington, DC: American Public Health Association; 2004.

Why Study Methods?

WHY METHODS MATTER

People have a natural tendency to look first to the "facts." In public health, those are often statistics: How many individuals have tuberculosis in the region? How many individuals acquire HIV annually? Answers to these questions provide immediate, necessary, and useful information. For many, this may be enough. For others, this may be only the beginning. How this information is ascertained relates directly to what the facts are. All numbers, all statistics, are extensions of the methods that collected them. To understand the underlying method is to go deeper, to understand how the statistics are right—and how they are wrong. For those interested in participating in a field that uses epidemiology—and that includes virtually every public health discipline—it is essential to be aware of the underlying methods and understand them. Not only does this enhance one's ability to use the statistics while implementing or analyzing studies, but also designs studies capable of yielding correct facts with an appropriate and valid interpretation.

To some, the word *methods* represents an abstraction not grounded in day-to-day life. It may seem that to discuss methods is to overlook tangible reality in favor of a philosophical in-quiry. But we all use methods in our day-to-day lives. Nearly every activity humans perform has some natural, organic progression implicit in it, demanding a systematic approach. For example, think about getting dressed each morning: What is your method? Do you proceed from outerwear to under-clothes—or the reverse? The implications of the latter (e.g., coat first) could be quite dramatic: The end result of this method is starkly different than the usual, orderly method in which one proceeds. Think, too, of cooking, an activity one does routinely and that demands order in following the recipe. In a recipe, the methods are documented and clearly laid out. In most instances, informed or minor deviations to the recipe result in a similar product. However, in other instances, and under certain conditions, even the most minor of deviations can result in disaster. Imagine, for example, a cake without the requisite leavening or eggs. Though mundane perhaps, each of these activities contains a method. A specific ordered set of steps was enacted to get you from point A (no clothes, no food) to point B (clothed, fed). This set of steps is systematic and re-peatable, and designed to do or create something. The recipe is documented, making it possible to repeat again and again with precision. With our studies, we will see protocols that are developed in this same model. Protocols allow us to systematically conduct studies that are clearly and precisely conducted, and may be repeated with different participants, at different locations, and at different times.

Methods are also used in science. Many are already familiar with the demanding methods entailed in hard sciences such as chemistry—a lab notebook, an explicit set of instructions with which to conduct an experiment, and documentation of each and every step along the way. In order to conduct an experiment, exactitude in documentation of the steps is essential. How much of the buffer was titrated? What was the specific and quantified result of the experiment? Precision in the system of action, and the documentation, is what makes the experiment possible, interpretable, and repeatable.

In epidemiology, methods are no different. We use our methodological toolkit to answer questions. We document our methods such that they are repeatable and testable, and so that we can assess and measure deviations in the methods themselves as well as the subject under study. How data are collected has a profound effect on the ultimate results. Methods matter. Looking at results or facts in a vacuum makes it nearly difficult to truly understand the phenomena under study. It makes it impossible to design or implement valid studies, work on them in the field, correctly interpret the findings, or translate the findings into public health recommendations.

The next chapters will provide instruction in epidemiologic methods as applied to infectious disease. The purpose of this chapter is to start you on your path to viewing infectious disease content material through an epidemiologic methods lens: looking at data, information, statistics, qualitative contexts, and considering the role of the methods in them. Once this foundation is established, it becomes easier to understand infectious diseases in the context of epidemiological methods. This allows you to move beyond the "facts" regarding a specific disease and gain an understanding of what the disease is, what independent variables (risk factors) are associated with it, what confounders (characteristics that are noncausally associated with the disease) may exist, and how the disease can be prevented or treated. Whether new, emerging, or re-emerging pathogens, understanding how to study them (or how others study them) makes all the difference in understanding what public health interventions are needed.

MEASURING OUTCOMES

In this section, we will look at several examples that describe how to dig deeper into methods. This will lay a foundation for the next chapters, which detail specific tools in infectious disease epidemiology.

Everyday, most of us are exposed to some amount of media regarding medications, either over-the-counter or prescription. This might be at our own healthcare provider's office, through reading a magazine, seeing a commercial, or using a brand name over-the-counter drug from the pharmacy. Generally, in order to be unleashed onto the shelves, newer medications have undergone a rigorous examination through clinical trials: studies that systematically review the safety and efficacy of the medication in humans. One level of methods is readily apparent here: the

epidemiologic methodology required to develop, implement, analyze, and interpret the clinical trial. (This, in fact, is a complete field unto itself, with researchers from clinical medicine, nursing, epidemiology, and biostatistics working to assess drugs and their safety, efficacy, and effectiveness.)

Let us now consider how the information was collected to establish the safety and efficacy of the medication you are hearing about or taking. Imagine you are a participant in a clinical trial of a new medication to treat bacterial sinusitis (a common bacterial infection in which the sinus passages are colonized by bacteria, often following a cold or upper respiratory infection).

The study is a randomized controlled clinical trial. (This means that you have been randomly assigned, like flipping a coin, to receive a new treatment to be compared to another treatment. The groups being compared might be a new treatment compared to the current standard of care, as in the example.) You have been prescribed two tablets to be taken twice daily—one active medication, one placebo—and neither you nor your physician knows which is which (this is a double-blind, placebo-controlled trial). You return to the clinic for a follow-up study visit. The research nurse inquires about your adherence to study treatment; she might use a specially designed instrument to systematically inquire about your adherence behavior (Figure 2-1). "Did you take all of your study medication since the last study visit?" she kindly inquires. As it happens, you were feeling better in the last day and, though you know you should not have done it, you did not take the whole dose yesterday morning—just one of the two pills you were supposed to. Worse, you do not recall which pill you did not take, the one in Bottle A or the one in Bottle B. How many of us do not disclose the truth when asked this question? There are powerful influences, both conscious and subconscious, that can cause one to be less than truthful: these can include not remembering, fear of appearing socially undesirable, and concern about being dismissed from the study.

Consider, too, something as basic as the way in which the question was asked: Did the nurse say, "Did you miss any of your doses?" or "Did you miss your last dose?" or "Did you miss any doses today?" or "Many people occasionally miss their study medicine; did you miss any of your doses since your last study visit?" Or perhaps any number of other variations. How the nurse asks the question will be associated with how you respond to the question. Her attitude and affect as she asks the question—her tone, inflection, and body language—will influence how you respond. The method of inquiry by which this datapoint was collected becomes important with respect to the data themselves that yield the results of this study. In addition, the method can also affect your subsequent behavior. If the socially desirable but inaccurate response is uttered, it

FIGURE 2-1 Example of an Instrument to Capture Baseline Adherence Information; the ACTG Adherence Baseline Questionnaire

ACTG Adherence Baseline Questionnaire

Date: _____

Patient ID: _____

How Administered? **Self** ☐ 1 **Interviewer** ☐ 2 **Both** ☐ 3

The answers you give on this form will be used to plan ways to help other people who must take pills on a different schedule. Please do the best you can to answer all the questions. If you do not wish to answer a question, please draw a line through it. If you do not know how to answer a question, ask your study nurse to help. Thank you for helping in this important study.

INSTRUCTIONS: Please answer the following questions by placing a circle around the appropriate number response.

A. How sure are you that:
(Please circle a response for each question.)

	Not at All Sure	Somewhat Sure	Very Sure	Extremely Sure
1. You will be able to take all or most of the study medication as directed?	0	1	2	3
2. The medication will have a positive effect on your health?	0	1	2	3
3. If you do not take this medication exactly as instructed, the HIV in your body will become resistant to HIV medications.	0	1	2	3

B. The following questions ask about your social support.
(Please circle one response for each question.)

	Very Dissatisfied	Somewhat Dissatisfied	Somewhat Satisfied	Very Satisfied
1. In general, how satisfied are you with the overall support you get from your friends and family members?	0	1	2	3

	Not At All	A Little	Somewhat	A Lot	Not Applicable
2. To what extent do your friends or family members help you remember to take your medication?	0	1	2	3	4

Several questions used at the beginning of a study to evaluate patient characteristics (beliefs, social support) that may be associated with medication adherence.
Source: AIDS Clinical Trials Unit/Division of AIDS/National Institutes of Health (ACTG/NIAID).

may be that you would no longer wish to participate in the study, perhaps out of embarrassment. Or perhaps you remain in the study, but in the future do not feel comfortable telling her the truth about your adherence behavior.

Although the type of analysis usually used in a randomized controlled trial (called intention to treat analysis) allows to be generated an estimate of the how well the drug works, attrition from the study can create enormous barriers to

Bacterial Sinusitis (RCT)

Acute bacterial sinusitis is one of the most common ailments for which people seeking care are prescribed antibiotics. If you have ever had this infection and inflammation of the sinuses, you are well aware that it can be excruciatingly painful and can drive one to the doctor. Like a terrible sequel to another illness, it often comes right on the heels of an upper respiratory infection. Some of the bacteria responsible for acute bacterial sinusitis include *Haemophilus influenzae, Moraxella catarrhalis, Streptococcus pneumoniae* (Figure 2-2), *Staphylococcus aureus,* and *Streptococcus pyogenes* (Figure 2-3). Improved treatment modalities for acute bacterial sinusitis are needed.[1-3]

Azithromycin is a commonly used antibiotic, recently formulated to be able to be administered in a single-dose regimen. One team of investigators conducted a multi-centered (meaning more than one clinic location was used), randomized (meaning that the participants were assigned by chance to the treatment condition), double-blinded (meaning that neither the patient nor the providers knew which treatment arm each patient was on) clinical trial. How did they do this? This is a very common clinical trial structure. Consenting adults were randomly assigned (also known as randomized, like flipping a coin) to receive either the treatment under investigation or the standard of care. The new treatment, the one under investigation, is the 2.0 g single dose of azithromycin microspheres; the standard of care is 500 mg once a day of oral levofloxacin, another antibiotic. Participants were randomized to receive either the single dose of the azithromycin microspheres plus a placebo of oral levofloxacin (investigational arm) for 10 days *or* a placebo for the 2.0-g dose and active oral levofloxacin for 10 days (standard of care arm). Participants were followed to day 17–24 to see if they had a clinical response to the medication—either cure (resolution of signs and symptoms or clinical improvement such that no further medications were required) or failure (clinical state that was worsened and required new or additional antibiotics). The investigators concluded that the new formulation of azithromycin as a single dose was safe and effective for the treatment of acute bacterial sinusitis. However, in the editorial commentary directly following the article,[4] a question was raised regarding the selected study design and the concern that the decision about the outcome of interest (test of cure at 17–24 days post dosing)

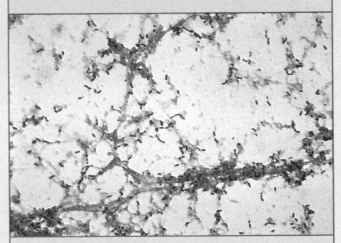

FIGURE 2-2 *Streptococcus pneumoniae*

Source: CDC/Dr. Mike Miller, 1978. Public Health Image Library. Accessed at: www.cdc.gov/phil.

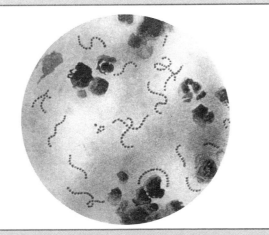

FIGURE 2-3 *Streptococcus pyogenes*

Source: CDC/Dr. Mike Miller, 1979. Public Health Image Library. Accessed at: www.cdc.gov/phil.

Bacterial Sinusitis (RCT)—continued

may not be the best way to assess the medication. Many people spontaneously resolve their sinusitis by 10 days, and beyond that, even more are likely improve after the window assessed in this study. In addition, there was no objective operationalization of improvement, which can present a problem. Even a clinical trial that follows appropriate recommendations for study design as did this one can be improved. Learning how to understand study designs and see their strengths and limitations is an important skill.

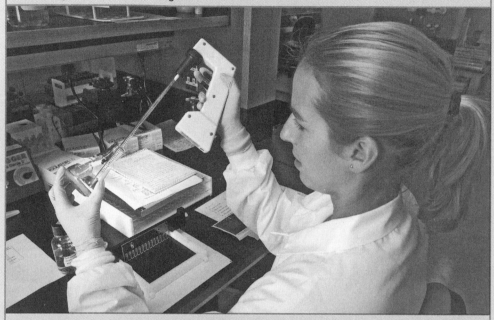

FIGURE 2-4 Processing specimens in the lab is an important part of many epidemiologic studies, including clinical trials.

Source: CDC/Dr. Maryann I. Daneshar, 2005. Public Health Image Library. Accessed at: www.cdc.gov/phil.

analyzing and interpreting the data in an accurate, comprehensive, and informative fashion. And clearly, false information creates barriers as well. Note how the methods of asking a clearly critical question about adherence can alter the study as a whole on several different levels. The amount of drug taken, your feelings about the study, your decisions to stay in the study or fully disclose your actual behavior may be impacted by a seemingly simple method: how one question was asked. All of this affects whether we end up believing the drug is effective—or not.

Had you stopped taking the drug or stopped participating altogether, or if the drug was found effective over the placebo, later analyses would attempt to evaluate patient adherence to medications and the action of the drug. But had you silently decided not to disclose your non-adherence, detecting this through any statistical or other analytic methods would be next to impossible. Thus, the method interacts with not only the data, but also the behavior of participants and with other ele-

ments of the study, potentially introducing bias (systematic differences that affect estimates under the study) into the study and, ultimately, into the conclusions.

Imagine now that you stay home from school due to your sinusitis. Mid-day, you receive a telephone call from a survey research firm. You have been randomly (through chance) selected to participate in a case-control study exploring the association between condom use with sex and human papilloma virus (HPV), thought to be the etiologic agent in development of cervical cancer.[2] Briefly, case-control studies compare people with and without the disease of interest (HPV) with respect to exposure (condom use). In case-control studies, cases are identified along with suitable controls, and antecedent exposures (those that happened before the disease) are assessed among participants in both groups. The two groups are then compared. This allows estimation of the relationship between the exposure and the disease and is especially useful in cases of rare (or relatively rare) diseases.

TABLE 2-1 How Asking a Question Matters

There are many different ways of asking about adherence to a medication, in our case, an antibiotic. Some are provided in the following table. Imagine if you are being asked this question, how the inflection of the interviewer's tone, or whether others are listening in on your interview, or how you feel may influence your response. Examples of considerations are given in the righthand column; more exist of course, so when you are working with adherence survey data, be sure to consider how the method of inquiry may impact the data you collect. When possible, collecting a biomarker (such as a blood level of the drug in question) is a great addition to the study. In addition to being an ideal outcome on its own, even if there are not sufficient resources to measure levels on all clients, it can be used to validate data obtained through interview.

Types of adherence questions	Examples of methodological considerations
Did you take your last dose of the medicine?	Which medicine? Does this refer to the doses that were prescribed, or the doses that the person wanted or intended to take?
When was the last time you missed taking any of your medications?	This might yield a non-specific response, such as, "the other day" or "not lately" unless carefully constructed close-ended responses are provided. (If this is a qualitative study, however, this may be modified to be a more appropriate open-ended question.)
How much of your medication did you take in the last week [100%, 75%, 50%, 25% 0%]?	How does the respondent decide how doses correspond to percentages? What if there is more than one medication type?
How much of your medication did you miss in the last week [100%, 75%, 50%, 25% 0%]?	As above. In addition, it may be easier for some to think about how many doses were missed rather than how many were taken. Some respondents may be more comfortable disclosing the number of doses they took opposed to number missed, despite its being more difficult to recall and/or calculate.
Did you have any trouble taking your medication?	This may be difficult to elicit truthful information, particularly if the person doing the interview is also the provider. In the event that there are barriers to adherence, it can sometimes be hard to tell one's own provider—even if they can articulate their concerns, which may also be difficult.
Did you take your medication as directed?	Does this mean on time? Right amount? Right time of day/night? With regard to food or rest? It is important for the question to be clear about exactly what it is asking.

You are asked several screening questions and it is determined that you are eligible to participate as a population-based control, because you had a Pap smear in the last 3 months and have never been diagnosed with cervical dysplasia (abnormal cervical cells that may progress to cancer). You respond to a 15-minute survey with questions about your demographics, routine screening, and clinical and sexual behavioral characteristics, and overall health and health utilization behavior.

What makes you different from a woman who would not be selected as a control for this study? One salient difference between you and someone else is that you were sick and home from your usual activities at the time the interviewer called. Individuals at work or school are in general healthier than those at home during the daytime. Other differences between you and someone not selected include: you have access to a phone, understand the questions, speak the language of the interviewer, and are willing to participate. Whatever the ultimate findings of the study, one must take into account the fact that the controls who are selected *can* differ substantially from those who could have been selected but were not. Methods matter. If we do not consider differences between those who enrolled in the study and those who were not, our internal validity—how accurately our study is evaluating this exposure/outcome relationship—may be limited. In addition, later applying (generalizing) our findings to a larger population may be difficult. This is another way methods come into play, and thinking about them becomes important. Things are not always as they seem: sometimes thinking about methods in infectious disease is a little bit like being a detective, ensuring that things are interpreted correctly starting with how the study was conducted. If you ignore the differences between cases and controls, and look only to the information on the surface, you might just draw the wrong conclusions: it could seem as if people who are at home are more likely to be ill and have the exposures of interest. This could be because those at home are sicker to begin with and thus more likely to have cervical dysplasia, HPV, and poor condom use—and have nothing to do with the research question in mind; this then prohibits drawing any conclusions about the relationship between condom use and dysplasia, as the investigators were hoping to do. Table 2-2 displays hypothetical differences between cases, controls, and persons not selected for the study.

Now that we are about to move on to the core set of methods used in infectious disease epidemiology, keep in mind that while we are seeking information, we also need to know how that information is collected. Always consider how the data

were gathered, the protocol for the study, who collected the information, how the questions were asked, who was included in the study and how they were selected, and which datapoints were analyzed. Later on we will discuss specific biases and how to assess them, but for now, when you learn about the epidemiologic toolkit, always think to the core of the question: How was what we collected affected by how we collected it?

Methods have an enormous impact on the data we can collect and how we will answer our research questions. Innovating and implementing creative methods to ascertain information about the outcomes under study with truth validity is a key methodological issue. How do we get to the truth? Without validity in our research designs or in the field, it is very difficult to correctly describe what is going on or accurately portray cases of diseases. Sometimes direct observation of behavior is not possible or not possible without distorting the behavior under study. This can be especially true with observation of sexual behaviors, adherence, illicit drug use or other behaviors that are sensitive, and about which people can be reluctant to share. Other times proxies are available, but still are less than accurate or very difficult to conduct (e.g., collection of used condoms). Developing a system, that can be a feasible and accurate proxy for self-report of sensitive data, is essential.

TABLE 2-2 Differences Between Cases, Controls, and Nonparticipants

Hypothetical differences between cases, controls, and persons not selected in a case-control study of condom use, HPV, and cervical cancer are shown. These differences may not be related to the exposure (condom use) or the outcome (HPV) at all—but may still affect how we are able to investigate this relationship.

Cases	Population-based controls	Persons not selected as controls
Has insurance	Sick when called and asked to participate, thus at home and not at school/work	No phone
Seeks gynecologic or STD-related care	Might wish to seek care, but not motivated on own	No insurance
Interested in and volunteers for research study	Interested in and volunteers for research study	Interested in research study but does not have time to participate because of work
Lives near research or clinical center	Knows about research center but has never been	Does not live near research or clinical center
May have increased/or decreased risk factors for HPV or cervical cancer	May have increased/or decreased risk factors for HPV or cervical cancer	May have increased/or decreased risk factors for HPV or cervical cancer
May have sought care and joined study because she does not use condoms	May have joined study because she does not use condoms	May be afraid to join study because she does not use condoms

Discussion Questions

1. What are three things you do each day that require a set method/order of events? List the steps to at least one of these methods.

2. Imagine you are in a study comparing individuals who go to college and those who do not with regard to acquisition of syphilis. Hypothesize at least five differences between these two categories of people, and how each might be related to each of the outcomes under the study.

REFERENCES

1. Brook I. Antimicrobial management of acute sinusitis: a review of therapeutic recommendations. *Infect Med.* 2002;19:231–237.

2. Heymann DL. *Control of Communicable Diseases.* 18th ed. Washington, DC: American Public Health Association.

3. Murray JJ, Emparanza P, Lesinskas E, Tawadrous M, Breen JD. Efficacy and safety of a novel, single-dose azitrhomycin microsphere formulation vs. 10 days of levofloxacin for the treatment of acute bacterial sinusitis in adults. *Otolaryngol Head Neck Surg.* 2005;133:194–201.

4. Dilemma in trial design: do current study designs adequately evaluate effectiveness antibiotic in ABRS? [Editorial]. *Otolaryngol Head Neck Surg.* 2005;133:201–203.

CHAPTER 3

Descriptive Infectious Disease Epidemiology

BACKGROUND

This chapter will discuss one of the most important foundations in epidemiology and public health: descriptive methods. Descriptive epidemiology was one of the earliest methodologies in the field, only relatively recently followed by others. Descriptive epidemiology continues to be a key way in which emerging and re-emerging pathogens are discovered and etiologic agents of outbreaks are identified. With increased usage of rapid computing resources, which make iterative modeling and statistical analysis available at the desktop, the last two decades saw a de-emphasis in descriptive epidemiology in favor of more sophisticated assessment of multivariable relationships. However, many researchers are now revisiting, expanding, and enhancing descriptive techniques. Those who specialize in outbreak investigations never ceased using and improving these important methods. These techniques help us better understand outbreaks and public health phenomena, allowing appropriate and beneficial value to be placed on more basic—and crucial—techniques.

Consider your reaction to the following scenario: You are healthy and young, seldom sick. You might not have an exten-sive education in biology or medicine, but you have a basic, layperson's-level knowledge of disease. You attend an orientation for your new job at the hospital, where you are hoping to gain experience in hospital information systems. During lunch, you eat with other attendees at the hospital cafeteria. Nutrition-conscious, you opt for the salad bar and have tossed salad plus a small scoop of pasta salad. By the early afternoon session, you are vomiting and have moderate to severe diarrhea—you feel acutely ill. Fortunately, the orientation comes to a close and you do not have to leave early, but you are quite exhausted. You nurse your sickness at home for 36 hours before feeling fully recovered from the gastrointestinal upset and associated dehydration.

Your sample size—that is, how many people you are studying—is only one. And yet, you make the following observations:

- You were healthy upon arriving at the orientation.
- You felt sick within 2 hours of eating lunch.
- You do not know if others who ate at the salad bar are ill, but realize this may not mean much. (You, yourself, did not beg off the sessions as a result of your discomfort.)

What do these observations tell you? They may mean a couple of things:

- You were sick before you got to orientation, but asymptomatic until the first presentation that afternoon.
- Something you ate made you ill.

If you opt to go with the idea that something you ate made you ill, what information can assist you in evaluating this question? You decide to consult some books at the library on communicable diseases, and find out that staphylococcal food intoxication (caused by *Staphlycoccus aureus* enterotoxin [See Figure 3-1]) can be found in meats, egg products, macaroni and potato salads, and cream-filled pastries and has a brief incubation period (the time from exposure to presentation of symptoms)—it can be as little as half an hour. (The range is 30 minutes to 8 hours after eating.)[1] Then you look to the local public health office to see their listings of public health inspections of restaurants and institutions. You see that your very employer has had five incidents of foodborne outbreaks, including two of staphylococcal food intoxication in the past 2 months in the cafeteria. You are now soundly in the camp of believing that something at the salad bar was the etiologic agent for your illness, though you are still uncertain which element you ate made you ill. Was it the salad? The pasta? The dressing? The drink? Something that touched something else, say a dish that had residue from another meal on it? The following week when you begin work, another new employee in your section who also was at the orientation sheepishly inquires if you got sick with vomiting and diarrhea at orientation following lunch. You discuss what each of you ate. It turns out that your friend ate a slightly different menu than you did, taking a turkey sandwich with mustard and a side of pasta salad. The only area of overlap was the pasta salad. Mystery solved. Though your sample size is still only two, and you lack "proof," you and your new friend feel fairly confident that you had food poisoning and that it derived from the hospital cafeteria's salad bar, specifically the pasta salad. Soon you will learn the formal steps in an outbreak investigation, but for now, let us turn our focus to the information gained in this example and how it was synthesized. The method—no matter how simple—is instructive in better understanding the utility of descriptive epidemiology as a core methodological concept.

What happened here? How and to what end did you synthesize your observations?

1. You considered the person, place, and time of the event; that is, the description of yourself and what you did, the description of where you were first ill and what you were doing immediately preceding that time, and the time it occurred relative to other events as well as in absolute terms. These are the three most salient features of an outbreak investigation or of any descriptive epidemiologic study.

2. You identified the dependent variable (the outcome)—gastrointestinal upset.

3. You identified a potential independent variable (the putative causative agent)—staphylococcal food intoxication from the pasta salad.

4. You developed a case definition for the dependent variable—not just any gastrointestinal symptoms, but specifically moderate to severe vomiting and diarrhea relatively quickly following exposure to the potential causative agent.

5. You calculated the time from putative exposure to symptoms—the 2 hours until you got sick.

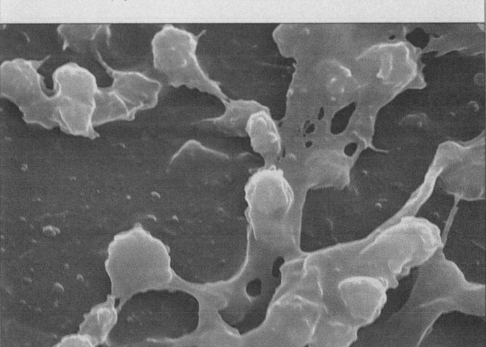

FIGURE 3-1 *Staphylococcus aureus* bacteria

This highly magnified electron micrograph depicts *Staphylococcus aureus* bacteria, which were found on an indwelling catheter. *S. aureus* is ubiquitous, and commonly found on the skin or in the noses of healthy individuals. Approximately 25% to 30% of the population is colonized in the nose with *S. aureus,* but without causing any infection.

Source: CDC/Dr. Rodney M. Donlan and Janice Carr, 2005. Public Health Image Library. Accessed at: www.cdc.gov/phil.

6. You performed a miniature literature review to investigate organisms that could have been associated with illness, based on your symptoms and timing.

7. You examined publicly available public health data to see the "story" of the hospital and see whether food poisoning is a reasonable explanation given the hospital's history.

The basics of descriptive epidemiology are apparent in this example:

- *Characterization of person, place, and time:* You were able to describe all facets of what occurred on these three axes: who was affected, what the environment was like, and when the event occurred. You also describe when it occurred in relation to later symptom development.

- *There was no intervention:* The situation was described to its fullest using available information. In this example, the resources were observations, library resources, and an exchange with a friend (data collection). Nothing was done or tested, no intervention provided.

- *Assessment of potential causes:* You used multiple resources to try to identify what could have been the cause. The Internet can be a good resource (when using reputable sources). Libraries, journals, and other more scholarly sources are even better.

- *Establishment of a working case definition:* You put together the person, place, and time characteristics that you identified, creating a solid and thorough description of what you experienced.

- *Hypotheses were suggested:* In many descriptive studies it is not possible to gather specimens. As in this case, one does not usually know they were going to get sick and cannot take samples due to situational constraints. Here, biologic specimens from the individuals affected were not obtained because the patient self-treated and did not self-refer for care or diagnosis. Specimens most likely would be taken later in a foodservice setting and, if additional cases emerged, possibly biologic samples from those affected as well. Still, even without these, a hypothesis was identified.

John Snow Mapping Cholera

John Snow used the quintessential epidemiologist skill: mapping. A serious outbreak of cholera took place in 1854 in London, England, following on the heels of an equally dangerous one in 1849. Cholera is an acute bacterial enteric disease caused by *Vibrio cholerae* (see Figure 3-2), primarily serogroups 01 and 0139. Cholera has a case fatality rate of 50% in the absence of treatment (meaning that approximately half of those infected will die if not treated). Death is primarily due to dehydration caused by severe diarrhea and vomiting.[1] Cholera is one of three diseases requiring notification under the International Health Regulations,[1] and is strongly linked to living conditions and access to clean water. Although epidemics and pandemics of cholera occur even today, often related to emergencies, disasters, and other impediments to accessing clean water, cholera is preventable and treatable.

John Snow used many of the descriptive and outbreak epidemiologic skills you will learn in this book to identify the cause of the outbreak of cholera in London. In the 1849 outbreak, there were more than 500 deaths due to cholera in a matter of 10 days.[2–7] At that time, water from the two water companies, Lambeth and the Southwark and Vauxhall,

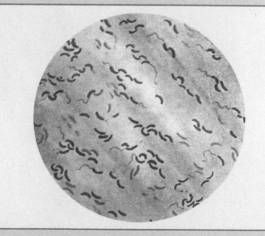

FIGURE 3-2 *Vibrio cholerae* bacteria

This Gram-stain depicts flagellated *Vibrio comma* bacteria, a strain of *V. cholerae*, the cause of Asiatic cholera.

Source: CDC/Public Health Image Library, 1979. Accessed at: www.cdc.gov/phil.

continued

John Snow Mapping Cholera—continued

used water from a polluted part of the Thames river (see Figure 3-3). The sewage pollution there was thought to be the cause of disease. After 1849, the Lambeth Company began using water from a less densely polluted part of the river. During the second outbreak in 1854, Snow identified that people supplied by the Lambeth Company were now much less likely to contract and die from cholera. Snow used maps to assess the water sources supplying those individuals with cholera and compared them to neighborhoods where there was less disease. Taken together, he was able to identify the source. Without the sophisticated testing that we have today, he went to the Broad Street pump and removed the handle—now an iconic public health action. This done, water from the contaminated source was no longer available. Quickly, the outbreak subsided. In addition to saving lives, this action supported Snow's hypothesis: If he had been mistaken about the cause, this intervention would have been unlikely to be effective.

The Broad Street pump is iconic in epidemiology in general and infectious disease epidemiology in particular. Snow used tools that we have available to us and that are the cornerstones of infectious disease epidemiology. He identified a potential source (water from the Southwark and Vauxhall Company), counted cases in relation to the outcome (contraction of cholera), mapped it (now we have geographical information systems [GIS] to help us in this endeavor), identified a hypothesis, tested the hypothesis, took public health action, and documented his findings. All things we do now! The actual numbers may be found in Table 3-1, so you may look at the data yourself.

FIGURE 3-3 Snow's London

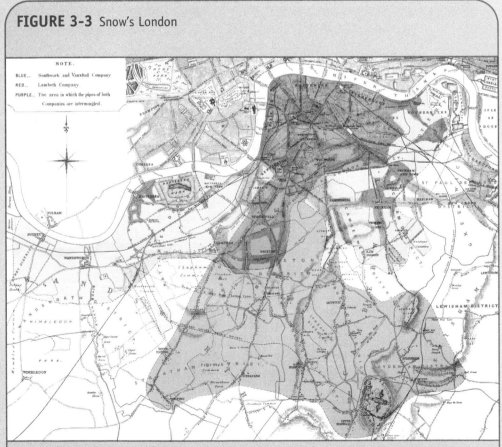

NOTE.

BLUE.. Southwark and Vauxhall Company.
RED.. Lambeth Company.
PURPLE.. The area in which the pipes of both
Companies are intermingled.

John Snow used mapping to depict the place elements of the cholera outbreak he was analyzing. This map is iconic—along with the broad street pump—of infectious disease epidemiologists. It did not take computers or complexity to identify the source of the cholera epidemic in London: just clear thinking and use of descriptive epidemiology.

Source: John Snow Web Site/UCLA Retrieved 12/25/2006 from http://www.ph.ucla.edu/epi/ snow.html.

TABLE 3-1 Cholera Data Analyzed by John Snow[2]

Proportion of deaths to 10,000 houses, during the first 7 weeks of the epidemic, in the population supplied by the Southwark and Vauxhall Company, in that supplied by the Lambeth Company, and in the rest of London.

Water Source	Number of Houses	Deaths from Cholera	Deaths in each 10,000 Houses
Southwark & Vauxhall Company	40,046	1,263	315
Lambeth Company	26,107	98	37
Rest of London	256,423	1,422	55*
Where do these data come from? → → →	*Service records*	*Death records*	*(Deaths/houses served)* × 10,000

Note: this number was originally published as 59 in Snow's actual table in On the Mode of Communication of Cholera.[4] It may have been the result of a typo, changes in underlying data from the census department, or the actual number of houses in each area.*

• Also noted in article by Carvalho FM, Lima F, and Kriebel D. Re: on John Snow's unquestioned long division. *Am J Epidemiol* 2004;159:422.

• *A public health intervention was suggested by your findings:* As a result of what you discovered, you may be able to work with hospital staff to improve food management techniques and ultimately reduce the risk of foodborne outbreaks in the future. One step that has not yet occurred in this scenario is that you would need to ensure that your findings are communicated to your local health department.

Some of the most exciting and important discoveries have been made (or initiated) through descriptive epidemiology. John Snow used mapping to deduce and identify the source of cholera in London during two outbreaks during the mid-1800s. Through mapping and thorough description of (and thought about) cases and exposures of cases as well as noncases, Snow enacted a public health intervention—the iconic removal of the Broad Street pump—and stopped the outbreak.

Many diseases have been identified through the work of keen clinicians: observations of evidence training, mapping, and more. For example, in 1981, a rare type of pneumonia was identified among five young, healthy, active homosexual males in Los Angeles. Even this small number of patients was sufficient to give rise to the suggestion that a new disease was in play—the disease that later came to be known as acquired immunodeficiency syndrome, or AIDS. It was keen observations and their juxtaposition with "normal" that allowed these cases to be recognized for the gravity they possessed; it would have been very easy for these cases to go below the radar of the clinicians.

Public Health Prevention Advice in the Pursuit of Avoiding Cholera

A Handbill from the New York Board of Health, 1832[5] Notice

Be temperate in eating and drinking,
avoid crude *vegetables* and *fruits*;
abstain from *cold water*, when heated;
and above all from *ardent spirits* and
if habit have rendered it indispensable, take much less than usual.

Sleep and clothe warm
Avoid labor in the heat of day.
Do not sleep or sit in a draught of air when heated.

Avoid getting wet.
Take no medicines without advice

There are many other examples of new, emerging, or rare disease entities being noticed by clinicians, epidemiologists, lab technicians, and patients themselves. In each of these cases observations of outcomes (the dependent variable, or the illness) and potential predictors (the independent variables, or the risk factors or causative agents), the relation between these, and a formal or informal comparison

Case Reports and HIV/AIDS

Noticing aberrations in population health and potential differences in presentation of disease are often the first steps towards stopping disease; recognition is critical. Case reports are often the product of one or two astute individuals noting that something is different, unusual, wrong, or just plain out of sorts. Almost always, what is amiss is in the person, place, or time characteristics of the events: a common disease in the wrong type of person (older, younger, sicker, healthier than usual); a disease common in the West but rare in the East appears in a new place; a disease that usually occurs in the winter is found in the summer. When someone notices this, it may be because they see patients in a clinic, like a healthcare provider, or perhaps they work at the emergency department and notice an influx of a certain type of patient who is not like the norm. Or a public health worker at the department of public health may notice increased surveillance reports that look too similar when submitted via passive reporting, or calls to a disease-specific help desk that raise suspicion of an emerging, re-emerging infectious disease, or an outbreak situation. There are many "clues" that can help us identify case reports and potential health scares.

In the summer of 1981, the world changed with the notice of five cases of *Pneumocysitis carinii* pneumonia (PCP) in June. These were disclosed in the *Morbidity and Mortality Weekly Report (MMWR)* as the case reports show in Figure 3-4.[8] This pneumonia is cased by a fairly ubiquitous parasite and is seen most commonly among immunocompromised and elderly persons. For PCP to be in young, health individuals was very rare. These five cases ushered in the era of HIV/AIDS (see Figure 3-5). Five young men, all "actively homosexual," were identified as having PCP (see Figure 3-6)—a small but significant cluster of a rare disease among healthy persons of this age cohort.

FIGURE 3-4   First case reports of PCP pneumonia—the ushering in of an era

1981 June 5:30:250—2

Pneumocystis Pneumonia—Los Angeles

In the period October 1980–May 1981, 5 young men, all active homosexuals, were treated for biopsy-confirmed *Pneumocystis carinii* pneumonia at 3 different hospitals in Los angeles, California. Two of the patients died. All 5 patients had laboratory-confrimed previous or current cytomegalovirus (CMV) infection and candidal mucosal infection. Case reports of these patients follow.

Patient 1: A previously healthy 33-year old man developed *P. carinii* pneumonia and oral mucosal candiasis in March 1981 after a 2-month history of fever associated with elevated liver enzymes, leukopenia, and CMV viruria. The serum complement-fixation CMV titer in Octobeer 1980 was 256; in May 1981 it was 32.* The patient's condition deteriorated despite courses of treatment with trimehoprim-sulfamethoxazole (TMP/SMX), pentamidine, and acyclovir. He died May 3, and postmortem examination showed residual *P. carinii* and CMV peneumonia, but no evidence of neoplasia.

Patient 2: A previously healthy 30-year-old man developed *P. carinii* pneumonia in April 1981 after a 5-month history of fever each day and of elevated liver-function tests, CMV viruria, and documented seroconversion to CMV, i.e., an acute-phase titer of 16 and a convalescent-phase titer of 28* in anticomplement immunofluorescence tests. Other features of his illness included leukopenia and mucosal candidiasis. His pneumonia responded to a course of intravenous TMP/SMX, but, as of the latest reports, he continues to have a fever each day.

Patient 3: A 30-year old man was well until January 1981 when he developed esophageal and oral candidiasis that responded to Amphotericin B treatment. He was hospitalized in Febuary 1981 for *P. carinii* pneumonia that responded to oral TMP/SMX. His esophageal candidiasis recurred after the pneumonia was diagnosed, and he was again given Amphotericin B. The CMV complement-fixation titer in March 1981 was 8. Material from an esophageal biopsy was positive for CMV.

Patient 4: A 29-year old man developed *P. carinii* pneumonia in February in 1981. He had had Hodgkins disease 3 years earlier, but had been sucessfully treated with radiation therapy alone. He did not improve after being given intravenous TMP/SMX and cortico-steroid and died in March. Postmortem examination showed no evidence of Hodgkins disease but *P. carinii* and CMV were found in lung tissue.

Patient 5: A previously healthy 36-year-old man with a clinically diagnosed CMV infection in September 1980 was seen in April 1981 because of a 4-month history of fever, dyspnea, and cough. On admission, he was found to have *P. carinii* pneumonia, oral candidiasis, and CMV retinitis. A complement-fixation CMV titer in April 1981 was 128. The patient has been treated with 2 short courses of TMP/SMX that have been limited because of a sulfa-induced neutropenia. He is being treated for candidiasis with topical nystatin.

The diagnosis of *Pneumocystis* pneumonia was confirmed for all 5 patients antemortem by clocod or open lung biopsy. The patients did not know each other and had no known common contacts or knowledge of sexual partners who had similar illnesses. The 5 did not have comparable histories of sexually transmitted disease. Four had serologic evidence of past hepatitis B infection but had no evidence of current hepatisis B surface antigen. Two of the 5 reported having frequent homosexual contacts with various partners. All 5 reported using inhalant drugs, and 1 reported parenteral drug abuse. Three patients had profoundly depressed *in vitro* proliferative responses to mitogens and antigens. Lymphocyte studies were not performed on the other 2 patients.

Reported by MS Gottlieb, MD, HM Schanker, MD, PT Fan, MD, A Saxon, MD, JD Weisman, DO, Div of Clinical Immunology-Allergy, Dept of Medicine, UCLA School of Medicine; I Pozalski, MD, Cedars-Mt. Sinai Hospital, Los Angeles; Field Services Div, Epidemiology Program Office, CDC.

This is the actual report describing the first PCP cases that ultimately informed our recognition of the HIV/AIDS epidemic. This was in the June 5, 1981 issue of the Morbidity and Mortality Weekly Report.

Source: CDC, *Pneumocystis pneumonia-Los Angeles.* Morbidity and Mortality Weekly Report, 1981. 30: p. 250–2.

continued

Case Reports and HIV/AIDS—continued

FIGURE 3-5 Picture of HIV

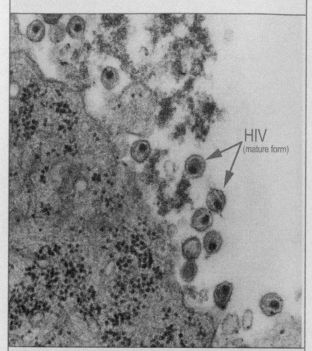

HIV
(mature form)

This highly magnified transmission electron micrographic (TEM) image revealed the presence of mature forms of the *human immunodeficiency virus* (HIV) in a tissue sample under investigation.

Source: CDC/Public Health Image Library, 1983.

FIGURE 3-6 Picture of PCP

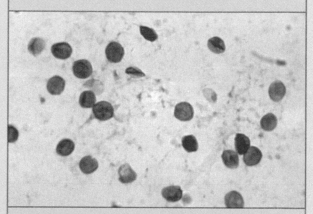

Pneumocystis carinii is a major cause of death in AIDS patients. Development of PCP pneumonia is classified as an AIDS-defining diagnosis, and the disease itself is considered an opportunistic infection.

Source: CDC/Public Health Library, 1971.

Just a month later, in July, the *MMWR* reported 26 cases of Kaposi's sarcoma (KS), a rare cancer, among young, healthy, homosexual males.[9] This is another case where the disease did not fit the usual characteristics, this time for person and place. The usual KS patients are elderly and immunocompromised. As with PCP, young, healthy cases in the United States were very rare. In addition, these cases had a very high case fatality rate (20%); usually cases are more chronic and do not result as often in death. And these cases were clustered unusually on two coasts of the United States, in New York and California.

In the second report, more information was provided, making its approach a case series study design. This report provides some denominator data, though limited: a historical comparator was used. "A review of the New York University Coordinated Cancer Registry for KS in men under age 50 revealed no cases from 1970–1979 at Bellevue Hospital and 3 cases in this age group at the New York City Hospital from 1961–1979."[9(p305)] This information highlighted that the 26 cases of KS occurring in such a short period of time and in such a small geographic area were, indeed, unusual. By August 1981, a report, indicating 108 people with one or both conditions (i.e., KS and/or PCP) and their basic demographics where available, was released.

A follow-up study was performed of cases of KS and/or PCP between June 1, 1981, and April 12, 1982.[10] In this study, detailed demographic, clinical, and behavioral data were collected from each patient or their proxies (for those who had died); this study found the data consistent with the possibility of a new sexually transmitted infectious organism that leads to acquired immune deficiency (as happened to be the case), but also the possibility that it could be another factor, such as drugs, commonly used by homosexual men at the time (i.e., amyl nitrate or "poppers"). These steps follow directly from those in all descriptive epidemiologic studies, where the cases were evaluated, described, and then the description suggests hypotheses and appropriate next steps to the researchers.

AIDS has since become a pandemic, with its worst human tolls now among heterosexuals in most parts of the world also among injection drug users and males engaging in homosexual behavior. The fastest rising incidence rates in the United States are among African American and Latino individuals and young men and women. Adolescents are a population of special concern, with adolescent behavior and developmental staging a barrier to any types of services, including prevention, testing, counseling, or treatment.[11–14] Fortunately, earlier transmission of HIV taking place through blood, the blood- and tissue-products supply has all but ceased with improved screening, at least in the United States.

The intensive detective work to solve the mystery of AIDS epidemiologically, as well as in the laboratory, has been well chronicled in a variety of books, articles, films, and other documents. As we watch the future unfold, we hope that we will have new and improved methods of control to add to those that we already have (such as highly active antiretroviral treatment, perinatal prophylaxis, circumcision, and others)—including the long-hoped-for promises of being able, one day, to prevent HIV transmission with vaccines.

between people with and without the disease helped identify and sometimes alleviate a public health threat. Descriptive epidemiology provides a method to examine datapoints, and uses specific methodologies. The formal study methods that use descriptive epidemiology include case studies, case reports, ecologic studies, and outbreak investigations to formalize and document observations.

DESCRIBING DATA

Presented with an outbreak situation such as we saw with HIV, most of us can collect and assimilate a vast amount of information using a method similar to a recipe example; even without training. But having a method, a recipe, transforms it from a hunch to a science. The utility in applying a system or a method, to this process is straightforward: It ensures that the process is logical and orderly, is documented, and provides guidance so it can be done again exactly (i.e., is replicable in the future). A good system is fully organized in all aspects with always the same exact steps to be conducted again in the future. While in the example of the pasta salad, you might have been able to arrive upon the right food culprit, but as the complexity of the public health concern increases, this becomes more and more difficult.

The first step in any detective work is careful organization of data. Before being able to implement a study—whatever study design is selected—one has to be able to describe the data. There are many ways to describe data. The overarching goal of doing so is to become well acquainted with each of the datapoints, alone and in relation to each other. The value of this step cannot be overestimated. Even compared with sophisticated computing techniques, sometimes just "sitting" with one's data allows a profile of what is going on to emerge. Remember, though, that we are *looking* at the data at this point, like a detective looking for clues. We are not drawing conclusions about causality or developing assertions about associations. We cannot adjust for factors that may obscure our understanding of the underlying relationships (as in confounders and effect modifiers). We are getting to know our data.

Whether you have ten people or thousands in your sample (the group to be included in your study), the basic steps are similar and the goals are the same: You want to describe information with respect to person, place, and time. The goal of descriptive epidemiology is not to tell us *why* something happens, but to provide information that can later be used to understand why, and understand what to do with the situation at hand. At times, all that is needed is a good, hard look at the data—qualitatively and quantitatively—to characterize the phenomenon of interest; but in general, additional study methods are required to adequately understand why something is happening. Descriptive epidemiology helps us understand

what we are dealing with, *how much* of it we are encountering, and *what* we should do about it.

There are three primary goals of descriptive epidemiology:

1. *To describe and evaluate trends in health outcomes or behaviors:* Outcomes of interest may include known, emerging, re-emerging, or previously unknown disease entities, health related behaviors, healthcare utilization, and other public health outcomes of interest. Descriptive epidemiology of diseases is straightforward: describing what characteristics are found in effected or diseased individuals, including looking for (but not proving relation to) potential causal agents. Description of healthcare utilization may include recognition that specific subpopulations are not receiving or accessing care, healthcare disparities are occurring, or negative health behaviors are increasing (e.g., increased reports of unsafe sex, failure to vaccinate, etc.).

2. *To provide data for planning needs:* An understanding of who is affected by the disease of interest, where and when they are affected, how long they are affected, and how many are affected is essential for planning and resource allocation. For example, in the event of an outbreak, estimates of how many individuals are infected can assist in planning the proper number of personnel required to respond, number of hospitalizations expected, central locations of highest need, and expected duration of the epidemic. In the early moments of an outbreak (or any health-related acute situation), these estimates are crucial.

3. *To suggest future research needs:* Descriptive epidemiology is just the beginning; often, additional studies are required to follow up on the initial work. Analytic studies employ individual-level data and comparison groups in order to identify etiology, risk factors, cost issues, programmatic profiles, and other variables that may contribute to outcomes of interest. Outcomes can be either negative (e.g., foodborne disease) or positive (e.g., condom use). Data from descriptive studies are almost without exception only the first step, pointing the way towards the analytic method required, the needed sample size, and whether a given study design can appropriately answer future research questions.

PERSON, PLACE, AND TIME

Methods for descriptive epidemiology are straightforward; the primary goal is to to comprehensively characterize the person, place, and time of the events under study:

- *Person:* This refers to the characteristics of the individuals affected by the disease of interest. Who are they? Are they mostly male? Female? A specific age group? A certain race/ethnicity? Religion? Are certain types of people specifically *not* affected by the outcomes of interest? What unites the affected individuals? What do they have in common; what characteristics do they *not* have in common? We want to paint a picture of the type of person who has the disease under study, knowing as much as is possible about that person. Standard person characteristics include:

○ Age
○ Educational level
○ Gender
○ Health status (co-morbidities as well as characteristics of the disease of concern)
○ Location of residence
○ Marital status, past and current
○ Race, ethnicity (It is important to recognize, however, that these are often "proxy" variables and may have less importance unto themselves. Race and ethnicity are broad, and the outcomes with which they are associated are frequently more strongly associated with other factors, such as behavior, economic status, and location of residence, than meaningful in and of themselves.)
○ Religion, spirituality, community
○ Socioeconomic status, access to healthcare services, educational and employment opportunity
○ Behavior (This is particularly important when a specific risk factor is under study. For example, in a suspected food poisoning outbreak, what did each person eat? Sexual behavior? Drug using behavior? Healthcare seeking behavior or access to care?)

• *Place:* Where did the events take place? Country? State? County? Zip code? Census tract? Venue? Restaurant? Where were the events in relation to each other? Were there other events proximal to each other, or were they in isolation? Did the events take place in urban, suburban, or rural areas? Forested? Industrial? We want to paint a picture of the location where the disease was contracted. In this world rich with accessible travel, it is important to identify the place associated with where the disease was contracted—not where it was identified. For example, someone traveling might be well upon leaving Africa but direly ill upon landing in Sweden. The characteristics of place that are necessary are those in Africa where the disease was acquired, not in Sweden where it was diagnosed. (Unless, of course, the disease was contracted *on* the plane, in which case that is the location of disease acquisition!) As rapid air travel has made the world smaller, this may be difficult, but in order for the descriptive epidemiology and description of place to be of use, it is essential. Standard place characteristics include:

○ Location where the disease was acquired (country, state, city, zip code, block, etc.)
○ Descriptive of location (type of housing, such as house, apartment, rural, urban, suburban, running water, sewage)
○ Surrounding characteristics of the environment (Desert? Industrial? Smoky? High pollen counts? Toxins in the air? Infectious agents proximal to the location of identification? Venue? School? Job?)

• *Time:* When did the events occur? When did symptoms first appear? When was the first diagnosis made? We want to paint a picture of timing of the disease under study, knowing as much as is possible about the persons with the disease. Standard time characteristics include:

○ Date (month, day, year) of event, including day of week
○ Clock time of event, of first appearance of signs and symptoms, of diagnosis
○ Relation to sun/darkness
○ Relation to timing of events, such as sewage release cycles or other relevant events, depending on the topic under investigation
○ Relationship of each event to each other as far as time and space. Geospatial clustering is when several cases occur in one area, or have one geographic characteristic in common. (For example, cases might be spaced far apart, but all along the same interstate freeway.) Temporal clustering is when several cases occur in a relatively brief period of time; how close the cases need to be identified to one another is dependent upon the disease being investigated.

To facilitate descriptive analysis, data on person, place, and time characteristics generally are collected and documented in a systematic fashion. Again, methods matter! Imagine you were gathering data about a suspected foodborne outbreak of salmonella at a large catered event. Which of these two do you think would be preferable?

• Interviewers contact all the guests by phone and chat with guests about what they ate, hoping that the interviewer and the interviewee are able to recall all the food items possible and any possible symptoms they may have had and when they had them, or
• Have a systematic inventory of all the foods present at the event, with the same questions administered to each guest (see Figures 3-7 and 3-8)? Questions in the inventory could cover specific foods and drinks consumed, list amounts in a common fashion, identify specific combinations of food, and include other foods eaten in the suspect time period, but not deriving from the catered event. A structured symptom inventory can then be

FIGURE 3-7 FoodNet surveillance form

Foodborne Diseases Active Surveillance Network (FoodNet) Case Report Bacterial Form

Local Case ID (Medical Record #): _____   Isolated Bacteria: _____

Patient's name: _____
    Last   First

Address: _____   Phone No: (   ) _____ - _____
        Number/Street   City   State   ZIP

PHLIS ID # (Patient-Specimen): ☐☐☐☐☐☐☐☐-☐☐☐☐☐☐☐☐☐-☐☐☐-☐☐
                                          Site ID   Patient ID   Spec ID Aliquot ID

Local ID: _____-☐☐☐☐

NEDSS ID: PSN1-☐☐☐☐☐☐-☐☐-☐☐   **CAS1-**☐☐☐☐☐☐☐-☐☐-☐☐
                Patient ID   State   Installation   Investigation ID   State   Installation

1) COUNTY (residence of patient): _____ _____	2) SEX: ☐ Male ☐ Female ☐ Unknown	4a) RACE: (original categories) ☐ White ☐ Black ☐ American Indian/ Native Alaskan ☐ Unknown ☐ Asian or Pacific Islander	4a) RACE: (additional FN categories) ☐ Asian ☐ Pacific Islander or Native Hawaiian ☐ Multi-racial ☐ Other
	3) DATE OF BIRTH: _____/_____/_____ month day year		5) ETHNICITY: ☐ Hispanic ☐ Non-Hispanic ☐ Unknown
6) SPECIMEN COLLECTION DATE _____/_____/ 200____ month day	7) AGE:_____ years 8) IF < 1 YEAR, AGE: _____ months	9) SUBMITTING LAB: _____ _____ Laboratory	9a) SUBMITTING PHYSICIAN: _____ Phone: ( ) _____ -_____

Informant _____   Date Report Received in Lab _____/_____/ 200____
                                                                                    month   day

10) SOURCE OF SPECIMEN: ☐ Stool ☐ Blood ☐ CSF ☐ Urine ☐ Unknown ☐ Other site (specify):_____

11) ISOLATED BACTERIA:

☐ *Salmonella* (serogroup _____) serotype_____)   ☐ *Vibrio* (species_____)

☐ *Shigella* (serogtype/species_____)   ☐ *Yersinia* (species_____)

☐ *Campylobacter* (species_____)   ☐ *Listeria monocytogenes* (serotype_____)

☐ *E. coli*   Pregnant? ☐ Yes ☐ No ☐ Unknown

    Biochemically identified? ☐ Yes ☐ No ☐ Unknown   Outcome of Fetus?
    O157 positive? ☐ Yes ☐ No ☐ Unsure/Not Tested   ☐ Abortion/stillbirth
    O Antigen Number _____   ☐ Induced abortion
    H7 positive? ☐ Yes ☐ No ☐ Unsure/Not Tested   ☐ Live birth/neonatal death
    H Antigen Number _____   ☐ Survived-clinical infection
    Isolate non-motile? ☐ Yes ☐ No ☐ Unsure/Not Tested   ☐ Survived-no apparent illness
    Shiga toxin-positive? ☐ Yes ☐ No ☐ Unsure/Not Tested   ☐ Unknown
    National database PFGE Pattern _____   ☐ Other Bacteria (specify:) _____

continues

FIGURE 3-7 FoodNet surveillance form—continued

Foodborne Diseases Active Surveillance Network (FoodNet) Case Report Bacterial Form

Data Entry: ☐ NEDSS   ☐ PHLIS   ☐ STATE SYSTEM   ☐ CASE-CONTROL STUDY   ☐ EPI INFO

A. Hospital Follow-up:

12) PATIENT STATUS AT THE TIME OF SPECIMEN COLLECTION:

☐ Hospitalized *(go to 14)*   ☐ Unknown *(go to 14c)*
☐ Outpatient *(go to 13)*

13) IF OUTPATIENT, WAS THE PATIENT SUBSEQUENTLY HOSPITALIZED?

☐ Yes *(go to14)*   ☐ No *(go to 14c)*   ☐ Unknown *(go to 14c)*

14) IF PATIENT WAS HOSPITALIZED
(that is, if answered "Hospitalized" to #12 or "Yes" to #13):

Hospital name:_____

Date of first admission: _____/_____/ 200____
month   day

Date of last discharge: _____/_____/ 200____
month   day

14a) TRANSFERRED TO ANOTHER HOSPITAL?

☐ Yes   ☐ No   ☐ Unknown

14b) If Yes, TRANSFER HOSPITAL NAME:

14c) HOW WAS THE INFORMATION (from #12,13, or 14) **DETERMINED?**

☐ Patient/relative contacted
☐ Physician contacted or chart review/medical records review
☐ Did not follow up
☐ County provided information

15) OUTCOME: ☐ Alive   ☐ Dead   ☐ Unknown

15a) HOW WAS THIS INFORMATION (from #15) **DETERMINED?**

☐ Patient/relative contacted
☐ Physician contacted or chart review/medical records review
☐ Did not follow up
☐ County provided information

B. Health Department Follow-up:

If the isolate was further characterized by the State Lab, please update #11.

16) DID THE STATE LAB RECEIVE THE ISOLATE?

☐ Yes   ☐ No   ☐ Unknown

16a) If Yes, STATE LAB ISOLATE ID NUMBER:

_____

17) DID THE PATIENT TRAVEL OUTSIDE THE U.S. WITHIN THE LAST

- 30 days if infected with *S.* Typhi or *Listeria*
- 7 days if infected with other bacterial pathogen

☐ Yes *(go to 17a)*   ☐ No *(go to 18)*   ☐ Unknown *(go to 18)*

17a) Date of departure from the U.S.: _____/_____/ 200____
month   day

Date of return to the U.S.: _____/_____/ 200____

18) WAS CASE FOUND DURING AN AUDIT?

☐ Yes   ☐ No   ☐ Unknown

19) WAS THE CASE PART OF AN OUTBREAK?

☐ Yes *(go to 19a)*   ☐ No *(go to 20)*   ☐ Unknown *(go to 20)*

19a) IF OUTBREAK RELATED, WAS IT A FOODBORNE OUTBREAK?

☐ Yes *(go to 19b)*   ☐ No *(go to 20)*   ☐ Unknown *(go to 20)*

19b) CDC EFORS NUMBER: _____

20) WAS CASE ENROLLED IN A CASE-CONTROL STUDY?

☐ Yes   ☐ No   ☐ Unknown

If No, Reason: _____

Reason Code: _____

21) IS CASE REPORT COMPLETE?   ☐ Yes   ☐ No

21a) If Yes, DATE CASE REPORT COMPLETED:

21b) INITIALS OF PERSON COMPLETING CASE REPORT:

_____

Comments_____
_____
_____
_____
_____
_____
_____
_____
_____
_____

This is the case report form for bacterial outbreaks of foodborne disease. Note that the data are collected systematically for all aspects of person, place, and time. These data are then submitted to FoodNet for surveillance of foodborne outbreaks.

Source: CDC/FoodNet[16]

FIGURE 3-8 Example of standard foodborne disease outbreak case questionnaire

Questions about water consumption could include:

From what sources of water did you drink during the seven days before you became ill?

Municipal tap water	❑ Yes	❑ No	❑ DK	❑ Refused
Well water	❑ Yes	❑ No	❑ DK	❑ Refused
Untreated surface water	❑ Yes	❑ No	❑ DK	❑ Refused
Bottled water	❑ Yes	❑ No	❑ DK	❑ Refused
If yes, brand	❑ Yes	❑ No	❑ DK	❑ Refused
Other, specify	❑ Yes	❑ No	❑ DK	❑ Refused

In the seven days before your illness did you eat at any of the following types of commercial food establishment?

Restaurant	❑ Yes	❑ No	❑ DK	❑ Refused
Fast-food	❑ Yes	❑ No	❑ DK	❑ Refused
Cafeteria	❑ Yes	❑ No	❑ DK	❑ Refused
Deli	❑ Yes	❑ No	❑ DK	❑ Refused
Ready-to-eat food from supermarket	❑ Yes	❑ No	❑ DK	❑ Refused
Street vendor	❑ Yes	❑ No	❑ DK	❑ Refused
Concession stand at outside event	❑ Yes	❑ No	❑ DK	❑ Refused
Snack bar	❑ Yes	❑ No	❑ DK	❑ Refused
Gas station	❑ Yes	❑ No	❑ DK	❑ Refused

Specify all of above

Name of establishment _____

Address of establishment _____

Date eaten ____ / ____ / _____   Time eaten _____

Foods eaten _____

_____

_____

_____

Local health departments adapt a standard foodborne disease outbreak questionnaire specific to their needs and that of the outbreak under study. Any number of questions will be asked, and a specific food inventory (and other exposures as well, if applicable, such as petting zoo or swimming pool exposure for *E. coli*).

Source: Author.

obtained, eliciting specific symptoms, severity, timing of first onset and resolution, treatments (e.g., over-the-counter medications for diarrhea, hospitalization for dehydration), and resolution.

Clearly, the latter would be systematic and would obtain higher quality data capable of identifying the cause of the salmonella outbreak—or at least providing valid clues.

Instruments for collection of descriptive data should be developed and—to the extent possible (noting that in a public health emergency sometimes speed in response is more important than perfection)—pretested to assess validity and reliability, and pilot tested before use.[15,16]

These data collection forms are the basis for collecting descriptive information. The data are obtained through a variety of means (by interview, self-interview, computer-assisted

Describing Data

An example of how data on each person may be translated from the data collection form into analyzable data, in this line listing format

Some of the specific techniques mentioned here will be further evaluated when you take biostatistics (or other statistics) courses. Taking the following steps once you have collected line listing of data is important, in order to get to know your data:

1. *Calculate the frequencies of categorical variables.* This will inform you of how the sample is distributed among different categories of independent variables. Summary data of your outcomes are especially important because they reveal the proportion of missing data, which can impact your study enormously. Some examples of frequencies:

Demographic and clinical characteristics of women diagnosed with sepsis postoperatively (N = 110).

	n	%
Gender		
Female	73	66.4
Male	37	33.6
Age (years)		
<18	15	13.6
18–35	28	25.5
36–45	56	50.9
>45	11	10
Past medical history		
No significant medical problems	8	7.3
Mild	59	53.6
Moderate	41	37.3
Severe	2	1.8
Past Surgical History		
No abdominal surgeries	38	34.6
One prior abdominal surgery	39	35.4
Two or more prior abdominal surgeries	33	30.0
Body mass index (BMI)		
Underweight (<18.5 kg/m^2)	4	3.6
Normal (18.5 to 24.9 kg/m^2)	48	43.6
Overweight (25 to 29 kg/m^2)	34	30.9
Obese (>30 kg/m^2)	21	19.1
Unknown	3	2.7

2. *Calculate measures of central tendency (mean, median, mode) and dispersion (standard deviation or variance) for continuous variables.* How are variables distributed? Do they follow a normal distribution (that is, like a bell curve)? Or are they skewed left or right? Are the tails heavy or skinny? This can be assessed visually to some degree, and tested quantitatively as well. Some examples of measures of central tendency and dispersion:

Characteristics of participants with cryptosporidium (N = 136)

	Mean	Median	Mode	Standard deviation
Age (years)	25.4	24.0	23.0	5.79
BMI (kg/m^2)	23.7	23.5	23.4	21.25
Baseline CD4 (absolute count) at study entry	419.0	365.0	368.0	331.25

continues

Describing Data

3. *Plot the continuous data one variable at a time, using box plots, stem and leaf plots, or other graphic displays at your disposal.* This describes the data variable by variable. In addition, it helps identify where there are out of range values or missing values, and gives a general description of your continuous data.

Stem-and-leaf plot for age (age of index)

```
1f | 45555
1s | 6667777777
1. | 88888888888888888899999999999999
2* | 00000000000000000000000111111111111111
2t | 222222222222222222222233333333
2f | 4444444444444444444444445555555555555555
2s | 66666666666666667777777777
2. | 88888888899999999999
3* | 0000000000011111111111
3t | 2222222222222222333333333
3f | 4444444444455555555555555555555
3s | 666666666777777777777
3. | 8888888888888889999999
4* | 0000011111111111111
4t | 2222222333333333333333
4f | 44444444555555
4s | 666777
4. | 8888999
5* | 0000000011111
5t | 333
5f | 444
5s | 6666777
5. | 8899
6* | 11
6t | 3
6f |
6s | 66
6. | 9
7* |
7t |
7f | 55
7s | 7
```

A histogram describing the age of the index patients.

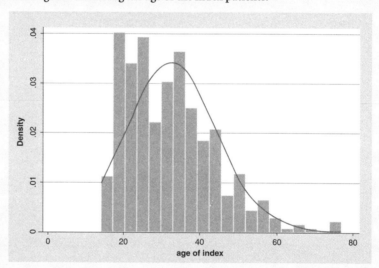

4. *Plot the data in a scatterplot, placing the dependent (outcome) variable on the Y-axis (the vertical axis) and the independent (potential predictor) variable on the X-axis (the horizontal axis).* What do the data look like? How do they relate to each other? Is there any discernable pattern or relationship between the independent variables and dependent variable under study? Is there any discernable pattern between independent variables? (Remember that we are still looking for "clues"; not seeing a pattern does not mean there is *not* one, just as seeing one does not mean there *is* one!)

Using a scatterplot showing the relationship between age and CD4 count, we can see here that it looks as if CD4 counts are higher the younger the participant is. This is not enough to *prove* anything or provide statistical testing on its own, but it does give one a feel for the relationship. If you plot this first, you will know what to expect when you analyze your data. For example, if you found the opposite from what this picture suggests (i.e., CD4s increase with age) you might want to do some quality checking.

continues

Describing Data

Data in a Scatterplot

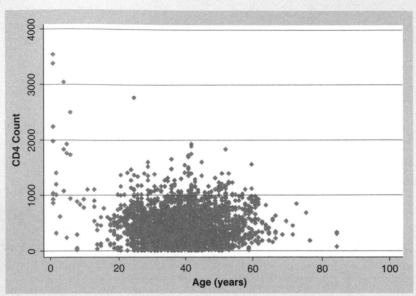

5. *Look at outliers, datapoints that stand out from the rest of the distribution.* For continuous variables, this can be quantified by looking at datapoints that extend beyond a set level (e.g., two standard deviation above or below the mean). What are they? Get to know each of these outliers. Investigate them. Are they data entry errors? Documentation problems? Or are they true? There are a number of techniques available to diagnose outliers and treat them appropriately. However, sometimes, if the data are correct, the outlier can be a substantive "clue" towards figuring out the problem at hand. Each might represent an acute case, a pronounced relationship, or something "different" that can be extremely useful.

Box and whisker plot of baseline CD4 count.

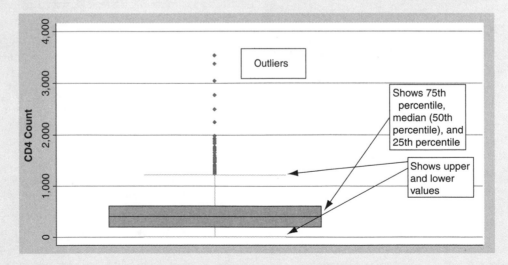

self-interview) from the guests and other potentially exposed individuals. The information is then transformed into a line listing. For example, the box below shows how part of a line listing might take data collected on form in Figure 3-8 and analyze it. The box also displays ways that line listed data can be analyzed and visualized. (Note that many more questions would be asked; this is just an example.)

SPECIFIC METHODS

As stated earlier, the most important thing about descriptive epidemiology is getting acquainted with your data. The techniques outlined above do this, though it is important to recognize that understanding the data requires more than just tabulating and printing: Interpretation is key. Looking at the quantitative information provided in the steps above—as well as reviewing it qualitatively and holistically—and then taking the analysis a step further is important: The interpretation of the information obtained is vital. Looking at the disease under study, the potential causes under exploration, and what makes the data suggest that it is one cause over another, and then combining the evidence with previous knowledge of infectious disease, are what make descriptive epidemiology an incredibly useful methodological tool.

Several specific descriptive designs use the data collection methods, including—as you will see in almost every epidemiologic techniques descriptive and analytic alike—systematic data collection. These include case reports, case series, ecological studies, and outbreak investigations. Together they comprise the descriptive epidemiologic methods' core. These study designs transform the data you collect and have gotten to know into interpretable information.

Case Reports

Case reports are an essential link between clinical medicine and public health. Continuing clinical education often uses the format of case reports in order to facilitate communication between providers or to teach students. However, these are somewhat different than case reports as a descriptive epidemiologic method. Here, an astute clinician notices something "odd" in the presentation of a specific patient or in the appearance of a cluster of "unusual" events. What makes something odd or unusual, though? What piques the awareness of the provider and helps him or her take note of the event? There are several hallmarks that might capture one's attention:

- Presentation of a known disease in an unusual population; for example, PCP is relatively common among older, immunocompromised populations, but seldom seen in young, healthy populations.

- Presentation of a previously unrecognized syndrome or disease.
- Presentation of a disease more or less severe than previously seen, or with a different characteristic than noted before (such as genetic resistance to a drug, failure to be treated with standard of care treatment, etc.).
- Presentation of a disease that was transmitted in a mode not generally seen or suspected.
- A cluster (temporal or geospatial) of diseased individuals that is unusual in some way.

Case reports are often communicated within one facility, but may also be disseminated to peer-reviewed journals, governing bodies overseeing clinical care (e.g., hospital review boards), or government entities (e.g., Centers for Disease Control and Prevention, Ministries of Health). These then are shared as needed with other practitioners and public health agencies. Similar cases may be sought or diagnostic procedures recommended in the event that providers see cases in the future. This helps launch public health into action should the need arise.

Case Series

Case series are similar to case reports, except that there is usually more than one case of the disease, where in a case report there is generally just one. In addition, frequently case series attempt to identify denominator data, though the method of obtaining these denominator data is often relatively crude. For example, a provider, who is seeing six cases of *Trichomonas vaginalis* (a sexually transmitted disease) that did not respond to metronidazole (the usual treatment) after adherent patients tried several cycles of treatment, may do in-depth case reports on the six patients. The provider then might identify how many cases of metronidazole-resistant *T. vaginalis* had occurred over a specified time period at that clinic. This number becomes the numerator, and the number of people exposed to metronidazole with *T. vaginalis* the denominator. Together these data suggest a rate (though it is not actually one), though it is crude for the following reasons:

- *The data are retrospective in nature.* Documentation for this specific research question was not likely to have been collected systematically. Other patients may have had the same clinical presentation and not been captured, or they may have been included in dataset but not documented in the same way. So information can be missing or differentially ascertained on the individuals in question.

- *The availability of the clinic records may be less than optimal.* The ability to review all records for status with regard to *T. vaginalis*, metronidazole treatment, or other outcomes may be minimal. For example, medical charts may be out because the patient is frequently sick, because they are never sick, or for reasons unknown. This means that those individuals on whom data may be collected may differ from those on whom data cannot be collected.
- *The clinic-based population provides only an estimate of the individuals who were able to access care at that particular clinic.* There are may be others who did not have access to the clinic, had no insurance, or ability to seek care. Others may not have had signs or symptoms that encouraged them to seek care, or they may have been previously treated with metronidazole, but—for whatever reason— not returned for follow-up care despite actual need. This means that the underlying rates at the clinic are not equivalent to those of the underlying population.

Still, estimation of metronidazole-resistant *T. vaginalis* rates at the clinic, no matter how crude, can be helpful in assessing whether this is a rare event—or just appears to be increasing or actually might be. In addition, case series typically begin to employ a more systematic data collection tool than case reports, increasing the data's reliability and validity.

Ecologic Studies

Ecologic studies differ from other types of descriptive epidemiology in that individuals are not the unit of analysis. In this type of study, we analyze data on the *group* level. These studies are very important for several reasons:

- They frequently generate important hypotheses that need further, analytic research.
- They make comparisons between large groups of people—say, inhabitants of different countries—that would otherwise be impossible.
- They can be done without the benefit of substantial resources; often publicly available information is sufficient to conduct, analyze, and interpret an ecologic study.

Geographic comparisons are common with ecologic studies, but not the only possible approach. Other comparisons could include classes, schools, genders, races, or other grouping variables. Often data are provided that are descriptive of the outcome or exposure, and then linked with additional descriptive data on the alternate axis. For example, one could link data on unsafe sex (see Figure 3-9) and condom sales to investigate their (non-causal) relationship.

Here is a more vivid example. Imagine we have statistics on the number of cases of condoms sold by county in two states for a period of 10 years, as well as the reported rates (adjusted for the age differences of the underlying population structures) of three STDs, gonorrhea, chlamydia, and syphilis, for the same period of time. Associations between the independent variable—condom sales (exposure)—and the dependent variables—each of the three STDs (outcomes)—can be calculated. This is valuable information. These data may shed some light on the relationship between condom sales and the outcome STDs: Do counties with high condom sales rates have increased or decreased STD rates? Are the condoms associated with prevention of STDs on the aggregate level? They also may inform us on changes seen in this relationship over time. As the condom sales increased, did the STD rates increase or decrease? Over time, ecologic studies can be useful in evaluating various hypotheses about the relationship under study.

Ecologic studies are not without limitations, however, though they are very important and have stimulated many important public health research studies and subsequent accomplishments. Ecologic designs have been integral in understanding overall relationships in a number of areas of research. For example, in HIV, they suggested that circumcision may be associated with reduced rates of HIV acquisition. This finding in the aggregate stimulated observational studies, and, finally, three large randomized controlled trials of circumcision in Africa.[17,18] Thanks to the results just released from the trials in Uganda and Kenya,[18] which stopped early due to the efficacy of the procedure, it is clear that the ecologic studies generated an important hypothesis that may ultimately have an enormous public health impact. The results indicate a strong protective effect of the operation, but it took confirmation from the randomized trials to establish an individual-level estimate of the association.

The primary limitation of ecologic studies is called the *ecologic fallacy*. This fallacy emerges because we do not know if the association seen on the aggregate (group) level holds on the individual level. For example, despite our statistics that characterize the *group's* behavior, we know nothing about the individuals making up the group. Suppose counties that have the highest condom sales have the lowest STD rates. This supports the hypothesis that increased condom use is associated with decreased STDs. But we can never know if the people with the lowest STD rates are the ones using the condoms. It could be that:

- *The STD rates are high in the area.* People have heard this, learned from the safer sex social marketing campaign, and begun to purchase more condoms. That does

FIGURE 3-9 Burden of disease attributable to sexual and reproductive health risks (%DALYs in each region)—Unsafe sex

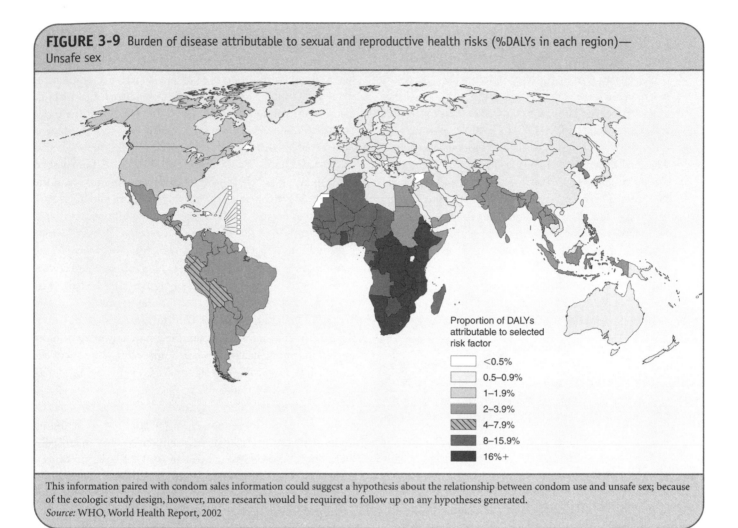

Proportion of DALYs attributable to selected risk factor

	<0.5%
	0.5–0.9%
	1–1.9%
	2–3.9%
	4–7.9%
	8–15.9%
	16%+

This information paired with condom sales information could suggest a hypothesis about the relationship between condom use and unsafe sex; because of the ecologic study design, however, more research would be required to follow up on any hypotheses generated.
Source: WHO, World Health Report, 2002

not mean they use them, however. The rates could be decreasing for other reasons, such as increased STD screening by the local public health clinic.

- *Many people do use condoms.* However, they are not having sex with people with STDs but rather people without. The people with the STDs are having unprotected sex, but they are having it with people getting treated already for STDs, thus the appearance of decreased STDs is artificial and independent of condom use.

- *We do not know which came first: the high condom sales or the low STD rates.* Maybe the low STD rates preceded the high condom sales, which occurred for an unrelated reason.

These are just potential explanations; there could be many others that the data would not reveal due to the ecologic fallacy. Another problem with ecologic studies is that it is not possible to be sure about temporality. Knowing which event came first, the dependent or the independent variable,

usually remains unknown until a stronger study design can evaluate the research question on the individual level. Still, these are very important hypotheses-generating studies, and can be very valuable in suggesting associations that need further study.

Taking Public Health Action

We will soon discuss the next steps in study design development; descriptive studies are merely the beginning of getting to know your data and deciding upon appropriate next steps. In general, after describing the data—the outbreak, the cluster, the cases, the individuals—under study, the next step is to identify a study design that is capable of demonstrating a causal link between a characteristic (the *independent variable*, such as the organism) and the outcome (the *dependent variable*, such as the disease). Descriptive analyses cannot do this, although they are extremely useful in generating hypotheses that may be studied later. Although public health practitioners and

TABLE 3-3 Descriptive Epidemiology Summary Table

Design	Description
Descriptive epidemiologic designs	Studies that describe public health events with a detailed investigation into person, place, and time characteristics generally involve no formal comparisons between groups. Hypothesis is generated not tested.
Case reports	An unusual event is identified in one person. Generally report a new disease, a disease in a new type of patient or population, or something otherwise unusual. Description of the particular person with regard to person, place, and time—and details of condition—is provided. Hypothesis is generated, not tested.
Case series	A group of case reports is assembled, with cases that represent a similar condition or situation. Where possible, data are provided to indicate usual frequency of event, either through estimates of rates or historical data. Hypothesis is generated, not tested.
Ecologic studies	Collect aggregate data on exposures and aggregate data on outcomes provided for geographical areas, or other population-level groupings. Hypothesis is generated, not tested.
Outbreak investigations	Specialized type of descriptive epidemiologic design that assesses acute disease or other public health events. Outbreak investigations attempt to identify source of emerging or re-emerging disease (or other public health emergencies), stop them, and prevent them in the future. Hypothesis is generated, not tested, although information derived from these can often be used to immediately stem threats to public health.

policies in general like to be sure of the cause of a particular outbreak, one important premise of public health is that action can and should be taken when it is evident that it can protect the health of individuals and the health of the public. This is important: Whenever in the investigative process it becomes clear that there is a strong likelihood that a specific cause or behavior is associated with a specific health-threatening outcome, public health action to reduce exposure to the source should be undertaken. For example, in the case of a city water filtration system with excessive cryptopsporidium[1]—a parasite that causes severe diarrhea among immunocompromised individuals—immediate action should be taken. Extensive epidemiologic studies can be completed, as indicated, to show definitively that there is a problem, where the source is, and so on, at the same time as actions are taken to immediately *stop* exposure. In a foodborne outbreak at a restaurant, for example, if 30 individuals have become ill from an obvious and demonstrated source, corrective action must be taken immediately. In this sort of situation, it would be rare for it to be advisable to wait for a lengthy study: People are sick and additional infections must be prevented. Descriptive epidemiologic studies sometimes provide enough information to suggest a rapid intervention to protect public health, and it is worth undertaking such action—at least until the understanding of the problem is refined with more exacting study designs. This should be tempered, though, with appreciation for the rights of individuals. Public health action that can harm the rights of individuals in anyway should be carefully considered before implementation. If the public health action could restrict freedom, cause discrimination or stigma about the disease or the exposure, or physically or emotionally harm to those at risk for the disorder, it is preferable to be absolutely sure about the situation at hand before taking action.

Descriptive epidemiology has historically been one of the most important types of study. Before we use the sophisticated techniques outlined in upcoming chapters, description is critical. Understanding each and every datapoint with information on exposures, outcomes, and confounders, each and every person that is affected, and how the disease (or other outcome) manifests with regard to person, place, and time is very important. Once we have this vital information and understand what is going on with the public health issue at hand, we can proceed to test hypotheses and try to better understand the relationships between exposures and disease.

Taking Rapid Public Health Action: The Good, the Bad, and the Ugly

Taking public health action as quickly as possible is important. However, equally important is recognizing that sweeping actions can have negative as well as positive consequences. A good example is the actions surrounding discovery of severe acute respiratory syndrome (SARS).[19–21]

When people became suddenly and severely ill with respiratory symptoms in 1999, the syndrome and method of transmission (droplet) were rapidly identified some time prior to a complete understanding of the causative agent, a coronavirus (see Figure 3-10). Several public health interventions were quickly taken: Affected and potentially exposed individuals were sought, quarantined, and treated. Certain flight restrictions from geographically affected regions were implemented. This rapid response may have limited the number of deaths from SARS. Once the causative agent was found in the laboratory and the disease better understood, some of these restrictions were lifted.

However, it is essential that public health personnel are also aware there can be hazards of too rapid a response. Because of generalized hysteria, for a short time people stopped flying in commercial airplanes, began wearing masks whenever they were in public in affected parts of Asia, and scorned those with coughs or SARS-like symptoms. Some of these actions were reasonable in close proximity to an ill individual: Handwashing, masks, and quarantine make sense in case some are already ill. But the

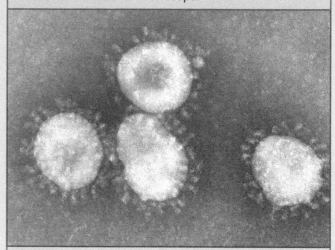

FIGURE 3-10 Coronaviruses are a group of viruses that have a halo, or crown-like (corona) appearance when viewed under a microscope.

The coronavirus is now recognized as the etiologic agent of the 2003 SARS outbreak. This virus is a cousin of what we consider the common cold. Only in SARS, it is substantially more acute and deadly, though equally contagious.

Source: CDC, 1971; Public Health Image Library/Dr. Fred Murphy.

majority of persons coughing were ill with garden-variety colds, not SARS. The high level of intensity of response could have been capable of scaring individuals and prevent those who may have been ill from seeking care than reduce transmission of this serious virus. A tempered public health response might have been negative—reacting too late to the situation resulting in more deaths—but it also may have provided time to understand the virus's characteristics and develop responsible social marketing campaigns to help people into care without stigmatizing them. To be sure, hindsight is always "20/20," and at the time, it was impossible to know what we were dealing with and taking a conservative approach, most likely to protect the public's health is the best approach. But recognition that rapid action can have negative consequences as well as positive is important to note. At the same time, experience with SARS has a direct bearing on how we will handle avian flu, should this become pandemic. Active engagement in public health protection, using information gained from outbreak investigations, is necessary. In addition, ecological studies, based on trends in non-avian flu[22–24] following September 11, 2001, suggest that the normal patterns of flu may have been significantly altered when air travel was curtailed in the United States following 9/11. In a case such as SARS or avian flu, stopping air travel, quarantine, and more extreme measures may make sense as far as stemming the epidemics. More data are needed however, and methodology to understand the impact of regulations is important. The limitations of ecologic studies mean that hypotheses regarding the efficacy of airline travel regulations, for example, need more in-depth hypothesis testing before we understand for certain their benefit.

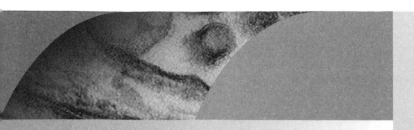

Discussion Questions

1. What are the three most essential elements of descriptive epidemiology? Why are they important in the task of describing infectious disease phenomena?

2. Go to www.cdc.gov/foodnet/ and select one foodborne outbreak. Describe its characteristics with regard to person, place, and time.

3. What are the descriptive epidemiologic study designs? Name them, and describe their strengths and limitations.

4. List at least three ways that data can be described quantitatively.

REFERENCES

1. Heymann DL. *Control of Communicable Diseases*. 18th ed. Washington, DC: American Public Health Association; 2004.

2. UCLA Department of Epidemiology. John Snow. Available at: http://www.ph.ucla.edu/epi/snow.html. Accessed December 25, 2006.

3. Tufte E. *Visual and Statistical Thinking: Displays of Evidence for Decision Making*. Cheshire, CT: Graphics Press LLC; 1997.

4. Snow J. On the Mode of Communication of Cholera by John Snow. 2nd edition, much enlarged. 1855. Reprinted in: Frost WH, ed. Snow on Cholera. New York, NY: The Commonwealth Fund; 1936.

5. Smith GD. Commentary: behind the Broad Street pump: aetiology, epidemiology and prevention of cholera in mid-19th century Britain. *Int J Epidemiol*. 2002;31:920–932.

6. Friis RH, Sellers TA. *Epidemiology for Public Health Practice*. 3rd ed. Boston: Jones and Bartlett; 2004.

7. Department of Epidemiology, Michigan State University. The John Snow archive and research companion. 2006. Available at: http:// www.matrix.msu.edu/~johnsnow/index.php. Accessed December 31, 2006.

8. CDC. Pneumocystis pneumonia—Los Angeles. *MMWR*. 1981;30: 250–252.

9. CDC. Kaposi's sarcoma and Pneumocystis pneumonia among homosexual men: New York City and Los Angeles. *MMWR*. 1981;30:305–308.

10. CDC. A cluster of Kaposi's sarcoma and *Pneumocystis carinii* pneumonia among homosexual male residents of Los Angeles and range counties, California. *MMWR*. 1982;31:305–307.

11. CDC. HIV prevalence, unrecognized infection, and HIV testing among men who have sex with men—five U.S. cities, June 2004–April 2005. *MMWR*. 2005;54(24):597–601.

12. CDC. HIV/AIDS surveillance report, 2004. 2005. Available at: http://www.cdc.gov/hiv/stats/hasrlink.htm. Accessed November 1, 2005.

13. CDC. HIV/AIDS surveillance report: cases of HIV infection and AIDS in the United States, 2005. 2006. Available at: http://www.cdc.gov/hiv/topics/ surveillance/resources/reports/2005report/pdf/2005/SurveillanceReport.pdf. Accessed December 1, 2006.

14. Marston C, King E. Factors that shape young people's sexual behaviour: a systematic review. *Lancet*. 2006;368:1581–1586.

15. CDC. CDC surveillance summaries: surveillance for foodborne-disease outbreaks—United States, 1993–1997. *MMWR*. 2000;49(SS-1):1–72.

16. CDC. FoodNet. 2005. Available at: www.cdc.gov/foodnet/surveillance.htm. Accessed December 10, 2006.

17. Auvert B, Taljaard D, Lagarde E, Sobngwi-Tambekou J, Sitta R, Puren A. Randomized, controlled intervention trial of male circumcision for reduction of HIV infection risk: the ANRS 1265 trial. *PLoS Med*. 2005;2(11): 1112–1122.

18. National Institute of Allergy and Infectious Diseases. Adult male circumcision significantly reduces risk of acquiring HIV—trials in Kenya and Uganda stopped early. 2006. Available at: http://www3.niaid.nih.gov/news/newsreleases/2006/AMC12_06press.htm. Accessed February 7, 2007.

19. CDC. Outbreak of severe acute respiratory syndrome—worldwide, 2003. *MMWR*. 2003;52(11):226–228.

20. CDC. Update: outbreak of severe acute respiratory syndrome—worldwide, 2003. *MMWR*. 2003;52:241–248.

21. Gostin L, Bayer R, Fairchild A. Ethical and legal challenges posed by severe acute respiratory syndrome: implications for the control of severe infectious disease threats. *JAMA*. 2003;290:3229–3237.

22. Brownstein JS, Wolfe CJ, Mandl KD. Empirical evidence for the effect of airline travel on inter-regional influenza spread in the United States. *PloS Med*. 2006;3:e401:1826-e401:1835.

23. Viboud C, Miller MA, Grenfell BT, Bjornstad ON, Simonsen L. Air travel and the spread of influenza: important caveats. *PLoS Med*. 2006;3:e503: 2159-e503:2160.

24. Brownstein JS, Mandl KD, Wolfe CJ. Air travel and the spread of influenza: Authors' Reply. *PLoS Med*. 2006;3:e503:2160-e503:2161.

CHAPTER 4

Outbreak Investigations

LEARNING OBJECTIVES

By the end of this chapter, you will be able to:

- Describe the purpose of outbreak investigations.
- List the main steps in an outbreak investigation.
- Articulate what information outbreak investigations can and cannot provide.
- Describe and know how to develop epidemic curves.
- Recognize main types of outbreaks in their graphic representation.

OUTBREAK INVESTIGATIONS—DESCRIPTIVE EPIDEMIOLOGY WITH A SPECIFIC PURPOSE

Countless books, articles, presentations, and reports have been written about outbreak investigations and how to conduct them. This chapter will not make you an expert in the conduct of outbreak investigations. The aim of this chapter is to utilize the outbreak investigation as a special case in which we can use descriptive epidemiology skills while foreshadowing what is to come with our analytic epidemiology toolkit. Outbreak investigations offer a unique opportunity to understand the immediate interface between research and public health intervention, as we work to find threats to public health, eliminate them, and prevent them from recurring. At this point of overlap, we can see the power of methods and some of the many ways they can be put to good use.

What is an outbreak investigation? Outbreak investigations are not methodologically different from other epidemiologic study designs. The primary difference is usually that they are more urgent and time-sensitive than other studies,

and they generally have more immediate constraints than other studies. Outbreak investigations have had tremendous impact not only on the health of individuals, but on our understanding of disease as well.[1–18] Because they often investigate emerging or re-emerging infectious agents that may have never before been encountered, there is sometimes a conspicuous lack of information about the diseases under study. When the disease is well-known, the degree of acuity may be high, either because the disease is highly infectious (e.g, influenza), readily transmitted to others (e.g., foodborne outbreaks), or dangerous (e.g., antibiotic resistant nosocomial infections). Each of these points can be important; but perhaps the most salient difference between other epidemiologic study designs and outbreak investigations is that with almost every other type of study we know (more or less) what we are studying. In outbreak investigations, we sometimes will, but often we do not. Other epidemiologic study designs, which we will go into some depth about in the next chapters, are generally not undertaken until a solid foundation has been laid with descriptive studies—descriptive studies generate hypotheses and analytic studies test hypotheses. With outbreak investigations, there is newness and there are unknowns. This is the detective work that epidemiologists are most recognized for, and there are countless examples of epidemiologists whose outbreak investigations resulted in many, many lives saved. Historically, outbreak investigations have helped improve public health in general as well as to improve methodology that is used in epidemiology as a whole.

Before elucidating the steps in an outbreak investigation, let us consider some vocabulary. The terms *epidemic* and *outbreak* are similar and overlapping, yet are used in subtly different ways. Outbreak implies a cluster of cases that are either temporally or geospatially proximal; it has a more local feeling to its use of, whereas *epidemic* suggests something more alarming, longer, and perhaps more widespread. When speaking to the public about a health issue, using the term *outbreak* instead of *epidemic* might be prudent—it raises less fear in people and allows them to focus on the characteristics of the cases instead of the fear of the epidemic.

There are many definitions of outbreaks, but they may be thought of most simply as the occurrence of an illness with a frequency clearly in excess of what is normally expected in a defined, well-delineated local area or region. Note that there are key pieces of this definition: It is geographically bounded and it requires knowledge of the baseline frequency and a clear demonstration that there are more cases than usual.

An *endemic* is when a disease continues at the same level of incidence for a prolonged period of time in a specific area; for example, certain areas are endemic for diseases like cholera or malaria, which means they have sustained high levels of incidence for these diseases. This may be contrasted with other regions, where even one case of these diseases constitutes an epidemic to be taken extremely seriously. In some ways, the definitions of epidemic and endemic may seem at odds: Why do we need a term to describe high rates of disease, if the local rates are always so high, why is not that the norm and thus the baseline? If the definition for epidemic requires that a disease rate is clearly in excess of normal, would this not suggest that the high rate has become the baseline? Indeed, this is the very reason why we need a separate term to describe high rates that exceed what they should be and extend for a prolonged period of time. Though the disease might be found at increased rates all the time, this does not imply that we do not want to reduce the disease burden. Take malaria, for example, millions die of malaria each year, and there are many countries with endemic malaria. Still, this remains a significant health concern, even though, sadly, the high rates are the norm for some regions. *Pandemics* are epidemics that extend across continents and around the globe. The current fear that avian flu (H5N1) could become pandemic means that this one strain of influenza would create illness across borders and around the world. The 1918 flu is one of the most recognizable pandemics, infecting and killing millions.[14,19–25]

The steps in an outbreak investigation progress logically, integrating study design—that is, descriptive and analytic methods, detective work, and public health action. The following steps are those most commonly taken in outbreak investigations of infectious disease. The beauty of this methodology is that it can be applied with very little modification to other public health concept areas. For example, cancer, environmental insults, occupational hazards, mental health or behavioral issues, and more can be treated to some degree with the same approach used and developed in infectious disease.

STEPS IN AN OUTBREAK INVESTIGATION

The basic six steps of an outbreak investigation are discussed in the following sections.

1. Define the Purpose of the Investigation

This step is common to each and every study. Like all research endeavors, the purpose of the investigation needs to be clarified from the start. All outbreak investigations share the same immediate overall goals: stop illness and promote health. However, the specific purpose of each investigation needs to be clarified further than that. What is the primary purpose of the investigation, the specific goals? This differs from study to study. In an acute foodborne outbreak such as that at a restaurant, the goal is usually to identify the causative agent, the vehicle, the source, and the food-handling deficit that allowed the disease to be spread. In an outbreak of a new infection causing rapid and severe illness with a high mortality rate, such as severe acute respiratory syndrome (SARS), the goal may be to identify the agent (Is it old? New? If new, what is it? Do we have or can we adapt a diagnostic test for the agent? Is there a treatment for the illness?) and take immediate public health action to halt its spread.

2. Establish the Existence of the Epidemic

This is where your descriptive measure come into play. We always need to first ensure that there really is an epidemic. Imagine you are examining a potential outbreak of syphilis among adolescent males who have sex with males (MSM). Before assuming that the increase in rates is due to a true outbreak, more information needs to be gathered. Perhaps there was a secular change that makes it appear that there is an outbreak, when there actually is not. Syphilis, like some other diseases, tends to have a natural history with periods of disease increase over years. Perhaps there was improved surveillance resulting in more cases. In order to answer these questions, rates of the disease under study need to be compared to some usual baseline. In outbreak investigations, we might want to compare the number of cases to what we expect based on any number of things, such as the usual cases for a given time period in that area, or the distribution of cases over prior years. After adjusting for the population (the denominator), is there a true, nonartifactual increase in the number of cases? If one looks at the same time period over several years, is that increase still evident? For example, if one looks at summer months, there are generally more cases of chickenpox than in other months; if one looks at winter months there are generally more cases of influenza than in other months. So, comparisons of the adjacent time periods as well as prior years to identify patterns are important. One can also look at age-, gender-, and race-adjusted rates to see if there are differences in the subpopulations experiencing the disease and if this can point to an alternative explanation beyond that of a true outbreak.

3. Develop a Case Definition

Preliminary information about the cases assists in the development of a case definition that carefully operationalizes what a case is. A case definition is an explicit set of criteria against which people may be measured to see if they are cases or not. Case definitions are used to determine if a person meets a strict definition of the disease in question. The case definition operationalizes the disease under study, allowing a systematic approach that finds like persons and categorizes them all similarly. Then their case/noncase status can be studied to identify differences between the categories, and find predictors. Often cases are divided into the categories of definite, probable, or possible. When this approach is used, each of these levels has its own definition as well. This step is very similar to the development of inclusion and exclusion criteria, a crucial element in observational as well as experimental analytic epidemiology studies. For the purpose of outbreak investigations, case definitions are usually wide in scope, so that more people will be considered a case than truly are. When relatively little is known about the disease entity being studied, it is important to be sure that cases that could help identify the etiologic agent are not overlooked. This is referred to as "casting a wide net." This means that there will be some false positives (people who are considered cases but truly are not) and fewer false negatives (true cases that are not identified because the case definition was too narrow); this helps us to be sure that we do not neglect to count cases that can help us to understand the outbreak.

4. If Laboratory Methods Are Available, Confirm the Diagnosis

Evidence of the infectious agent thought to be causing the outbreak is optimal, if it can be obtained. If no laboratory methods are available for the specific pathogen (as often there would not be if the disease is new or unknown), then alternative or surrogate measures can be used. For example, imagine the development of a new form of infectious liver disease—similar to but not hepatitis B. Liver enzymes (assays that show how well the liver is functioning) could be used as clinical markers of the disease, and these could be used to focus on the disease and define it until microbiological assays become available. Other forms of clinical information—patient report, physical exam, lab results, diagnostic radiology, medical record, pathology—can be used in the absence of diagnostic confirmation or, when confirmation is available, in addition to it, to ensure that the full range of presentations is incorporated.

SARS: Example of a First Case Definition

With SARS, a new infectious disease that had not been previously encountered, real detective work had to be done in order to determine the cause and suggest public health action. The first case definition casts a wide net to try to minimize the number of true cases missed (while allowing more false positive cases). It was clear that it would be preferable to include too many cases and test them than to include too few. Use of this preliminary case definition helped identify true cases and, in turn, helped figure out what the pathogen—the new coronavirus—was.

The following is the CDC's preliminary case definition for severe acute respiratory syndrome (SARS) (as of March 19, 2003)[26,27]:

Suspected Case

Respiratory illness of unknown etiology with onset since February 1, 2003, and the following criteria:

- Documented temperature >100.4°F (>38.0°C)
- One or more symptoms of respiratory illness (e.g., cough, shortness of breath, difficulty breathing, or radiographic findings of pneumonia or acute respiratory distress syndrome)
- Close contact (defined as having cared for, having lived with, or having had direct contact with respiratory secretions and/or body fluids of a person suspected of having SARS) within 10 days of onset of symptoms with a person under investigation for or suspected of having SARS or travel within 10 days of onset of symptoms to an area with documented transmission of SARS as defined by the World Health Organization (WHO).

This case definition uses clinical findings to operationalize the disease, as there was, at the time, no knowledge of the virus causing the disease. Note how this case definition, like most, shows description based on person, place, and time.

What Does a Case Definition Look Like?

In an effort to improve systematic application of case definitions, in 1990, the CDC created a listing of case definitions associated with notifiable infectious conditions.[5,8,11,28] These were amended in 1997, and we are still operating using these versions. As much as is possible, we want to create the best case definitions we can, and reduce the need for subsequent changes: any change to a case definition can have an enormous impact on surveillance. Changing a case definition can result in an artifactual increase or decrease in cases, which can be confusing at times. Case definitions can be presented in a variety of formats; those by local healthcare agencies may differ from the national- or international-level ones. However, they all have a basically similar structure, as shown in Figure 4-1, based on those from the CDC.[5,8]

FIGURE 4-1 Case definition structure

Definition of Terms Used in Case Classification

Clinically compatible case: a clinical syndrome generally compatible with the disease, as described in the clinical description

Confirmed case: a case that is classified as confirmed for reporting purposes.

Epidemiologically linked case: a case in which a) the patient has had contact with one or more persons who either have/had the disease or have been exposed to a point source of infection (i.e., a single source of infection, such as an event leading to a foodborne-disease outbreak, to which all confirmed case-patients were exposed) and b) transmission of the agent by the usual modes of transmission is plausible. A case may be considered epidemiologically linked to a laboratory-confirmed case if at least one case in the chain of transmission is laboratory confirmed.

Laboratory-confirmed case: a case that is confirmed by one or more of the laboratory methods listed in the case definition under Laboratory Criteria for Diagnosis. Although other laboratory methods can be used in the clinical diagnosis, only those listed are accepted as laboratory confirmation for national reporting purposes.

Probable case: a case that is classified as probable for reporting purposes.

Supportive or presumptive laboratory results: specified laboratory results that are consistent with the diagnosis, yet do not meet the criteria for laboratory confirmation.

Suspected case: a case that is classified as suspected for reporting purposes.

Source: CDC[5,8]

Other categorization systems sometimes used include the definite/probable/possible designations that are more frequently used by clinicians, and map roughly to confirmed/probable/suspected. What is most important when dealing with case definitions is that the exact criteria listed are met—there is no squeaking in or out. The utility of any case definition depends upon the exactitude with which it is used. This also holds true for inclusion and exclusion criteria in a study: If the criteria cannot be met or defined exactly as to whether someone is or is not eligible, then including them in the sample can be detrimental to the overall study. (This is why in multicentered clinical trials there is almost always a highly controlled exemption procedure, whereby any deviations from the eligibility criteria—no matter how seemingly small—must be cleared by the organizing body. This not only ensures the subject's safety, but also the integrity of the study.)

Figure 4-2 provides a straightforward case definition for rabies.[5,8]

Figure 4-3 shows a complex one for syphilis, with more than one level (suspected, probable, possible, definite), multiple phases, and requiring laboratory confirmation in conjunction with clinical presentation.[5,8]

continues

What Does a Case Definition Look Like?—continues

FIGURE 4-2 A case definition for rabies

RABIES, ANIMAL

Laboratory criteria for diagnosis
- A positive direct fluorescent antibody test (preferably preformed on central nervous system tissue)
- Isolation of rabies virus (in cell culture or in laboratory animal)

Case classification
Confirmed: a case that is laboratory confirmed

RABIES, HUMAN

Clinical description
Rabies is an acute encephalomyelitis that almost always progresses to coma or death within 10 days after the symptom.

Laboratory criteria for diagnosis
- Detection by direct fluorescent antibody of viral antigens in a clinical specimen (preferably the brain or the nerves surrounding hair follicles in the nape of the neck), or
- Isolation (in cell culture or in a laboratory animal) of rabies virus from saliva, cerebrospinal fluid (CSF), or central nervous system tissue, or
- Idenitification of rabies-neutralizing antibody titer ≥5 (complete neutralization) in the serum or CSF of an unvaccinated person.

Case classification
Confirmed: a clinically compatible case that is laboratory confirmed

Comment
Laboratory confirmation by all of the above methods is strongly recommended.

Source: CDC[5,8]

FIGURE 4-3 A complex case definition, for syphilis

SYPHILIS (All Definitions Revised 9/96)

Syphilis is a complex sexually transmitted disease that has a highly variable clinical course. Classification by a clinician with expertise in syphilis may take precedence over the following case definitions developed for surveillance purposes.

Syphilis, primary

Clinical description
A stage of infection with *Treponema pallidum* characterized by one or more chancres (ulcers); chancres might differ considerably in clinical appearance.

Laboratory criteria for diagnosis
- Demonstration of *T. palllidum* in clinical specimens by darkfield microscopy, direct fluorescent antibody (DFA-TP), or equivalent methods

Case classification
Probable: a clinically compatible case with one or more ulcers (chancres) consistent with primary syphilis and a reactive serologic test (nontreponemal: Venereal Disease Research Laboratory [VDRL] or rapid plasma reagin [RPR]; treponemal: fluorescent treponemal antibody absorbed [FTA-ABS] or microhemagglutination assay for antibody to *T. pallidum* [MHA-TP])

Confirmed: a clinically compatible case that is laboratory confirmed

continues

FIGURE 4-3 A complex case definition, for syphilis—continues
FIGURE 4-3 A complex case definition, for syphilis—continued

Syphilis, secondary

Clinical description
A stage of infection caused by *T. pallidum* and characterized by localized or diffuse mucocutaneous lesions, often with generalized lymphadenopathy. The primary chancre may still be present.

Laboratory criteria for diagnosis
- Demonstration of *T. pallidum* in clinical specimens by darkfield microscopy, DFA-TP, or equivalent methods

Case classification
Probable: a clinically compatible case with a nontreponemal (VDRL or RPR) titer ≥4

Confirmed: a clinically compatible case that is laboratory confirmed

Syphilis, latent

Clinical description
A stage of infection caused by *T. pallidum* in which organisms persist in the body of the infected person without causing symptoms or signs. Latent syphilis is subdivided into early, late, and unknown categories based on the duration of infection.

Case classification
Probable: no clinical signs or symptoms of syphilis and the presence of one of the following:
- No past diagnosis of syphilis, a reactive nontreponemal test (i.e., VDRL or RPR), and a reactive treponemal test (i.e., FTA-ABS or MHA-TP)
- A past history of syphilis therapy and a current nontreponemal test titer demonstrating fourfold or greater increase from the last nontreponemal test titer

Syphilis, early latent

Clinical description
A subcategory of latent syphilis. When initial infection has occurred within the previous 12 months, latent syphilis is classified as early latent.

Case classification
Probable: latent syphilis (see Syphilis, latent) in a person who has evidence of having acquired the infection within the previous 12 months based on one or more of the following criteria:
- Documented seroconversion or fourfold or greater increase in titer of a nontreponemal test during the previous 12 months.
- A history of symptoms consistent with primary or secondary syphilis during the previous 12 months.
- A history of sexual exposure to a partner who had confirmed or probable primary or secondary syphilis or probable early latent syphilis (documented independently as duration < 1 year).
- Reactive nontreponemal and treponemal tests from a person whose only possible exposure occurred within the preceding 12 months

Syphilis, late latent

Clinical description
A subcategory of latent syphilis. When inital infection has occured >1 year previously, latent syphilis is classified as late latent.

Case classification
Probable: latent syphilis (see Syphilis, latent) in a patient who has no evidence of having acquired the disease within the preceeding 12 months (see Syphilis, early latent) and whose age and titer do not meet the criteria specified for latent syphilis of unknown duration.

Syphilis, latent, of unknown duration

Clinical description
A subcategory of latent syphilis. When the date of initial infection cannot be established as having occurred within the previous year and the patient's age and titer meet criteria described below, latent syphilis is classified as latent syphilis of unknown duration.

Case classification
Probable: latent syphilis (see Syphilis, latent) that does not meet the criteria for early latent syphilis, and the patient is aged 13–35 years and has a nontreponemal titer ≥32

continues

FIGURE 4-3 A complex case definition, for syphilis—continued

Neurosyphilis

Clinical description
Evidence of central nervous system infection with *T. pallidum*

Laboratory criteria for diagnosis
- A reactive serologic test for syphilis and reactive VDRL in cerebrospinal fluid (CSF)

Case classification
Probable: syphilis of any stage, a negative VDRL in CSF, and both the following:
- Elevated CSF protein or leukocyte count in the absence of other known causes of these abnormalities
- Clinical symptoms or signs consistent with neurosyphilis without other known causes for these clinical abnormalities
Confirmed: syphilis of any stage that meets the laboratory criteria for neurosyphilis

Syphilis, late, with clinical manifestations other than neurosyphilis (late benign syphilis and cardiovascular syphilis)

Clinical description
Clinical manifestations of late syphilis other than neurosyphilis may include inflammatory lesions of the cardiovascular system, skin, and bone. Rarely, other structures (e.g., the upper and lower respiratory tracts, mouth, eye, abdominal organs, reproductive organs, lymph nodes, and skeletal muscle) may be involved. Late syphilis usually becomes clinically manifest only after a period of 15–30 years of untreated infection.

Laboratory criteria for diagnosis
Demonstration of *T. pallidum* in late lesions by fluorescent antibody or special stains (although organisms are rarely visualize in late lesions)

Case classification
Probable: characteristic abnormalities or lesions of the cardiovascular system, skin, bone, or other structures with a reactive treponemal test, in the absence of other known causes of these abnormalities, and without CSF abnormalities and clincal symptoms or signs consistent with neurosyphilis
Confirmed: a clinically compatible case that is laboratory confirmed

Comment
Analysis of CSF for evidence of neurosyphilis is necessary in the evaluation of late syphilis with clinical manifestation.

Syphilitic Stillbirth

Clinical description
A fetal death that occurs after a 20-week gestation or in which the fetus weighs >500 g and the mother had untreated or inadequately treated* syphilis at delivery

Comment
For reporting purposes, syphilitic stillbirths should be reported as cases of congenital syphilis.

Source: CDC[5,8]

Figure 4-4 shows a more straightforward case that depends only upon laboratory classification, although the clinical description is given in order to categorize it.[5,8]

Finally, Figure 4-5 shows a definition for plague that is intermediate in complexity between Hansen's disease and syphilis.[5,8]

continued

What Does a Case Definition Look Like?—continued

FIGURE 4-4 A straightforward case definition, for Hansen's Disease (leprosy)

HANSEN DISEASE (Leprosy)

Clinical description
A chronic bacterial disease characterized by the involvement primarily of skin as well as peripheral nerves and the mucosa of the upper airway. Clinical forms of Hansen disease represent a spectrum reflecting the cellular immune response to *Mycobacterium leprae*. The following characteristics are typical of the major forms of the disease:
- *Tuberculoid:* one or a few well-demarcated, hypopigmented, and anesthetic skin lesions, frequently with active, spreading edges and a clearing center; peripheral nerve swelling or thickening may also occur.
- *Lepromatous:* a number of erythematous papules and nodules or an infiltration of the face, hands, and feet with lesions in a bilateral and symmetrical distribution that progress to thickening of the skin.
- *Borderline (dimorphous):* skin lesions characteristic of both the tuberculoid and lepromatous forms.
- *Indeterminate:* early lesions, usually hypopigmented macules, without developed tuberculoid or lepromatous features.

Laboratory criteria for diagnosis
- Demonstration of acid-fast bacilli in skin or dermal nerve, obtained from the full-thickness skin biopsy of a lepromatous lesion

Case classification
Confirmed: a clinically compatible case that is laboratory confirmed

Source: CDC[5,8]

FIGURE 4-5 A case definition that is intermediate in complexity, for plague

PLAGUE (Revised 9/96)

Clinical description
Plague is transmitted to humans by fleas or by direct exposure to infected tissues or respiratory droplets; the disease is characterized by fever, chills, headache, malaise, prostration, and leukocytosis that manifests in one or more of the following principal clinical forms:
- Regional lymphadenitis (bubonic plague)
- Septicemia without an evident bubo (septicemic plague)
- Plague pneumonia, resulting from hematogenous spread in bubonic or septicemic cases (secondary pneumonic plague) or inhalation of infectious droplets (primary pneumonic plague)
- Pharyngitis and cervical lymphadentis resulting from exposure to larger infectious droplets or ingestion of infected tissues (pharyngeal plague)

Laboratory criteria for diagnosis
Presumptive
- Elevated serum antibody titer(s) to *Yersinia pestis* fraction 1 (F1) antigen (without documented fourfold or greater change) in a patient with no history of plague vaccination or
- Detection of F1 antigen in a clinical specimen by fluorescent assay

Confirmatory
- Isolation of *Y. pestis* from a clinical specimen or
- Fourfold or greater change in serum antibody titer to *Y. pestis* F1 antigen

Case classification
Suspected: a clinically compatible case without presumptive or confirmatory laboratory results
Probable: a clinically compatible case with presumptive laboratory results
Confirmed: a clinically compatible case with confirmatory laboratory results

Source: CDC[5,8]

5. Find Cases and Describe Them By Person, Place, and Time

Once the existence of the epidemic has been confirmed and the case definition has been developed, the next step is to begin the arduous process of finding cases and describing them by person, place, and time; usually these data are collected using a format called a line listing. All possible avenues are then explored to find cases and noncases; the specific methods used depend on the disease and the context under study. For example, with food poisoning, persons might include patrons of a restaurant in which there was a potential food outbreak, guests at a party, public health offices, emergency rooms, hospitals, private provider offices, health plans, community groups, and more. If there are persons who were at the same event but did not get sick, they might be included in order to help elucidate the exposure of interest. Individuals are then measured against the case definition and assessed for their symptoms to see if they meet the criteria and may be considered a case. An in-depth interview, preferably in person, is conducted to systematically collect all information about their illness (when did they get sick, with what symptoms did they get sick, where did they get sick, where had they been when they began to show symptoms, and so forth) as well as their behavior (what had they eaten, had they taken medication, had they taken drugs, were they exposed to environmental agents, and so forth). The type of illness under study helps to narrow the focus of the questions. For example, a skin infection would have a markedly different panel of predictor and outcome questions than would a gastrointestinal infection.

All persons interviewed would be categorized as a case or noncase, and their data entered into a line listing in a database for analysis. Sometimes, depending on the needs of the outbreak, a case definition with multiple levels, such as definite, probable, possible, insufficient evidence, or others may be used. This is particularly helpful when there are many cases that present clinically appearing to meet the criteria but lacking in biological or laboratory confirmation. The line listing is incredibly useful for a variety of reasons. Graphs can be made very simply from your line listing of the number of cases (on the vertical or Y-axis) vs. time (on the horizontal or X-axis); this creates an epidemic curve that allows us to understand the characteristics of the epidemic. Did it come up fast out of nowhere, peak, and then decline? Did it come in waves? Each of these has a specific meaning and offers a clue to the underlying cause of the outbreak. Recall that outbreak investigations are a form of a descriptive epidemiologic study. Thus, all the skills we learned in descriptive epidemiology regarding how to portray the data come into play here. In addition, you can graph the incubation time (the interval from time of infection to time of onset of clinical illness), that provides a good signature for the disease under study. These are additional clues in understanding the disease.

Graphing Epidemics— the Unit of Time Matters

Here is an example of where the units of measurement in your X-axis really matter. In Figure 4-6, you can see that the unit of measurement is the day. This makes sense. You can see the point source and the sharp upsurge in cases, followed by a linear and rapid decline.

In Figure 4-7, however, we have a case of a salmonella outbreak on an airplane. We have the same pattern, so it is easy to see the point source of the outbreak. But here our unit of measurement is 3-hour periods. If we looked at days, we would see all the cases within 2 days, so this is an important point to be made.

Note for both of these outbreaks that there are some cases before the general outbreak begins to escalate. This may be people who staff the church lunch, parents at the birthday

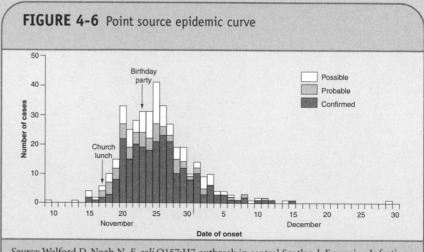

FIGURE 4-6 Point source epidemic curve

Source: Walford D, Noah N. *E. coli* O157:H7 outbreak in central Scotland. Emerging Infectious Diseases—United Kingdom. *Emerg Inf Dis* 1999;5:189–94.

continued

Graphing Epidemics—the Unit of Time Matters—continued

party, or the pilots and co-pilots eating the meal in advance of everyone else.

These two—and many foodborne outbreaks, in fact—are point source outbreaks in which there is one exposure, and it rises and falls relatively quickly. A propagated outbreak is one in which you can see waves as people transmit the infection to one another. Note in Figure 4-8 how the axis counting the cases is in weeks, not days or hours as above.

FIGURE 4-7 Salmonella point source airplane epidemic curve on a flight from London to the United States, by time of onset, March 13–14, 1984

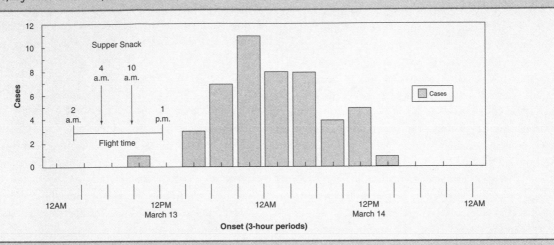

This is another point source outbreak, but this time on board an airplane, and taking place over a number of hours rather than days.

Source: CDC[4]

FIGURE 4-8 Cases of bloody diarrhea, by week, Cameroon

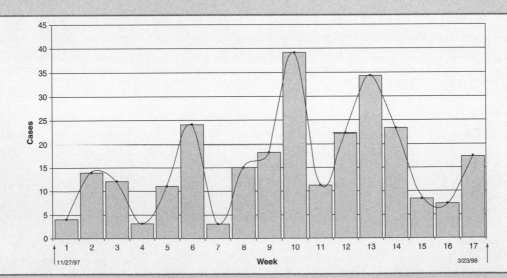

This is a clear example of a propagated outbreak. Notice the upswells in waves as each generation of the area infects a subsequent generation.

Source: Cunin P et al. An epidemic of bloody diarrhea: Escherichia coli 0157 Emerging in Cameroon? *Emerg Inf Dis* 1999;5:2.

Ultimately, using any and all available data—laboratory, diagnostic, clinical, interview, line listing, graphs of time of onset and cases, incubation time—the goal is to generate a hypothesis. From this, a direction regarding which public health action to follow can be taken and/or a hypothesis can be further tested. As discussed, if there are serious implications of the disease/exposure under study and enough is known to take public health action, such as closing down a restaurant, making recommendations about vaccination, or halting global travel, public health measures may be enacted. Often an analytic study will be performed, using study designs discussed in the next chapters. Frequently, a case-control study will be performed, but other designs—such as a cross-sectional, retrospective cohort, or prospective cohort—may be conducted following an outbreak investigation, depending on the research question under study and the data and resources available. As stressed before, where public health is imminently threatened, public health action should be taken first.

6. Implement Control and Prevention Efforts

At this point, after gathering data and describing the situation, you would use the information and knowledge gained from the investigation to stop the current outbreak and prevent future ones. Data gleaned from the investigation will also generally contribute in some fashion—from surveillance systems to ways to monitor the disease or exposure that was targeted. If the outbreak happens from an infectious organism that has already been under surveillance, then additional surveillance mechanisms may be added, or augmented. If the problems are on a local level, such as a restaurant not adhering to food-handling regulations (e.g., inadequate running water, insufficient hand-

> ## Summary of Steps in an Outbreak Investigation
>
> 1. Define the purpose of the investigation.
> 2. Establish the existence of the outbreak.
> 3. Develop a case definition.
> 4. Confirm the diagnosis.
> 5. Describe the cases by time, place, and person, using a line listing.
> 6. Implement control and prevention efforts.
> 7. Prepare and disseminate a report/document.
>
> Later you will:
>
> 8. Develop a hypothesis and evaluate against established facts.
> 9. Plan/conduct an analytic study.
>
> Note that each of these steps is greatly impacted by the methodologic choices made: the purpose of the investigation drives the choice of methodology, the creation of the case definition, how the cases are confirmed or operationalized, how the data are collected and analyzed. The way the findings are reported on then influence what actions are taken, and how future studies are conducted.

washing, food not maintained at proper temperature), these may be enforced on a local level. For example, if it were a restaurant, it might be shut down temporarily until the problem could be corrected. If the outbreak was of a new organism, new

> ## SARS: Face Masks and Travel Advisories
>
> One important aspect to note about the swiftness of public health intervention in the shadow of SARS: the personal component. Pictures abounded in the media of all kinds of people in Hong Kong wearing face masks on the street, empty streets because people feared the disease, and people being turned away from airplane flights when they had a cough or other nonspecific symptoms of SARS—which could represent symptomatology of a variety of illnesses, including the common cold of which the more deadly coronavirus is a cousin. The travel advisories, advice to seek medical help with the presence of certain signs and symptoms, and other public health interventions that were speedily put into place, were effective in stopping what could have been a terrible epidemic; to date, we have not seen a re-emergence of SARS, and this is a testament to the proficiency with which the outbreak was addressed. It also bodes well for the international efforts devoted currently towards the potential for an avian flu (H5N1) outbreak. Should other outbreaks come to pass, we may be able to take effective action instead of allowing the virus to take hold. But it is important to remember that such action is not without unanticipated effects: There are those who were discriminated against due to where they were from, symptoms or other diseases they had, and fears in general. Would we want to have lessened the actions that were taken? Absolutely not. But noticing that there are consequences in terms of social realms is important. As public health professionals, we can make sure that we communicate effectively to the media in order to reduce public alarm and the chances for abuse of individuals.

SARS: First Cases

An international effort that included the World Health Organization (WHO) and the Centers for Disease Control and Prevention (CDC) was initiated in 2003. This collaboration was developed to identify the cause and stem the transmission of a severe acute respiratory syndrome, often fatal, that had not been seen before. Although you may not recall the first cases of AIDS in 1981, most of you will recall this tense public health moment.[27] By March 26, 2003, there had been 1,323 suspected and/or probable cases from around the world, with 49 deaths (case fatality = proportion of people infected that die = 49/1323 = 3.7%), with attack rates among contacts of cases (also called secondary attack rates) in excess of 50%. The virus, later identified as a new coronavirus, caused acute symptoms, including shortness of and rapid breath, pneumonia, sore throat, fever and chills, body aches, and abnormal laboratory findings. Active global surveillance and public health intervention followed immediately upon identification of the first case. The SARS epidemic was more deftly handled than almost any epidemic previous to it. With the first cases identified in February 2003, global alerts and surveillance began by February 11, 2003. By mid-March, substantial progress had been made.

- Travel advisories were instituted for those planning travel to Hong Kong, China, and other destinations where the disease was known to exist.
- Travelers were advised to seek medical attention if they developed SARS-like symptoms.
- A case definition for suspected cases of SARS (a preliminary case definition that came before its laboratory diagnosis) was created and disseminated.

Swift global public health action resulted in a stemming of the pandemic. By year's end, there were no additional cases, and we have been fortunate: As of this writing there have been no additional serious SARS outbreaks.

Describing Outbreaks: Person, Place, and Time

One of the biggest outbreaks of Ebola virus hemorrhagic fever took place in Kikwit, the Democratic Republic of Congo, in 1995.[10,29,30] Ebola virus hemorrhagic fever (ebolavirus)—in the family filoviridae[15]—strikes quickly, and can devastate a community within days. Highly contagious, the virus causes diffuse bleeding and systemic, respiratory, and cardiac symptoms, with death within a matter of days (in the 1995 outbreak: mean, 10.1 days; range, 3 to 21 days).[10] During this outbreak, 316 people were infected, with a case fatality rate of approximately 80% (i.e., about 80% of those who contracted the disease died from it). One way to improve one's skills at descriptive epidemiology is to look at articles and outbreak investigations that have already been conducted and see if you can pick out the descriptions of person, place, and time from the narrative. To practice, take the articles cited here about Ebola outbreaks and identify person, place, and time in each as we do here for the 1995 outbreak:[10,31,32]

- *Time:* The cases began as early as January 1995, although these were not noted to be part of the outbreak until later, when patients were being seen in the larger hospital environment, and healthcare workers became ill. The CDC made the diagnosis of Ebola hemorrhagic fever on May 10, 1995.
- *Place:* Kikwit is a rural town on the banks of the Kwilu River in the Democratic Republic of Congo, population approximately 400,000.[10,33]
- *Person:* Persons ranged in age from 1 to 70 years old, were slightly more likely to be female, and had for the most part previous contact with an infected individual. Hospital healthcare workers were among the infected. Bwaka and colleagues conducted an extensive review of clinical characteristics associated with the outbreak to characterize the patients.[10] Through this systematic investigation, insight about the specific clinical manifestations of the 1995 outbreak were made possible. This extensive chronicling of symptoms, and a comparison between those who did and did not die, allowed hypotheses to be generated regarding how future outbreaks could be managed.

Knowing the characteristics of an outbreak is not enough: documenting them for the future, as was done here, is essential.

Which Diseases Are Reportable?

In the United States, reporting of certain infectious diseases is mandatory. This means that labs, hospitals, providers—anyone—that diagnoses a reportable condition is mandated to submit it as per their local or state health guidelines and procedures. In turn, the state health departments submit reports to the National Notifiable Diseases Surveillance System (NNDSS).[8] The Council on State and Territorial Epidemiologists (CTSE) collaborates with the CDC in an effort to ensure that all reports are appropriately submitted to the CDC. Some conditions are also reportable to the World Health Organization, because they have international as well as domestic implications.[8] These include cholera, associated coronavirus (SARS-CoV) disease, plague, yellow fever, West Nile virus, paralytic polio, and smallpox.

surveillance techniques might be needed—and new infrastructure developed in order to address it. It is essential to document all the details of the research and implementation activities that have taken place. This allows future researchers and public health professionals to do several things: Evaluate what did and did not work, replicate your methods, and compare their findings to yours. Science is a dialogue, with each of us hearing and responding to each other, so detailed and professional documentation of methods is crucial. Information can then be contributed to the scientific and public health communities so that lessons learned are passed on to others and may be built upon.

DATA COLLECTION

Specific methods are important. Systematic data collection and methods to reduce bias in collection of data, both interview data as well as data abstracted from medical records, are key components in ensuring validity of results. The most crucial element of data collection for outbreak investigations is that data need to be collected systematically and rigorously. In looking for cases, if a catchment area is defined and specific persons exposed are supposed to be pursued, it is essential to omit certain categories of persons who for any reasons will introduce bias into your investigation, as it would into any study. In addition, interviews need to be conducted in a culturally sensitive, professional manner by well-trained interviewers who know how to minimize bias and ensure that all interviews are conducted in the same exact way.

Some methods are specific to outbreak investigations and generally are reserved for them, whereas other methods are part of the more general epidemiologic toolkit and can be used in a variety of contexts. These outbreak-specific methods include systematic data collection designed for outbreaks, line listings to generate epidemic curves, graph interpretation, assessment of incubation times, and synthesis of information to yield a working conclusion.

You will be learning a lot about systematic data collection in the coming chapters. How we ask questions and whether we ask them systematically and consistently between interviewers, between participants, and even between questions on a survey tool or data collection protocol are critical to coming to valid conclusions. If we ask people the same questions differently—or ask them different questions altogether—it will not be possible to trust the findings that the outbreak investigation yields.

Let us take another look at the example in Chapter 3 that portrayed a catered event at which there was a suspected salmonella outbreak. The line listing is the end result of the systematic data collection. How does it start? First, the public health practitioners needed to learn about the outbreak from either the group running the event or attendees of the function. Imagine in this case it was a large charitable organization that was having a fundraising event. Prior to the event, volunteers were invited to have the catered dinner, because they were expected to interact with donors during the evening. As a result, the volunteers were the first to have the food, the first to become ill, and also—because they worked together and were friendly after the event—the first to perceive that there was a potential problem, when more people got ill than they thought should have happened by chance. The epidemiologists, at the office of public health who took the report, initiated an outbreak investigation. Why? Because foodborne outbreaks of some types are reportable. We need to keep track of the number and type of foodborne outbreaks in order to be able to track emerging pathogens and to improve the safety of the food supply.

Once the outbreak investigation is initiated, and after a case definition is developed or adapted by the local public health practitioners, template forms are identified and used for data collection. FoodNet is a large surveillance system that collects comprehensive data on food safety and foodborne outbreaks.[34,35] Other types of outbreak investigations will have their own form databank; if necessary, the investigators would make a case report form specific to the outcomes they are investigating and the potential exposures. Although there are many interesting and important nuances regarding data collection forms, some of which we will get to later, the most crucial is that there is a systematic approach to collection of data. Haphazard data collection, in which questions are not asked in the same way to each person and/or responses are not recorded in the same way, makes it difficult to trust what we find or extract a valid interpretation from it. In an outbreak investigation, specific information is required; for example, what each person exposed ate, in what quantity, whether they were sick, and, if sick, when they began to be sick and with which symptoms. It would be easy to accidentally collect data on all people who were sick, what they ate, a profile of their symptoms, and so forth. But this would not tell us much. It would only provide information on those who were sick without giving us anything to compare with. The data collection tool needs to collect data on all persons exposed to the event irrespective of illness status. This will point us to an understanding of what caused the sickness.

EPIDEMIC CURVES

Information contained within the line-listed data is taken and transformed into a graphic depiction, and an epidemic curve is generated. Unlike the data collection discussed in the previous section, the epidemic curve includes only those who became ill. Along the *X*-axis (the horizontal axis) is time; along the *Y*-axis (the vertical axis) is the number of cases. This allows exploration of the characteristics of the epidemic, and helps identify what might be the source. Figures 4-6, 4-7, and 4-8 are good examples of epidemic curves derived from line-listings.

What does an epidemic curve show? If one is lucky, the characteristics of the curve reveal clear clues to the underlying disease. This does not always happen, however; sometimes the curve suggests characteristics that could relate to a handful of diseases. Sometimes the curve may not suggest a specific disease. It may be that the data themselves are flawed, capturing information inaccurately or incompletely. It can also mean that there is no pathogen yet identified or that we know of described by the curve. More often than not, methods may be the problem at hand: If the data were not collected using a systematic method that reduces bias, it is conceivable that the resulting epidemic curve will be less than useful in identifying the etiology of the outbreak.

Given a comprehensive, systematically collected line listing, an epidemic curve can suggest the incubation time and the mode of transmission of the underlying pathogen.

Here is how, using as an example a famous *Staphylococcus aureus* and *albus* outbreak at a church supper in 1940 in Oswego, New York.[36] This quintessential foodborne outbreak is used by the Epidemic Intelligence Service (EIS) as one of its many case studies that train the highly skilled group of EIS officers. Many in attendance at this church supper became ill, and *Staphylococcus aureus* and *albus* were found in the vanilla ice cream and believed to be the cause of the outbreak.

The data went from the line-listed state to a graphic state, with cases plotted by their time of onset.

CDC-EIS, 2003: Oswego—GI Illness Following a Church Supper (401-303)
Line listing from investigation of outbreak of gastroenteritis,
Oswego, New York, 1940

ID	AGE	SEX	TIME OF MEAL	ILL	DATE OF ONSET	TIME OF ONSET	Baked Ham	Spinach	Mashed potatoes	Cabbage salad	Jello	Rolls	Brown bread	Milk	Coffee	Water	Cakes	Van ice cream	Choc ice cream	Fruit salad
1	11	M	unk	N			N	N	N	N	N	N	N	N	N	N	N	N	N	N
2	52	F	8:00 PM	Y	4/19	12:30 AM	Y	Y	N	N	N	Y	N	N	Y	N	N	Y	N	N
3	65	M	6:30 PM	Y	4/19	12:30 AM	Y	Y	Y	N	N	N	N	Y	N	N	Y	Y	N	N
4	59	F	6:30 PM	Y	4/19	12:30 AM	Y	Y	N	N	N	N	N	N	Y	N	Y	Y	Y	N
5	13	F	unk	N			N	N	N	N	N	N	N	N	N	N	N	Y	N	N
6	63	F	7:30 PM	Y	4/18	10:30 PM	Y	Y	N	Y	N	N	N	N	Y	N	Y	N	N	N
7	70	M	7:30 PM	Y	4/18	10:30 PM	Y	Y	Y	N	Y	Y	Y	N	Y	Y	Y	Y	N	N
8	40	F	7:30 PM	Y	4/19	2:00 AM	N	N	N	N	N	N	N	N	N	N	N	Y	Y	N
9	15	F	10:00 PM	Y	4/19	1:00 AM	N	N	N	N	N	N	N	N	N	Y	N	Y	N	N
10	33	F	7:00 PM	Y	4/18	11:00 PM	Y	Y	Y	N	N	Y	Y	N	N	Y	N	Y	Y	N
11	65	M	unk	N			Y	Y	Y	N	Y	Y	N	N	N	N	N	Y	N	N
12	38	F	unk	N			Y	Y	Y	N	N	Y	N	N	Y	N	N	Y	Y	Y
13	62	F	unk	N			Y	Y	N	Y	Y	Y	Y	N	N	Y	N	N	N	N

Source: CDC[36]

To a graphic state, with cases plotted by their time of onset as in Figure 4-9 through 4-11. Note that two epidemic curves were created, one that was with half-hour time blocks on the X-axis, the other with one-hour time blocks. Depending on the pathogen, the unit of time can be very important; selection of the wrong time unit or failure to explore this as a factor may decrease your ability to see the true "picture" of what is going on. When each case became a case—that is, when he/she began exhibiting symptoms—the case number was plotted. This step is repeated until all of the cases are listed. It is essential to collect in the line-listing the exact time at which the case first experienced the symptoms in question. This will not only make the outbreak investigation more thorough, but also will enable identification of the proper time increment for use in the epidemic curve graphing. For example, in the case of an outbreak on an airplane (as in Figure 4-7 earlier in the chapter), the food was served on the flight and individuals became ill within hours. If the time interval selected for the epidemic curve were days, the entire outbreak would have been missed. Thus, if exact time were not collected, it would be impossible to construct a curve that would be at all informative. Similarly, if cases took place in a more spread out fashion, it may be more useful to plot them by week or month rather than day or hour. Without collecting the data at the time of the initial interview, chances for that data collection may ultimately be lost. Getting all of the information at one time is necessary, because there may not be a second chance. As time moves forward, people

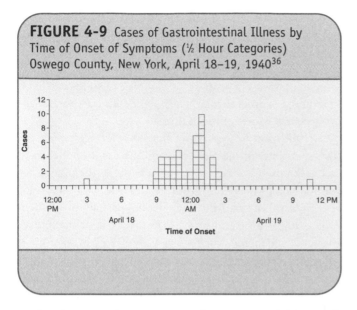

FIGURE 4-9 Cases of Gastrointestinal Illness by Time of Onset of Symptoms (½ Hour Categories) Oswego County, New York, April 18–19, 1940[36]

tend to disappear, become more reluctant to participate, and, most importantly, forget their outcomes or exposures.

Time between infection and onset of symptoms is used as a clue to try and understand which organisms are the potential culprits. In order to decide which units to use for the graphing of incubation time, one guideline is that the units should be between one-eighth to one-third as long as the incubation period of the disease in question.[36] The case study[36(p14)] points out the following about understanding the graph of the incubation time, which can be difficult to see.

- The graph of incubation periods is not symmetric or normally distributed; two peaks are revealed.
- Those who ate later had shorter incubation times. Individuals who ate early had a median incubation time of 5½ hours where those eating later had median 3

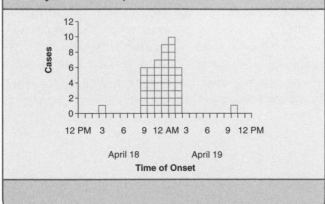

FIGURE 4-10 Cases of Gastrointestinal Illness by Time of Onset of Symptoms (Hour Categories) Oswego County, New York, April 18–19, 1940[36]

hours. This gives a hint that the infectious organism at work must worsen over time; this is consistent with an enterotoxi producing organism such as *Staphylococcus aureus*. But, it could be for other reasons, too. The case suggests that younger people may eat later and more, thus conferring on them a higher dose.

- The authors note that only 22 of the 46 cases provided enough information to calculate incubation periods. This is clearly a methodological question: what to do with those for whom the onset time is missing?

How do you calculate the range in incubation times from looking at this graph? Easy: Just look at the minimum and the maximum. Here the minimum is 3.0 hours and the maximum is 7.0 hours. The range is 4.0 hours ($7.0 - 3.0 = 4.0$). This allows you to consult a book on infectious diseases and their characteristics and consider candidates for the outbreak's cause.

In the point source epidemic curves in this example, the curve has a steep increasing slope and a gradual decline. When it declines it declines, however; it does not go up and down after the initial downward trend. And generally, at the right-hand tail, when it is over, it is over—there are no additional "bursts" of cases. This type of epidemic curve suggests a point source outbreak, also known as a common-vehicle exposure or common source outbreak. This means that there was one source of the pathogen, such as a contaminated food source. If this is the case, you may ask, why didn't all the cases appear at the same time? There are several reasons for this, though the specifics vary depending upon the disease under investigation.

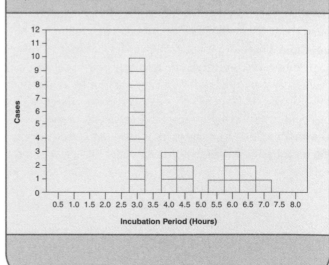

FIGURE 4-11 Cases of Gastrointestinal Illness by Incubation Period in Hours Oswego County, New York, April 18–19, 1940[36]

- Not everyone may have been exposed at the exact same moment. Over the duration of a supper, there may have been individuals who prepared the food; those who ate at the beginning, middle, or end of the event; plus those who took food home with them to consume at a later time.
- People may have eaten different amounts of the offending food source.
- People come in different sizes and shapes. Body mass has a great deal to do with the level of symptomatology an individual may exhibit, thus an adult may become ill slower than a child, or a petite woman faster than a large man.
- Host characteristics differ from person to person. Individuals who are immunocompromised may be more susceptible to the pathogen's effects, as may an elderly person or an infant.
- Memories are not perfect. It may be that a case does not accurately recall when he or she first experienced the symptoms. Or it may be that symptoms that are relatively benign or similar to more usual experiences may not precipitate the person's noting the time they first occurred, skewing the curve.

The distribution of the disease onset provides a range of when the exposure could have taken place. First, look at the center of the visual peak of the curve, because that provides a rough average time of exposure. From that, a range—first to last—of exposures can be generated. Given all the potential causes of the outbreak, one can then look at the range and see what sources were within it. Events that take place too far on either side can be noted, while more attention paid to exposures within the range. Does this mean *for sure* the events are in the range? Of course not. The range is only as good as the data that created it, and the data are only as good as the methods that collected them. Thus odd answers or ranges beg the question: Is it a methodological problem or could it be a new infectious disease or variant about which we are not yet aware?

Point source outbreaks are relatively easy to detect, especially if they are the result of a single exposure, as shown in this example. If, however, the event is repeated, due to either multiple exposures to the same food, a periodic exposure such as something that happens every week due to some underlying routine, or a continuous exposure, the curve will be more difficult to decipher. Another complication is if the outbreak is transmitted person to person. Still more difficult is when a combination of these characterize the outbreak, such as a common source outbreak that is then transmitted person to person (also known as a propagated outbreak). Experts will likely be required in order to interpret the epidemic curve and identify potential causes of the outbreak.

In addition to evaluating the shape of the curve, the start/stop times of the outbreak, and the number of cases at each point on the curve, it is possible to assess the time in between different waves of the outbreak. The evaluation of this serial interval can inform the epidemiologist about what exactly is happening and how the outbreak is being spread. Graphing the incubation time visually describes the time it takes to transmit the agent to a successive wave of persons if there are secondary cases (when one person spreads the disease to others). This is useful in further narrowing down what the infectious agent could be. Using the same data provided in the line-listing can also give a clue to the nature of the etiology of the outbreak by looking at the incubation time of the illness. If there are data available regarding time of exposure to the source as well as when symptoms first started, then the incubation time can be plotted as well. The same plotting method as above would be used, only graphing the distribution of incubation times to suggest what might be the average (the mean) incubation time as well as the minimum and the maximum incubation times.

Every infectious disease has its own qualities that make it recognizable: the combination of specific symptoms, including which are most common, the incubation time, and the duration of illness. By looking at each of these in the epidemic curve and the incubation time curve, we obtain some information about what these qualities are.

One thing that is very exciting about infectious disease epidemiology is that it requires several simultaneous skills: the ability to think on one's feet, to use a set of tools designed to systematize and describe those affected, and a creative mind that thinks outside of the box. One must consider the contexts at work, the exception as well as the rule, and use all the available data to solve a mystery. Outbreak investigations are just the beginning, primarily using description and keen thinking. Analytic methods become even more exciting, as we go from description to comparison as our major task.

Salmonella Outbreak

Alfalfa sprouts are delicious, a wonderful addition to a healthful sandwich. Heap on gourmet cheeses, tomatoes, and some thick wheat bread, and you have a common sight in restaurants and health food stores. Unfortunately, because of the way that they are produced, alfalfa sprouts have been linked to a variety of outbreaks of *Salmonella enterica* and *Escherichia coli* O157:H7.[37] Foodborne transmission is responsible for as much as 90% of disease burden of salmonellosis.[38] It can cause serious gastroenteritis, and has been linked to deaths in some patients; *E. coli* O157:H7 has been linked to an alarming number of deaths. Why are alfalfa sprouts so susceptible to contamination with bacteria? As seeds, they are soaked in water and then housed to germinate in a warm environment, which is suitable for their growth as well as that of the pathogens.

There was a sharp increase and rapid decrease of cases in this epidemic curve, similar to the *E coli* O157:H7 outbreak we saw in Figure 4-6. This is helpful in identifying it as a point source outbreak. For more information about this outbreak and how it was used to assess the effectiveness of a decontamination process, please see the chapter on case-control studies.

Unfortunately, *Salmonella* outbreaks are common. In 2006, there was an outbreak of another salmonella strain, *S. typhimurium*.[17] The outbreak was reported to have caused 182 cases in 21 states. The source was believed to be tomatoes, and the outbreak was contained due to the effective investigation.

FIGURE 4-12 Cases of salmonellosis and shigellosis, by year, 1974–2004, United States[38]

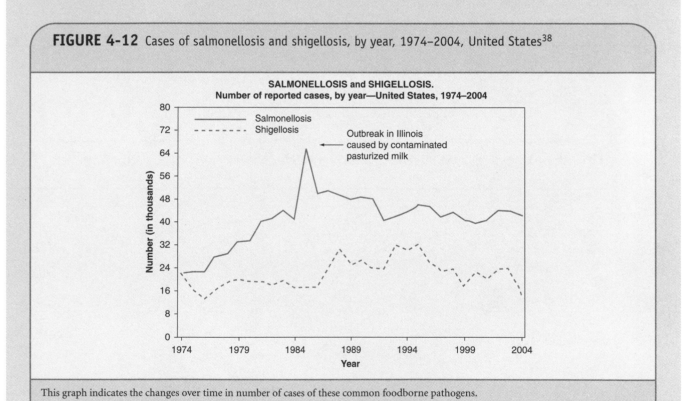

This graph indicates the changes over time in number of cases of these common foodborne pathogens.

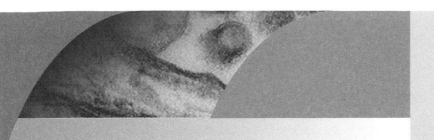

Discussion Questions

3. Why do you think there were cases very early on? What clues do those cases give you?

4. What explanation can you give for the cases at the far end of the epidemic curve? Why are they there following a slight gap in time?

Figure 4-13 shows a famous epidemic curve from the Legionnaires' convention in 1976.[39] This was the first time that this acute bacterial upper respiratory infection had been seen in such a large outbreak (at the American Legion conference in Philadelphia). The organism lingers in static water, such as in air conditioners.

1. Who do you think the nonconventioneers were?

2. Why did the epidemiologists developing this curve feel it was important to divide conventioneer from nonconventioneer?

FIGURE 4-13 Legionnaires' Disease by Date of Onset, Philadelphia, July 1–August 18, 1976[39]

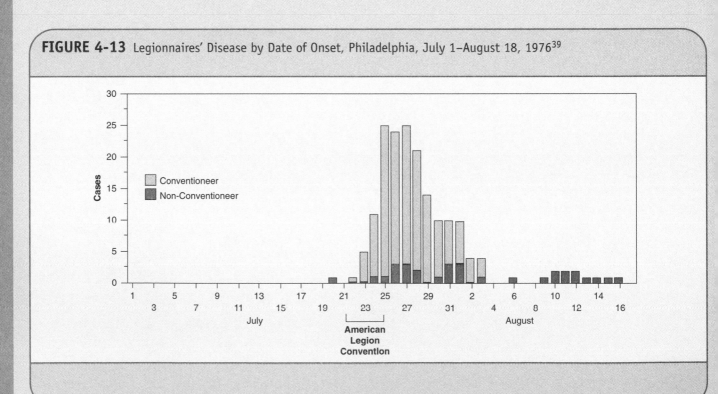

REFERENCES

1. Centers for Disease Control and Prevention. Kaposi's sarcoma and pneumocystis pneumonia among homosexual men: New York City and Los Angeles. *MMWR.* 1981;30:305–308.

2. Centers for Disease Control and Prevention. Pneumocystis pneumonia—Los Angeles. *MMWR.* 1981;30:250–252.

3. Centers for Disease Control and Prevention. A cluster of Kaposi's sarcoma and *Pneumocystis carinii* pneumonia among homosexual male residents of Los Angeles and range counties, California. *MMWR.* 1982;31:305–307.

4. Centers for Disease Control and Prevention. Salmonellosis in passengers on a flight from London to the United States, by time of onset, March 13–14, 1984. Available at: http://www.cdc.gov/excite/fi14.html. Accessed November 30, 2003.

5. Centers for Disease Control and Prevention. Case definitions for infectious conditions under public health surveillance. *MMWR.* 1990;39 (RR-13):1–50.

6. Centers for Disease Control and Prevention. Preliminary report: foodborne outbreak of *Escherichia coli* O157:H7 infections from hamburgers—western United States, 1993. *MMWR.* 1993;42:85–86.

7. Centers for Disease Control and Prevention. Update: multistate outbreak of *Escherichia coli* O157:H7 infections from hamburgers—western United States, 1992–1993. *MMWR.* 1993;42(14):258–263.

8. Centers for Disease Control and Prevention. Case definitions for infectious conditions under public health surveillance. *MMWR.* 1997;46 (RR-10):1–64.

9. Reingold AE. Outbreak investigations—a perspective. *Emerg Infect Dis.* 1998;4(1):21–27.

10. Bwaka M, Bonnet M-J, Calain P, et al. Ebola hemorrhagic fever in Kikwit, Democratic Republic of the Congo: clinical observations in 103 patients. *J Infect Dis.* 1999;179(Suppl):S1–S7.

11. Centers for Disease Control and Prevention. CDC surveillance summaries: surveillance for foodborne-disease outbreaks—United States, 1993–1997. *MMWR.* 2000;49(SS-1):1–72.

12. Nelson K. *Infectious Disease Epidemiology.* Gaithersburg, MD: Aspen.

13. Bukholm G, Tannæs T, Britt Bye Kjelsberg A, Smith-Erichsen N. An outbreak of multidrug-resistant *Pseudomonas aeruginosa* associated with increased risk of patient death in an intensive care unit. *Infect Control Hosp Epidemiol.* 2002;23:441–446.

14. DeHart RL. Health issues of air travel. *Ann Rev Public Health.* 2003; 24:133–151.

15. Heymann DL. *Control of Communicable Diseases.* 18th edition. Washington, DC: American Public Health Association.

16. Centers for Disease Control and Prevention. FoodNet. 2005. Available at: www.cdc.gov/foodnet/surveillance.htm. Accessed December 10, 2006.

17. Centers for Disease Control and Prevention. Salmonellosis—outbreak investigation, October 2006. November 3, 2006. Available at: www.cdc.gov/ncidod/dbmd/diseaseinfo/salmonellosis_2006/outbreak_notice.htm. Accessed December 25, 2006.

18. Centers for Disease Control and Prevention. Pandemics and pandemic threats since 1900. 2006. Available at: www.pandemicflu.gov/general/historicaloverview.html. Accessed December 25, 2006.

19. Moser M, Margolis H, Bend TR. An outbreak of influenza aboard a commercial airline. *Am J Epidemiol.* 1979;110:1–6.

20. Brownstein JS, Wolfe CJ, Mandl KD. Empirical evidence for the effect of airline travel on inter-regional influenza spread in the United States. *PLoS Med.* 2006;3(10):e401.

21. Centers for Disease Control and Prevention. Avian influenza infection in humans (bird flu). 2006. Available at: www.pandemicflu.gov. Accessed December 25, 2006.

22. Centers for Disease Control and Prevention. Update: influenza activity—United States, October 1–December 9, 2006. *MMWR.* 2006;55(50): 1359–1362.

23. Kilbourne ED. Influenza pandemics of the 20th century. *Emerg Infect Dis.* 2006;12(1):9–14.

24. World Health Organization. Cumulative number of confirmed human cases of avian influenza A(H5N1) reported to WHO. 2006. Available at: www.who.int/csr/disease/avian_influenza/country/cases_table_2006_12_27/en. Accessed December 25, 2006.

25. Taubenberger J. 1918 influenza: the mother of all pandemics. *Emerg Infect Dis.* 2006;12(1):15–22.

26. Centers for Disease Control and Prevention. Outbreak of severe acute respiratory syndrome—worldwide, 2003. *MMWR.* 2003;52(11):226–228.

27. Centers for Disease Control and Prevention. Update: outbreak of severe acute respiratory syndrome—worldwide, 2003. *MMWR.* 2003;52:241–248.

28. Centers for Disease Control and Prevention. Summary of notifiable diseases—United States, 2004. *MMWR.* 2004;53(53):1–80.

29. Centers for Disease Control and Prevention. 1994 revised classification system for human immunodeficiency virus infection in children less than 13 years of age. *MMWR.* 1994;43(RR-12):1–28.

30. Centers for Disease Control and Prevention. Outbreak of Ebola hemorrhagic fever. *MMWR.* 1995;44:381–382.

31. Centers for Disease Control and Prevention. Outbreak of Ebola viral hemorrhagic fever—Zaire, 1995. *MMWR.* 1995;44(19):381–382.

32. Centers for Disease Control and Prevention. Update: outbreak of Ebola hemorrhagic fever. *MMWR.* 1995;44:468–475.

33. Centers for Disease Control and Prevention. Update: outbreak of Ebola viral hemorrhagic fever—Zaire, 1995. *MMWR.* 1995;44(25):469–479.

34. FoodNet. Available at: www.foodnet.org. Accessed December 2, 2006.

35. Mead PS, Slutsker L, Dietz V, et al. Food-related illness and death in the United States. *Emerg Infect Dis.* 1999;5(5):607–625.

36. Centers for Disease Control and Prevention, Epidemiology Program Office. Case Studies in Applied Epidemiology Number 401-303. Oswego—An Outbreak of Gastrointestinal Illness Following a Church Supper—Instructor's Guide. Available at www.cdc.gov. Accessed December 31, 2006.

37. Gill CJ, Keene WE, Mohle-Boetani JE, et al. Alfalfa seed decontamination in a Salmonella outbreak. *Emerg Infect Dis.* 2003;9(4). Available at: www.cdc.gov/nicdod/EID/vol9no4/02-0519.html. Accessed December 25, 2006.

38. CDC. "Summary of notifiable diseases—United States, 2004 (Published June 16, 2006)." *M MWR.* 2004;53(53):1–80.

39. Centers for Disease Control and Prevention Legionnaires' disease by date of onset, Philadelphia, July 1–August 18, 1976. *MMWR.* 1976;25:38.

Rates and Measures

COUNTING AND COMPARING CASES— A CORNERSTONE OF INFECTIOUS DISEASE EPIDEMIOLOGY

How we count cases of disease and communicate those counts is a key skill in infectious disease epidemiology, as well as other areas of epidemiology. Rates and measures are the nuts and bolts of how we understand and communicate disease frequencies. The purpose of this chapter is to introduce the essential concepts of rates and measures so they are at the ready for you to apply in the area of infectious disease epidemiology. This is not comprehensive coverage of this topic: I encourage readers to consult one of the many fine general epidemiology textbooks to learn more about rates and measures. However, this is an introduction to contextualizing this important concept within the arena of infectious disease.

Here is an example involving hepatitis C to make this more vivid (see Figure 5-1). Hepatitis C is most commonly spread via injection drug use (IDU). Approximately 90% of those with hepatitis C have no symptoms while the disease is in its acute state, so many people go without their disease being detected; as many as 80% develop chronic infection. Of those, half may go on to develop cirrhosis of the liver or liver cancer.[1,2] Hepatitis C is highly infectious when compared with HIV—comparing single needle stick exposures, the risk of acquiring hepatitis C is estimated at approximately 3% compared with 0.3% for HIV. (Note that this is still less than the 30% transmission risk associated with hepatitis B.)[1,2] Studies of injection drug users suggest that between 50% and 95% of injection drug users have hepatitis C.[1]

Imagine there are two cities with outbreaks of hepatitis C. In the past year, local hospitals in County A have reported 15 cases of acute hepatitis C, and those in County B have reported 13 cases. You begin with your descriptive epidemiology, as discussed in Chapter 3. You wisely describe the characteristics of all individuals with hepatitis C with respect to person, place, and time. You count them. You plot them on maps. You describe their gender, their age, their income level, their use/nonuse of injection drugs, co-morbidities (illnesses they have along with hepatitis C), their family members or household contacts' hepatitis C status, and their occupation. You use laboratory studies to confirm they have hepatitis C and identify whether it is acute or chronic. You confirm the date and time of infection and the proposed method of infection. Now what?

You have at hand several things to consider. You have two outbreaks, or what seem to be bonafide outbreaks, in two different cities. There is a public health situation at hand. You are not sure why each of the outbreaks has occurred. Specific public health action at this point is uncertain at best. You need to go one step beyond pure description. You need to see if you can figure out what is causing this public health situation and what

FIGURE 5-1 This transmission electron micrograph (TEM) revealed numerous hepatitis virions, of an unknown strain of the organism

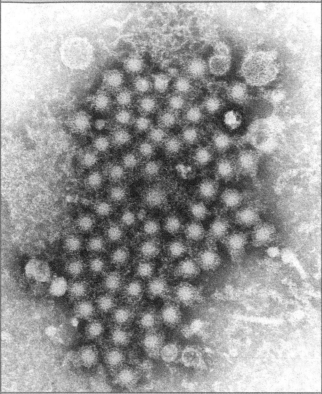

With the five known strains of hepatitis, this virus can cause acute and chronic manifestations of the disease, as well as result in carcinoma of the liver.

Source: CDC/Public Health Image Library.

you can do about it. As we saw in Chapter 4, before going further with your investigation one of the first things to do is to establish the existence of the outbreak. You will need a way to compare the two cities in question in order to evaluate this, as well as compare each city to its own baseline rates immediately preceding the events as well as over similar time periods in previous years. You need to compare these cities. In this chapter you will learn the basics of rates and measures that are used to describe the disease you are investigating.

Comparisons are essential in order to make sense of the situation at hand. In addition, they may be able to lead to clues about what is going on. But comparisons cannot be made on the

basis of absolute numbers, such as those described above. In order to make comparisons, you must have information about the underlying populations—the cities in this case—as well as the cases themselves. Do you recall deriving common denominators when you were in grade school—making two fractions have the same denominator in order to compare or manipulate them? This is exactly the same. You need to make a common denominator for each of the cities in order to compare them, as well as be sure that you have the ability (with common denominators) to compare each city with its own previous data. To do this, use rates and measures, the next step in describing your data.

You investigate further and find out that the population of County A is 784,712 and the population of County B is 1,500,546 (see Table 5-1). What do you think now? In order to calculate the county-specific rates, you divide each County's rate by its population, multiply by a common factor, and then can you compare rates between the cities.

By including the denominator in your evaluation, you can now see that County A actually has quite a big problem, and County B's is within its normal range (0.5 to 1.0 per 100,000 annually) which was not much different than its prior years. While high, County B has a large IDU population, and hepatitis C is fairly common. County A, on the other hand, generally has very few cases of hepatitis C and its current rate of 1.91 per 100,000 is, indeed, alarming. The previous years ranged from 0.2 to 0.4 per 100,000. You begin your investigation and focus, thus, on County A. What has happened? You discover after meeting with local infectious disease physicians that a new drug treatment center has opened up in County A. Upon intake, the new clients (who came from areas within and outside of County A) were given a hepatitis C screening test. Thus the increase in cases reflects the increased access to care of drug users who were already infected with hepatitis C and are now diagnosed and able to seek treatment. This increase would be considered artifactual, that is, appearing to be an epidemic when in fact it is not. The difference between an artifactual epidemic and a true epidemic lies in the way the data are either classified or detected, not that there is an actual increase in the number of cases. Here this is

TABLE 5-1 Hypothetical County-Specific Rates for Hepatitis C, 2000

	Cases in 2000	Mid-year Population, 2000	Cases/Population	Rate per 100,000
County A	15	784,712	0.00001912	1.91
County B	13	1,500,546	0.00000866	0.87

the case, because the increase was due to a change in the way cases were identified (i.e., routine screening by the treatment facility). Although the epidemic was artifactual, however, it is important to note that even though it is not an epidemic of hepatitis C, the cases are all real.

Without rates you would not have been able to compare counties, compare previous periods with that in question, determine the presence of a real or artifactual epidemic, identify the location of the infectious outbreak, or identify changes and trends over time. Using the denominators to develop rates instead of only viewing absolute numbers was extremely important in this outbreak investigation. The absolute numbers here would have been useful in terms of quantifying resource need, but not in determining if a true epidemic were afoot. Without knowing if it were an actual epidemic (say there were a new strain of the virus that was more highly infectious, or there was an increase in the number if injection drug users, for example), it would not be possible to try to identify the source of the epidemic and take public health action to stem it. Even though the absolute numbers would be useful for the current moment, without knowing whether the number of cases should be expected to increase, stay the same, or decrease, future resource allocation would be difficult to determine. Having rates also provide a means of communicating your findings to those around you in a common language that was quickly understandable and generalizable by all.

STANDARDIZATION

Use of denominators allows us to compare "apples with apples and oranges with oranges," taking into account differences in underlying population size to identify the true magnitude of an outbreak, or of any public health concern. Similarly, standardization allows us to take into account differences in underlying population structure. Rather than focus on the calculations, which are covered in nearly every introductory epidemiology textbook, we will discuss briefly the purpose of standardization in order to make the process more intuitive.

If you want to compare between groups, two things are necessary: you need to ensure you are looking at directly comparable measures (e.g., rates, prevalence, *not* absolute numbers), standardize against a norm to ensure natural makeup of sub-population is not "weighting" your findings in the direction of the group, which simply has more representation. These methods of standardization are techniques in which one applies one population's rates to another's. There are two types:

- Direct standardization, where subpopulation rates are applied to a standard population, and

- Indirect standardization, where standard population rates are applied to a subpopulation.

This allows comparison between two (or more) groups that differ with respect to underlying population, most notably (though not exclusively by any means) age. Why would we worry about this? Certain variables can distort relationships between the independent and dependent variables. For example, age does this very commonly for one simple reason: Older people tend to die at higher rates than younger people. If we fail to account for the underlying population structure differences in two areas requiring comparison, we will have misleading results, and we will not be able to understand the predictors or outcomes under study. For example, imagine we have two counties that appear to be experiencing an increase in the rates of cervical cancer, caused by the infectious agent human papilloma virus (HPV). City A is smaller than its counterpart, and is home to several large retirement facilities for active seniors, whereas City B is a college town, with a younger population. Comparing even the rates (not absolute numbers) of cervical cancer between the two is helpful, but still does not provide an understanding of age-adjusted rates. Because the older population is more likely to die, simply by virtue of age, it is difficult to determine what is happening or whether the rates are out of the ordinary. As it happens, when the underlying population structure is taken into account, it becomes clear that rates are higher in the younger population compared to what would have been expected. Because more elderly individuals die, and more of them inhabit City A, this critical health problem in City B could have been easily overlooked.

Because we have stable standard population data available, we will use direct standardization for this example, based on its characteristics and those of the underlying population. In general, you use direct standardization when you can, and reserve indirect standardization for when:

- the numbers of deaths are too small in some of the age groups to be standardized; or
- you *want to* compare one population to a standard population.

We can see in this example that there are more cases among residents of City B—the younger women—and fewer among the older women, we may have a problem in how we interpret our findings. This is important to assess because it may indicate that there is an increase in the rates of HPV among the college women, which could be preventable with public health intervention; it could also mean that—as in the case of the hepatitis C example—there was a change in screening practices leading to improved cervical cancer detection via Pap smear. Benefits may be seen from adjusting for other characteristics, when data are available. These may include gender, race, ethnicity, as well as age.

What do we do?

- Take the population standard (e.g., census data) broken down by relevant age categories (if standardizing by age)
- Take the rate from City A and multiply it by the population standard for each age category
- Take the rate from City B and multiply it by the population standard for each age category (be sure you are using the same multiplier, per 100,000 for example)
- Multiply each category's rate by the standard population size for that category
- What will result is the number of expected deaths if the standard had the same number of deaths as the population in question. Do this for each city, to facilitate comparison between them.

Another way of looking at the above steps:

What if we do not have a stable population standard or cannot find a relevant data source by which to directly standardize? Indirect standardization works well. The difference here is we compare City A to another standard population, say state data, and City B to that same population. Then we compare what rates we would have found if each city had the same population as the state standard. We basically apply the standard's rates to the population of the city. Then we compare, using a standardized mortality ratio (SMR), as below.

Imagine we are looking now at deaths from cervical cancer. What do we do?

- Multiply the death rate from the standard by the population of City A or B
- Add up the actual deaths from City A or City B
- Divide the observed deaths by the expected deaths (that you obtain from above) and this yields the SMR.

Direct Standardization

Age Group	U.S. standard population	City A	Number of cases for City A	Death rate in City A	Expected number of deaths for standard population if had same death rate as City A
<15 years	Number of population in this age category from standard source, e.g., census data	Population of City A in this age stratum	Cases in this age stratum	City A cases/City A population	City A rate × number of population in this age category from standard source
15 to 44 years	Number of population in this age category from standard source, e.g., census data	Population of City A in this age stratum	Cases in this age stratum	City A cases/City A population	City A rate × number of population in this age category from standard source
≥44 years	Number of population in this age category from standard source, e.g., census data	Population of City A in this age stratum	Cases in this age stratum	City A cases/City A population	City A rate × number of population in this age category from standard source

Indirect Standardization

Age group	In City A or City B — Population (or person-years)	In City A or City B — Observed number of deaths	Death Rates/ 100,000	Number of deaths EXPECTED in the City A or City B Population if they had the same rates as the state population standard being used
<15 years	Population or person-years observed in either city in this age category	Observed deaths from cervical cancer in this age category	Death rate in state (or standard population) in this age category	Multiply state deaths × city population for this age category
15 to 44 years	Population or person-years observed in either city in this age category	Observed deaths from cervical cancer in this age category	Death rate in state (or standard population) in this age category	Multiply state deaths × City population for this age category
>44 years	Population or person-years observed in either city in this category	Observed deaths from cervical cancer in this age category	Death rate in state (or standard population) in this age category	Multiply state deaths × City population for this age category
		Add up observed deaths		Add up expected deaths

Another way of looking at the above steps:

Standardized mortality ratio =

$$SMR = \left[\frac{\text{\# observed deaths}}{\text{\# expected deaths}} \right] \times 100$$

If the SMR is >1.0 then the number of deaths exceeds those expected; <1.0 means it is less than expected. If you have two cities, as in this example, then you can compare each city's SMR, so you have a city-by-city comparison in addition to a comparison with the standard.

USES FOR ABSOLUTE COUNTS, PROPORTIONS, RATES, AND RATIOS

When we think about measures used in epidemiology, we generally think of four distinct types: absolute counts, proportions, rates, and ratios. In general, the latter three are the most informative. This is not to say that absolute counts do not play a role in public health. In fact, they can be valuable in assessing need and utilization, as well as in the initial investigation of an infectious problem. For example, imagine there are two hospitals that are planning infectious disease units for their new wings. Tuberculosis (TB) patients and others with serious and transmissible airborne infections require rooms with specific types of ventilation systems and isolation.[1,2] The hospital administrators and architects are meeting, and need to know how often this sort of room will be required per year. If it is an infrequent event, only one such room might be added; if it is common, more rooms will be required. This clearly has cost implications, and so cannot be taken lightly. Too few rooms would be a public health threat; too many rooms would be an unnecessary expenditure that would deprive other patients of services. The administrator of one hospital checks her database and sees that over the past 10 years, their one isolation room was used an average (mean) of 2.3 times per year (standard deviation 0.35, range 0–4), and at no one time were two patients in need of the same room. The administrator of the other hospital checks his database and sees that over the past 10 years, their one external ventilation room was used a mean 5.8 times per year (standard deviation 1.2, range 4–10), and there were 17 instances in which multiple patients needed the room simultaneously, requiring them to be transported to alternate hospitals. Clearly, this information is useful, even though it is only absolute counts. Although we still do not have a sense of whether there is a big problem with TB or other respiratory infections in each of the locations, and we could not yet compare their underlying rates to see what is taking place, the hospitals can now build new rooms appropriately. (There is a bit of information that one can infer here, however. Imagine that one year each of these hospitals has five TB patients. Even without knowing any more information, which of these hospitals has a bigger problem, the first or the second? Clearly the first. Five TB cases seems beyond their expected norm whereas for the second hospital, five is at the lower end of annual cases. Even a little information can help us identify trends and changes over time.)

Proportions, on the other hand, tell us what proportion of a population was affected. For example, if 54 children attended a day care where a rotavirus (a serious gastrointestinal infection causing diarrhea, frequently found in day care settings) outbreak occurred, and there were 16 cases, one could say that 29.6% (that is, 16/54 = 29.6%) of the students became ill. This is called the attack rate: of those infected, the number that became ill—a very intuitive measure. Note that the numerator is contained within the denominator. This is the hallmark of proportions. This proportion can and should be refined further to include elements of person, place, and time; for example, "within a 2-week period [time], 29.6% [proportion] of the day care attendees ages 6 months to 2 years [person] were newly infected [new cases] with laboratory-confirmed rotavirus [level of diagnostic certainty] at the Daycare Center [place]." Many of the specific measures you will learn in the next section are proportions, as are many of the infectious-disease-specific measures.

Rates are another type of measure that specifically must include the concept of time in the measure. (Many proportions do include time, but in order to be a rate, it *must* be included.) Rates describe the number of cases that occurred, divided by the population at risk. That the persons are at risk is an important element of identifying the appropriate number for the denominator. The hepatitis C scenario above defined a rate, for example. Rates are typically expressed as per a unit of population, a factor of 10 that makes the rate into a more manageable number. Rates are especially useful because they describe the risk of the outcome under study of happening over a specific period of time. Thus, in the above example, the risk of newly contracting hepatitis C cases in the 8-week time period described is 1.9 per 100,000 in City A and 0.87 per 100,000 in City B. Note that this assumes that all members of the population are at risk of acquiring hepatitis C. This may not be a good assumption, because not all persons may be at risk if they are immune or have another situation rendering them risk-free.

Finally, ratios are when the numerator is divided by the denominator, but the numerator is *not* contained within the denominator. For example, imagine there is a newly identified infectious disease. Little is known about the disease except for its clinical presentation, and no etiologic organism has yet been isolated. The absolute count of cases as well as the rate of the disease in several adjacent communities have been calculated to facilitate planning and comparison with other communities. In addition, public health practitioners in the area have noted that the adult male:female ratio of individuals contracting this disease is 3.4, indicating that for every one adult female with the disease, there are 3.4 adult males. For individuals less than 13 years, however, the male:female ratio is 1.1, indicating that for every girl with the disease there are 1.1 boys. Note that the numerator in each of these is not contained within the denominator; that is, male and female categories are mutually exclusive. This is the salient distinguishing characteristic between a proportion and a ratio. How can a ratio help us? In this hypothetical example, one might recognize that many more adult males than females in the affected communities work outside in agricultural positions, and yet the boys and girls under 13 years play outside in similar distributions. This may give one a hint: Is there something about being outside that is associated with the disease? Could it be vector borne? Could it be an infectious agent that is associated with the work of the men, perhaps an organism in the field? Ratios can provide insight into the etiology of an agent, what it might be, and how to address confounders in the analysis of the data. Ratios are a useful adjunct to absolute counts, rates, and proportions, yet seldom replace them.

INCIDENCE MEASURES

Incidence is one of the most important types of measures in epidemiology, particularly infectious disease epidemiology. Incidence measures tell us how many *new* cases of a disease occurred in a given time frame. They allow us to examine what is happening at the moment with regard to cases—not what has happened in a previous time period. When a problem is first identified, incidence is all one has: the number of new cases in the past month. But after that, things get increasingly complex, because there are cases who have the disease, some who had it but recovered, others who have it but are undergoing treatment, and so forth. Counting the new cases becomes trickier as time progresses, but doing so offers the only true measure of what the new cases look like and the best estimate of risk. Incidence measures are rates, and as such, involve two key elements:

1. The number of *new* cases during a specified period of time (numerator)
2. The number of people *at risk* of developing the disease over the *same* period of time (denominator)

Let us break this down a bit:

- *Numerator:* The number of *new* cases during a specified period of time. Determining which are new cases and which are existing cases is a crucial determination in the development of rates. In a textbook such as this, it is generally quite straightforward. As you will see, examples tend to provide exact numbers of new cases dur-

ing a given time period, allowing the reader to calculate the incidence simply. In real life, however, the distinction of new vs. existing cases can be difficult, and yet, it is this very distinction that yields a useful and accurate estimate of incidence. Individuals who have a history of the disease are not counted in the calculation of incidence rates, depending on their susceptibility to the disease, whether they are at risk of the disease. For example, if the disease renders them fully immune from the disease, then they will not be counted in the denominator of people at risk because they are not truly at risk. Some diagnoses, on the other hand, are possible to have time and again and remain at risk throughout.

One example of the difficulty of this measure is seen in sexually transmitted disease (STD) research. Imagine calculating the incidence of *Chlamydia trachomatis*, a bacterial STD especially common among adolescents and young adults. Unlike viral infections, individuals may have repeated cases of this bacterial infection, so counting them can be tricky. One can count initial new infections as well as subsequent infections, but keeping them separate and counting them accurately is easier said than done.

- *Denominator:* The number of people *at risk* of developing the disease over the *same* period of time. The denominator of an incidence measure includes the *population at risk* of developing the disease. For some diseases, this is rather straightforward. For example, in measuring the risk of ovarian cancer, the population at risk clearly only includes women, and among women, only those with ovaries. In infectious disease, however, we face challenges in identifying an appropriate denominator. Those at risk of developing the disease over the specified period of time need to be *susceptible* to the disease. How do we estimate that? It depends on the disease under study. Diseases such as measles that confer immunity following illness, and generally, following vaccination (94% to 98% vaccine efficacy following the first immunization, and 99% with a subsequent booster)[1,2] would render a different at-risk denominator than a bacterial infection that one could contract repeatedly. In the latter case, as we saw with the *C. trachomatis* example above, one could have multiple incidence measures with fluctuating numerators and denominators. Incidence— new first cases—of the STD could be calculated looking at the denominator of those who have never had the disease before and with the denominator of all sexually active individuals. (This, too, could be seen in multiple fashions. For example, if one had the data available, one could evaluate only those sexually active individuals having unprotected intercourse, and so forth.) An additional incidence measure could be calculated looking at the number of new *first subsequent cases* during the specified time period as the numerator, and the number of *sexually active individuals who had contracted* C. trachomatis *once before* during the specified time period. This could be calculated repeatedly, because repeated STD infections are extremely common.

- *Time period:* Crucial to the incidence is the time period specified. Like other rates, the time period must be the same for the numerator and the denominator, and must be specified clearly in order for the incidence rate to be correctly interpreted.
- *Multiplier:* In general, to make comparisons simpler and avoid very small or noninteger incidence rates, a multiplier is often used. We know that this does not alter the underlying value, because it simple divides or multiplies it by a factor (10 is usually selected), and the result is the division of the numerator by the denominator, multiplied by this factor. This makes presentation of the incidence rates and comparison simpler, and because the multiplier is applied to both the numerator and the denominator, it does not affect the incidence itself.

There are two types of incidence measures: cumulative incidence (CI) and incidence rate (IR), also known as incidence density (ID) or incidence density rate (IDR). Conceptually, they are similar. Both express the number of new cases in a population; they differ in only their denominator.

- *Cumulative incidence:* If you imagine following all people in a population over a specific period of time, then CI is a measure of risk described by:

$$CI = \frac{\text{the number of new cases of disease among those at risk of the disease in a population over the given time period}}{\text{the number of individuals in that population over the same time period}} \times \text{multiplier}$$

The assumption of being able to follow each individual in that population is seldom met, however, although the basic tenets of this measure must be. That is, if we cannot follow all individuals, we need to be able to make some assumptions about the stability of the population. Plus, most populations are dynamic—people come into and depart from the population constantly, so estimating the true denominator at risk can be an impossible task. Still, although we often make due with CI even when we know that we cannot meet this assumption,

we can do better. And there are better measures to use, such as incidence rate, when we can.

- *Incidence rate:* If we follow each member of our population to see specifically how long each person is observed for the outcome of interest, and make note of when they are being followed by the cohort and when they are not, then we can obtain a true rate. This measure is one that directly integrates time into the denominator of the measure. Our measure of risk is then described by:

$$IR = \frac{\text{the number of new cases of disease among those at risk of the disease in a population over the given time period}}{\text{person-time followed over the same time period}} \times \text{multiplier}$$

It is important to note the differences between these two measures. IRs are commonly used in longitudinal studies of infectious (or other) diseases, such as natural history studies, cohort studies, or clinical trials, which will be discussed in the next chapters. CIs are used when there is information about the mid-year population at risk but no individual-level information available.

An example of how to calculate CI and IR:

Epiland is a hypothetical city in the United States. In 1999, there was an increasing concern about a new, emerging disease there. This information is available to you:

Mid-year population of Epiland, 1999	950,000
New cases of emerging disease under study between 1/1/1999 and 12/31/1999	1,020
Prevalent cases of disease on 1/1/1999	1,403
Estimated population of Epiland on 1/1/1999	876,449

Essentially everyone is at risk of the new disease, and it appears that even those who have been infected once can be infected again. The public health physicians develop a protocol that they submit to the relevant institutional review boards and local agencies. They invite clinic attendees at high risk of the disease to participate in a study to find out risk factors for the disease. They follow participants over three years with quarterly visits. At each visit, detailed clinical and behavioral data are collected, as well as laboratory specimens to evaluate exposure to the disease of interest. Participants "accrue" follow up time as long as they do not miss a study visit. Once they develop the disease they no longer accrue person-years of follow up.

People in the cohort   750

Person-years under study of members of cohort
(average 2.76 years of follow up per person)   2,070

New cases of emerging disease over three years
of follow up   59

How to calculate CI for the emerging in Epiland, 1999:

$$CI = \frac{\text{the number of new cases of disease among those at risk of the disease in a population over the given time period}}{\text{the number of individuals in that population over the same time period}} \times \text{multiplier}$$

(here we will use 100,000, but it could be any factor applied to both numerator and denominator)

$$= [1,020/950,000] \times 100,000 = 107.4 \text{ per } 100,000$$

How to calculate IR for the emerging disease in the cohort study described:

$$CI = \frac{\text{the number of new cases of disease among those at risk of the disease in a population over the given time period}}{\text{person-time followed over the same time period}} \times \text{multiplier}$$

(here we will use 100,000, but it could be any factor applied to both numerator and denominator)

$$= [59/2,070] \times 100,000 = 2.85 \text{ per } 100 \text{ person-years}$$

Note that if one were rendered no longer susceptible to the disease after having it, the number at risk in the population would change from year to year, incorporating those who had already been ill. This would have the effect of reducing the number of the population at risk.

PREVALENCE MEASURES

Prevalence measures are used commonly and represent a blurring of information. Prevalence estimates merge existing cases with new cases, so that prevalence is a measure of how many people there are with a new or existing disease. There are two types of prevalence:

- *Point prevalence* is the number of existing or new cases at a given moment.
- *Period prevalence* is the number of existing or new cases over a stated period of time.

The denominator for each is the number of persons in the population over that same period of time. For example, in order to find the prevalence of *C. trachomatis* at a specific time,

say January 1, 2000, one would identify all cases on that day that were either new on that day or present on that day (irrespective of whether they had been diagnosed before), and divide that number by the number of persons in the population on that same day. Similarly, to calculate period prevalence between January 1, 2000, and December 31, 2000, one would identify all new and existing cases during that time period and divide that number by the number of persons in the population during that time period. For example:

How to calculate point prevalence of emerging disease, Epiland, 1/1/1999:

$$\text{Point prevalence }_{1/1/1999} = \frac{\text{new and existing cases on 1/1/1999}}{\text{population on 1/1/1999}} \times \text{multiplier}$$

$$= [1,403/876,449] \times 100,000$$
$$= 160.1 \text{ per } 100,000$$

How to calculate period prevalence of emerging disease, Epiland, 1/1/1999 through 12/31/1999:

$$\text{Point prevalence }_{1/1/1999 \text{ through } 12/31/1999} = \frac{\text{new and existing cases on 1/1/1999 + new cases 1/1/1999 through 12/31/1999}}{\text{estimated mid-year population for 1999}} \times \text{multiplier}$$

$$= [(1,403/1,020)/950,000] \times 100,000$$
$$= 255.1 \text{ per } 100,000$$

How to calculate prevalence of disease in study cohort:

$$\text{Prevalence of disease in cohort} = \frac{\text{number of cases over follow up}}{\text{number of participants}} \times \text{multiplier}$$

$$= [59/750] \times 100$$
$$= 7.9 \text{ per } 100 \text{ participants}$$

Why bother with prevalence when you have incidence? It is a natural question. They both contribute valuable and differing information. Incidence helps identify an epidemic, a health care disparity, an access issues, a diagnostic change, and much, much more. Prevalence helps quantify needs for care, such as how many people are living with a disease; observe changes in treatment (improvements, declines); and more. Often we might wish to have measured incidence, but we are not able to get a value of new cases or the number of persons at risk. One characteristic of prevalence and incidence is that their relationship is both intuitive and quantifiable. As more individuals become sick, they increase the prevalence, with new and existing cases increasing together. That is, until one of two things happens: there is a treatment such that the prevalence goes down or the disease is sufficiently serious and the sick die such that the prevalence goes down. In both of these options—cure or death—the same thing happens, though for different reasons: The duration of the illness is shortened. Figure 5-2 is a good illustration of this relationship. Here you can see that mortality rates for AIDS were steadily increasing parallel with AIDS incidence until the late 1990s. At that point, a new class of treatment—protease inhibitors (PI)—was introduced. PIs are the most effective drug to date, increasing the time between AIDS diagnosis and death. This increased the prevalence of AIDS, because more individuals were surviving the disease. Here we have a case in which incidence remained steady while duration and thus prevalence increased. This is mathematically expressed like this:

$$\text{prevalence (P)} = \text{incidence (I)} \times \text{duration (D)}$$

You can think of it this way: New cases of any disease or condition (infectious or otherwise) occur, and become incident cases. Once this happens, affected persons have the following outcomes:

- Cure/resolution/remission
- Continuing illness
- Death

Individuals who either die or are cured do not become prevalent cases; those with continued disease do. Thus as duration is shorter—due either to death or cure—prevalence is lower, holding incidence the same. Similarly, if duration is longer—due to longer times of living with the disease, improved treatment, decreased likelihood of death—prevalence is higher, holding incidence the same.

Several specific measures are often used to describe infectious diseases and their outbreaks:

- Case fatality rate (CFR) expresses as a proportion how many individuals infected with the disease die of the disease, and is a measure of disease severity. For example, of the 296 people who contracted Ebola virus in the 1995 outbreak in Kikwit, as of the update on June 30 of that year, 233 died[3]; thus the CFR was 79%. Why is this measure a rate and not just a proportion? Though it can be blurry without all the specific information explicitly provided, you will note that the CFR does contain an explicit or implicit measure of time. For CFRs, the time frame may be hard to find if it is in a narrative articulation of the measure, but it will be there. (The article or report may say something on the order of, "between January 1 and June 25, 1995 there were 100 people infected and 4 died" so that the specific time period is made clearer.) It also assumes that all individuals were diagnosed with the same disease and the same definition of that disease, and that they were all followed for the duration of the time period so that their ultimate vital status could be ascertained.
- Attack rates (AR) parallel the previous two measures, providing us with the number exposed to a disease who ultimately got the disease over a specified period of time. For example, if 50 children were exposed to rotavirus at a day care, and 20 became ill, the AR would be 40%.
- Vaccine efficacy (VE) has some of the same characteristics as the aforementioned measures, but

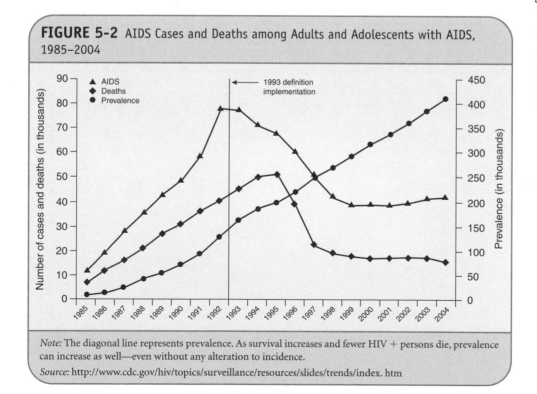

FIGURE 5-2 AIDS Cases and Deaths among Adults and Adolescents with AIDS, 1985–2004

Note: The diagonal line represents prevalence. As survival increases and fewer HIV + persons die, prevalence can increase as well—even without any alteration to incidence.

Source: http://www.cdc.gov/hiv/topics/surveillance/resources/slides/trends/index.htm

Case Fatality Rates

When we currently think of influenza pandemics, we generally think of at least two: the 1918 pandemic of the Spanish flu, which killed between 20 million and 50 million people globally, vastly more than the number killed in the world war that was just ending; and the avian flu, H5N1, which lies in wait and many fear will be the next flu pandemic.[4–10] Of course, in between there have been other pandemics (e.g., the 1957 Asian flu and 1968–1969 Hong Kong flu, most notably). And every year, thousands die of pneumonia and influenza, with the National Center for Health Statistics in 2000 ranking it seventh in all cause mortality for all ages and races (with 65,313 deaths), and fifth in the leading causes of death among persons ages 65 years and older.[11] But avian flu carries the fear of what could be the next strain to turn into a pandemic.[4,6–12]

Avian flu, a highly pathogenic avian influenza A (H5N1) virus, has occurred primarily among poultry in Asia; direct cases of transmission from poultry to humans have been seen, but very few human-to-human cases. Still, a strain that we humans are not well-acquainted with could yield us relatively helpless: Our shield of immunity is not primed against this strain, as with what happened in the 1918 flu (H1N1). If the avian flu shifted slightly to simplify human-to-human transmission, a swift pandemic could ensue; this remains a chief concern globally. Already, the World Health Organization (WHO), CDC, and other public health organizations are on the alert with active surveillance and intervention (e.g., reduction of infected poultry populations, vaccinations in development, strategic plans written, etc.).[4,6–11] Statistics are kept by the WHO and are available.[9] These provide a good opportunity to see case-fatality rates in practice (see Table 5-2).

How does one read this table? First, notice that the time period (required for a case-fatality rate) is annually, and the regions are countries. This is a very large geographical unit as well as a large time period, yet these are the data available to us, so we can calculate a case-fatality based on them, provided we are clear about what data we have. The case-fatality rate is calculated as:[13]

$$\text{Case-fatality rate} = \frac{\text{number of deaths during a specific time period}}{\text{number of cases during the same time period}}$$

So if we are interested, for example, in the case-fatality rate of Indonesia in 2006, our figure would be:

$$\text{Case fatality} = 45/55 = 81.8\%$$

TABLE 5-2 Cumulative Number of Confirmed Human Cases of Avian Influenza A/(H5N1) Reported to WHO (27 December 2006)*[9]

Country	2003		2004		2005		2006		Total	
	cases	deaths	cases	deaths	cases	deaths	cases	deaths	cases	deaths
Azerbaijan	0	0	0	0	0	0	8	5	8	5
Cambodia	0	0	0	0	4	4	2	2	6	6
China	1	1	0	0	8	5	12	8	21	14
Djibouti	0	0	0	0	0	0	1	0	1	0
Egypt	0	0	0	0	0	0	18	10	18	10
Indonesia	0	0	0	0	19	12	55	45	74	57
Iraq	0	0	0	0	0	0	3	2	3	2
Thailand	0	0	17	12	5	2	3	3	25	17
Turkey	0	0	0	0	0	0	12	4	12	4
Vietnam	3	3	29	20	61	19	0	0	93	42
Total	**4**	**4**	**46**	**32**	**97**	**42**	**114**	**79**	**261**	**157**

*Total number of cases includes number of deaths. WHO reports only laboratory-confirmed cases.
Source: World Health Organization (WHO)[9]

continues

Case Fatality Rates—continued

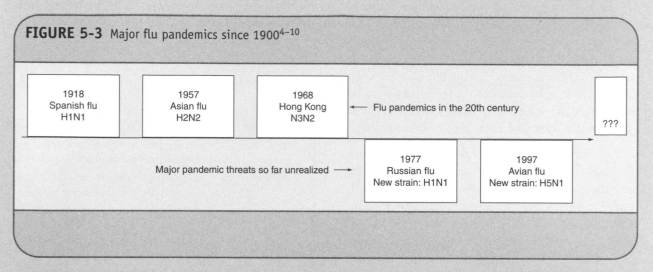

FIGURE 5-3 Major flu pandemics since 1900[4–10]

| 1918 Spanish flu H1N1 | 1957 Asian flu H2N2 | 1968 Hong Kong N3N2 | ← Flu pandemics in the 20th century | ??? |

Major pandemic threats so far unrealized ⟶

| 1977 Russian flu New strain: H1N1 | 1997 Avian flu New strain: H5N1 |

Note the notations at the bottom of the table, and that this only includes lab-confirmed cases. Avian flu is a serious diagnosis, and yet, many of its symptoms are like those of other viruses, and influenzas in particular. If you had to guess, do you think this number of cases under- or overestimates the true number of cases of avian flu to date?

What does the notation in Figure 5-3 mean? Influenza is a virus with three recognized types: A, B, and C. Two antigenic properties of the surface glycoproteins, hemagglutinin (H) and neuraminidiase (N), help to classify the influenza A subtypes; thus, when we note the combination, say H5N1, it denotes a specific subtype of influenza A.[2] Due to the recombining of antigens, called antigenic drift, these viruses shift constantly, changing over time. This is why there needs to be new vaccine compositions developed for the flu shot each year, providing the correct subtypes for each year. Though as humans we have developed immunity to subtypes that are common, we do not have defenses against avian flu, making us more vulnerable.

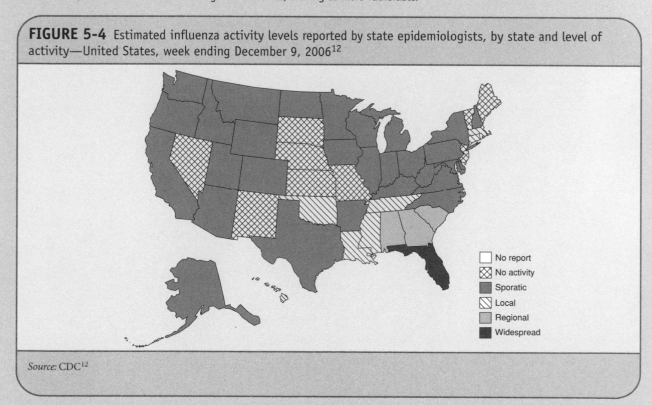

FIGURE 5-4 Estimated influenza activity levels reported by state epidemiologists, by state and level of activity—United States, week ending December 9, 2006[12]

☐ No report
⊠ No activity
■ Sporatic
▨ Local
▧ Regional
■ Widespread

Source: CDC[12]

assesses something different. VE tells us of those immunized against a specific disease, and how many of them did not develop that disease over a specified period of time. For example, the series of pertussis immunizations have a VE of 80% for the first 5 years, after which protection begins to wane.[2] If 100 children were immunized against pertussis, given the average VE over the first 5 years, an estimated 20% of the children would be susceptible to pertussis. (Note this does not mean they *would* get the disease, only that if exposed, they could be susceptible.)

Each of these measures has the same underlying assumptions: that the disease and outcomes are carefully operationalized, that the individuals are comprehensively followed forward in time, and that there is a specified time period under study.

Now that you understand some of the key ways of describing disease, we will move on to specific details of analytic studies, one of the most exciting aspects of epidemiology, and a context in which all the descriptive information learned in this and the last chapters can be put to good use. In analytic studies, you will learn the skills to compare exposed and unexposed persons, cases and non-cases, understand interventional approaches, and answer the research questions you will be able to articulate.

TABLE 5-3 Summary Table—Rates and Measures

Incidence	New cases per unit time
Prevalence	New and existing cases per unit time
Attack rate	Proportion of persons exposed to disease who become ill per unit time
Case fatality rate	Proportion of persons with disease who die from disease per unit time
Vaccine efficacy	Proportion of persons immunized who retain protection from disease per unit time

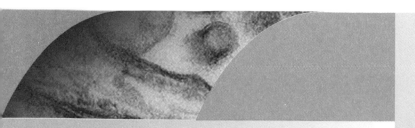

Discussion Questions

1. Go to www.who.int and investigate an infectious disease of interest to you. For that disease, find out the following:
   a. One epidemic curve
   b. Incubation time
   c. Clinical characteristics (including person, place, and time of those most affected)
   d. Case definition
   e. Means of diagnosis, clinical as well as with diagnostic procedures
   f. Case fatality rate

2. Go to www.cdc.gov and investigate another infectious disease of interest to you. For that disease, assess prevalence and incidence in the following year for a particular subpopulation (e.g., women 15–34 years of age). How are they different? Can you calculate (estimate) the duration of the disease from these data?

REFERENCES

1. Nelson K. *Infectious Disease Epidemiology.* Gaithersburg, MD: Aspen; 2001.

2. Heymann DL. *Control of Communicable Diseases.* 18th ed. Washington, DC: American Public Health Association; 2004.

3. Centers for Disease Control and Prevention. Update: outbreak of Ebola viral hemorrhagic fever—Zaire, 1995. *MMWR.* 1995;44(25):469–479.

4. Centers for Disease Control and Prevention. Avian influenza infection in humans (bird flu). 2006. Available at: www.pandemicflu.gov. Accessed December 25, 2006.

5. Centers for Disease Control and Prevention. Pandemics and pandemic threats since 1900. 2006. Available at: www.pandemicflu.gov/general/historicaloverview.html. Accessed December 25, 2006.

6. National Institute of Allergy and Infectious Diseases, National Institutes of Health. Focus on the flu: timeline of human flu pandemics. 2006. Available at: www3.niaid.nih.gov/news/focuson/flu/illustrations/timeline/timeline.htm. Accessed December 25, 2006.

7. Kilbourne ED. Influenza pandemics of the 20th century. *Emerg Infect Dis.* 2006;12(1):9–14.

8. Krause R. The swine flu episode and the fog of epidemics. *Emerg Infect Dis.* 2006;12(1):40–43.

9. World Health Organization. Cumulative number of confirmed human cases of avian influenza A(H5N1) reported to WHO. Available at: www.who.int/csr/disease/avian_influenza/country/cases_table_2006_12_27/en. Accessed December 25, 2006.

10. Taubenberger J. 1918 influenza: the mother of all pandemics. *Emerg Infect Dis.* 2006;12(1):15–22.

11. National Center for Health Statistics. www.nchs.gov. Accessed March 2, 2004.

12. Centers for Disease Control and Prevention. Update: influenza activity—United States, October 1–December 9, 2006. *MMWR.* 2006;55(50): 1359–3162.

13. Giesecke J. *Modern Infectious Disease Epidemiology.* London: Arnold Publishers/Oxford University Press; 2002.

CHAPTER 6

Laying the Foundation: How to Conduct a Study

LEARNING OBJECTIVES

By the end of this chapter, you will be able to:

- Understand key issues in the conduct of analytic studies.
- Develop a research question matrix.
- Identify and operationalize independent and dependent variables and potential confounders.
- Articulate steps required prior to study implementation.

RESEARCH QUESTIONS AND HYPOTHESES— STRUCTURING YOUR STUDY

Before introducing you to the toolkit of analytic epidemiologic studies and giving you the basic study designs, you need to know the basic structure of designing and conducting a study. This not only will help you in the event that you pursue a career in infectious disease (or other) epidemiology, but also will provide you with a vital tool in reading the literature and integrating science into your own public health practice. The essence of conducting every study is the same: The first step is always to identify your research question. The research question, and what evolves from it, are the basis for the entire study's design, conduct, analysis, interpretation, and dissemination. It is the roadmap that helps the study stay on track. Designing and using this roadmap is the same for experimental studies as it is for observational studies and evaluation.

Your research question derives in great part from a thorough understanding of the scientific literature in your area of inquiry. A comprehensive literature review is needed before embarking on any study. First you identify the question of interest, then phrase that question in a form that makes it testable. Once a testable hypothesis is generated, variables to operationalize the question are specified. Then the study is conducted to measure the exposure and outcome of interest. Once qual-

ity checks are conducted to ensure that the data were properly collected and analyzed, information gleaned from the study is interpreted and public health action is taken, as indicated by the study. Methods and findings are documented so that they may later be shared and the methods replicated. Information gained from your study will then be used as the basis for the next study, where unanswered questions may then be addressed. This is the cycle of science, as indicated in Figure 6-1.

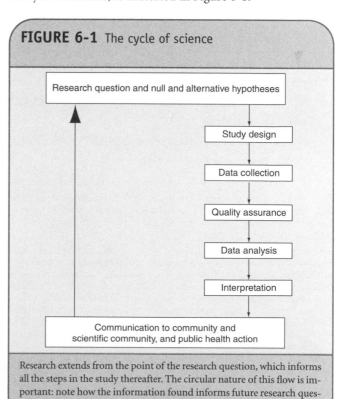

FIGURE 6-1 The cycle of science

```
Research question and null and alternative hypotheses
                    ↓
              Study design
                    ↓
            Data collection
                    ↓
            Quality assurance
                    ↓
             Data analysis
                    ↓
             Interpretation
                    ↓
Communication to community and
scientific community, and public health action
```

Research extends from the point of the research question, which informs all the steps in the study thereafter. The circular nature of this flow is important: note how the information found informs future research questions; this is crucial.

RESEARCH QUESTION DEVELOPMENT

What is a research question? The research question is just as simple as it sounds: It is the question you are asking of your research. For instance, is there an association between exposure to the dairy products at a buffet and vomiting? Is there an association between exposure to a new virus and severe respiratory distress? Is there an association between highly active antiretroviral treatment (HAART) for HIV and HIV viral load? This research question drives a more formal expression of the research question, called the null hypothesis (H_0). The H_0 is the statement of no difference, and provides the basis for statistical testing, which assesses the role of chance in the equation. Its counterpart is the alternative hypothesis (H_A), which expresses the opposite of the null hypothesis, and characterizes what we expect to find as the result of our study. Hypothesis testing is central to identifying if the relationship we find in our study's sample is due to the effects of chance alone or to a real relationship.[a] If we reject the H_0, then we allow that what we have found is unlikely to be due to the effect of chance alone;[b] that is, we reject the null and accept the alternative. All types of studies that are analytic in nature have research questions and hypotheses that drive their design and analysis; descriptive studies have research questions but generally not hypotheses that require rigorous testing; their focus is more on hypothesis generation. The following examples help to explain this construct:

Research question: Is there an association between HAART for HIV and HIV viral load?

H_0: There is no association between receipt of HAART and HIV viral load,

or viral loads among patients on HAART = viral loads among patients not on HAART.

H_A: There is an association between receipt of HAART and HIV viral load,

or viral loads among patients on HAART ≠ viral loads among patients not on HAART.

This research question could be addressed in more than one way: as you will see in the next chapter, an experimental design, which randomly assigns patients to receive HAART vs. the standard of care. Or a cohort study, as in chapters, in which patients who are on HAART are followed over time and compared with patients who are not on HAART. Each of these has unique purposes, strengths, and limitations, which will be discussed in the subsequent sections. The approach to the study's implementation, however, is the same irrespective of study design.

Here is another example, one that could be studied first with a description and then an observational study, either cohort or case-control, which you will shortly learn about:

Research question: Is there an association between exposure to the quiche at the buffet and salmonella food poisoning?

H_0: There is no association between receipt of quiche and salmonella

or salmonella rates among patients exposed to the quiche = salmonella rates among patients not exposed to the quiche.

H_A: There is an association between receipt of quiche and salmonella

or salmonella rates among patients exposed to the quiche ≠ salmonella rates among patients not exposed to the quiche.

This research question could not be studied in an experimental fashion, only descriptive and observational. Clearly, randomizing individuals to eat quiche that is laden with salmonella would not be ethical! Thus, this research question suggests a specific methodologic approach.

Research questions may be two-sided as above, or they may be one-sided, along with one-sided H_0 and H_A. These are identical to their two-sided counterparts, except that they specify a direction. For example, here are the one-sided null and alternative hypotheses:

Research question: Is HAART associated with decreased HIV viral loads?

H_0: Receipt of HAART is associated with increased or equal HIV viral loads

or viral loads among patients on HAART are ≥ viral loads among patients not on HAART.

H_A: Receipt of HAART is associated with decreased HIV viral loads

or viral loads among patients on HAART are < viral loads among patients not on HAART.

Note that in a one-sided H_0 and H_A, the equal sign remains in the H_0 (the ≤ or ≥) not in the H_A. The H_A is the

---

[a]You will learn more about such testing, also known as hypothesis testing, in other texts. This section will give introductory students sufficient information for understanding this chapter until they learn more in depth. Other students can use it as a refresher.

[b]This concept embraces the concept of statistical testing. This value, alpha, is the probability that we will obtain a value as extreme as or more extreme than we would by chance alone. We frequently—and arbitrarily—set a level of alpha at 0.05. This means that we will allow the possibility that 5% of the time we will believe we are seeing a difference even though it may not be there. This set point is increased or decreased as appropriate to one's study. For example, it may be that one is looking for safety values of a new medication, in which case having alpha = 0.01 is preferable. Alternatively, if one is hypothesis generating and there is no "cost" to accepting a difference is there when, in fact, it is not, alpha = 0.10 might be acceptable. Power (also known as 1 − beta) is the ability to find a difference if there is one. For example, if there is 80% power to detect a difference between treatment A and B, if there is a difference, then 20% of the time. If we see no difference there still may be one. Power is based upon the sample size, the difference one wishes to detect (increase power with increase differences), and variability.

statement that indicates a difference, whereas the null is the statement of no difference. Although there are statistical testing implications in this choice, for the purpose of this text, this is enough for you to understand.

The research question is the easy part: deciding what to ask. In most cases, this derives from research that has been done before or, sometimes, during acute public health needs. All research should begin with an extensive literature review to thoroughly understand what has been done in the past, how it was done, and what needs to be done in the future based on what research on the topic is currently underway. With experimental studies, the question is often whether a new treatment works better than the standard of care. With cohort studies, the question is generally whether a given exposure is associated with an outcome of interest. With case-control studies, the question is generally whether a given outcome is associated with an exposure of interest. For all of these, once the research question and the H_0 and H_A have been selected, the next step is operationalizing. Operationalization is when we define clear and workable variables that can be systematically collected and that are clearly defined enough to be consistent throughout all steps of the study, as well as generalizable to other studies.

How Many Strains of *E. coli* Are There Anyway?

Escherichia coli is a good example of an organism with a variety of strains. Fortunately, laboratory personnel are very good at operationalizing exactly what they are looking at; so must we be as epidemiologists. *E. coli* offers one of many good examples regarding why we need to be careful when we talk about infectious organisms, outcomes, and predictors: One word can have many meanings. The number of strains of any given organism can create confusion in the absence of clear definitions. When developing your research question, this is a good example of the need to define your variables clearly, even if you have laboratory data. Even when there is concrete evidence to support your choices, sometimes—as here—there may be many different possibilities. In behavioral research it is even harder: so often, one outcome or exposure may be described by infinite variables, thus clarity and clear operationalization is necessary.

A part of the normal intestinal environment, *E. coli* has several different strains that can cause virulent diarrhea and be quite dangerous, as seen in other examples. Here are the major categories of *E. coli* to consider.[1-6] If you were going to operationalize *E. coli*, you would need to be mindful, and operationalize it clearly with this in mind

- *Enteropathogenic E. coli:* This category is one of the oldest and most common causes of infant diarrhea worldwide. Commonly affecting infants while they are in nurseries, this type is spread via infant foods and formula, and typically occurs in children under 1 year of age. The diarrhea associated with enteropathogenic *E. coli* both is highly contagious and can be very dangerous due to its associated dehydration among children. This particular type of *E. coli* used to be seen in North America and Europe but is now largely confined to other parts of the world.
- *Enterotoxigenic E. coli:* As with enteropathogenic *E. coli*, this strain is generally associated with travel to developing countries, though it is increasingly being discovered in the United States as well. Mode of transmission is usually through contaminated food and sometimes water. This category of *E. coli* elaborates two specific toxins, hence the name of the category: heat labile or heat stable toxins; some elaborate both.
- *Enterohemorrhagic E. coli:* The most common of these is *E. coli* O157:H7. This category of *E. coli* expresses cytotoxins called Shiga toxins 1[c] and 2. Transmission is generally through ingestion of feces-contaminated food. Young children, the elderly, and those with compromised immune systems are most at risk. Progression to Hemolytic Uremic Syndrome (HUS) can occur in as many as 8% of cases.
- *Enteroinvasive E. coli:* This is a common endemic disease found in developing countries. Resembling the inflammatory response the body gives to shigella in the intestines, this disease can have incubation times as short as 10 hours. Contaminated food is the most likely source of transmission. Like other infections, antimicrobials are the usual treatment.
- *Enteroaggregative E. coli:* This is another source of infant diarrhea and, of concern, it causes persistent diarrhea among infants, which makes it dangerous. A relatively new emerged infection, enteroaggregative strains were identified in the 1980s. This strain has also been seen in industrialized countries among HIV+ persons.
- *Diffuse-adherence E. coli:* Little is known about this emerging category. It appears to be a more common cause of diarrhea among preschool children than infants or toddlers, unlike the other categories that are far more likely to cause disease among the younger set. More information about this category is sure to be forthcoming.

---

[c]Shiga toxin 1 is the same as that found in *Shigella dystenariae*, which can also progress to HUS.

SELECTION OF VARIABLES

The selection of variables to evaluate is an important decision. Rather than having vague independent and dependent variables, all types of designs in epidemiologic research, from descriptive to observational to experimental, require clearly identified variables. For example, imagine an experimental design evaluating the campaign to reduce exposure to mosquitoes during a West Nile Virus outbreak. Consider for a moment all the many ways that exposure to the campaign might be measured: number of people living near a social marketing campaign billboard, driving near the billboard, reporting in a survey that they saw the billboard, read the billboard, and took action based on the billboard, and so forth.

Operationalizing the variables of interest is a necessary step that needs to be done well. Without explicit operationalization, it would be easy to end up with information that is invalid. For example, consider all the ways that the outcome might be measured: purchase of DEET-based insect repellant, number of people coming to the emergency room fearing exposure, number of reported and confirmed cases of West Nile Virus, number of insect bites on the arms and legs, and so forth. Based on the research questions at hand as well as previous research, the investigator must be explicit about the variables under study. These need to be selected in a multidisciplinary fashion as well, to ensure that no one facet of the relationship or its study is being missed. We have not yet reviewed confounders or effect modifiers, but considering them at the inception of the study is necessary. If one gathers data on potential confounders and effect modifiers up front—variables that can obscure our understanding of relationships between exposures and outcomes or when different levels of exposures are associated with different effects in the outcomes, respectively—data may be collected on them. If no data are collected on these from the initiation of the study, it will become nearly impossible to ascertain data on them, as people move, environments change, and most people may not remember what was taking place in their lives at the time of original data collection.

Here's a slightly more complicated example. Consider the difference between the following operationalizations of the variables associated with the research question, "Is the substance abuse status of the client associated with unmet needs and immunocompromised system?" We need to operationalize the following variables:

- Substance abuse
- Unmet needs
- Immunocompromise

These all can be difficult. Imagine you work at an IDU clinic, and you want to assess the relationship between substance abuse

and needs. Do we want to consider substance abuse and unmet need at the start of the study? Within a certain time frame of the study (i.e., within 3 months of enrollment)? At the moment of the assessment? Do we want to allow these variables to change over time with the status of the participant (also known as time-dependent covariates)? All of this must be clearly specified—operationalized—in order for the definitions to be systematically applied to all participants by all research staff. Otherwise, the study will be conducted differently depending on the participant, the day, and the mood of the research staff! When we consider eligibility criteria for the study, this is especially important. If we had an exclusion for current injection drug users but would allow former injection drug users, provided they had not used drugs within the past year, then this would be a very different research population than one that would exclude anyone who had *ever* injected drugs.

How might these be operationalized?

- Substance abuse (independent variable)
  - History of ever using illegal drugs as assessed by study-specific drug inventory at baseline
  - Current (within 3 months of study enrollment) use of illegal drugs as assessed by study-specific drug inventory at baseline
  - Current (within 3 months of study enrollment) use of any substance as assessed by study-specific drug inventory at baseline, including tobacco, cigarettes, and prescription medications
  - Failure to maintain a drug-free time for three or more weeks as determined by substance abuse counselor
- Unmet needs
  - Self-report unmet needs at baseline in any one of the following domains using a specific instrument:
    - Activities of daily living
    - Social support
    - Family support
    - Health care provision
  - An index of 10 or greater on an acuity scale
  - Having lived in a homeless shelter, been in a transient living situation, had a hospitalization, or engaged in survival sex or commercial sex work at any time during the previous 12 weeks
  - Answering a question at baseline—"Do you have any needs that are not currently being met by your ancillary service care program at this time?"—as "yes" or "maybe"
- Immunocompromise
  - Having a CD4 cell count < 200 at baseline
  - Having a CD4 cell count < 350 at baseline
  - Having a drop in CD4 count of 100 or greater between any two visits of more than 12 weeks apart

○ Having or developing an AIDS-defining diagnosis over the duration of the study follow-up period

As these questions are answered and the protocol is being developed, it is helpful to describe this information in a concise table (see Table 6-1). The research question matrix is the answer to the problem of keeping all information regarding the study straight.

A TOOL TO HELP KEEP YOUR STUDY DESIGN IN ORDER: THE RESEARCH QUESTION MATRIX

This matrix may be modified as needed to incorporate the study's specific intention, research questions, hypotheses, and variables. For research, it is usually difficult to change any factors in the research design once the protocol is written and the project has been set up. In this case, the research question matrix serves as an actual roadmap. To be sure that you are on the right track and that you do not forget to measure anything, a research question matrix works to keep all of your research questions, exposures, and outcomes in order. On the other hand, in evaluation research, there is some fluidity in the research question matrix because evaluation is meant to inform the overall program in a feedback loop fashion. Once more

study planning has taken place, a data analysis plan, for example, or a quality assurance plan may be incorporated into this table for easy and ready reference.

From this overall structure, many steps can then be taken. The protocol can be written with the input of a multidisciplinary team. In the case of a drug study, a multidisciplinary panel might contain a physician, a nurse, a social worker (who is experienced in adherence to treatment), a psychiatrist, a clinical trials specialist, a biostatistician, a pharmacist, a pharmacologist, and more. Together this group of experts develops the protocol, which is then provided (in the case of a multicentered research group) to the governing bodies of the agency or study coordinating center. If it is a local study, then this information is given to several bodies to review. In some cases, it may go to a community advisory board (CAB) for review and input during development. At all facilities, it will go to an institutional review board (IRB) where the protocol will be reviewed to ensure safety for all participants as well as protection for the institution that is conducting the study.

Once approved by the IRB and any other committees that govern the local conduct of research, the study may be implemented. In the case of an experimental study, issues in implementation of the study should be completely developed and the study's implementation plan completely worked out. Nothing should be left to chance or "playing by ear." All planning should be done prior to the study being rolled out. A work plan should be constructed, which describes all elements of patient and data flow, with every aspect of the study considered fully and completely—from inclusion and exclusion criteria to data collection and quality assurance to data analysis. The steps should be clearly laid out and then systematically undertaken (see Table 6-2). Thinking through continuity of patient care and of research, and anticipating consequences of the research in advance reduces the number of problems that will occur.

After the entire protocol is mapped out on paper, multiple pilot exercises should be conducted, so that the protocol

TABLE 6-1 The Research Question Matrix

Research question	Dependent variable (outcome)	Independent variable(s)	Potential confounders	Potential effect modifiers
Is HAART treatment associated with decreased HIV viral load?	HIV viral load (RNA copies/mL by Roche assay < 400 copies/mL) within three months of treatment start	Treatment (non-HAART standard of care vs. HAART)	• Gender • Age • Adherence to study treatment	• Concomitant medications • CD4 count • Co-morbidities
Is HAART treatment associated with decreased HIV viral load?	HIV viral load (RNA copies/mL by Roche assay < 400 copies/mL) within three months of treatment start	Treatment (non-HAART standard of care vs. HAART)	• Gender • Age • Adherence to study treatment	• Concomitant medications • CD4 count • Co-morbidities

Organizing all of your research questions, variables, and potential confounders and effect modifiers is useful in being sure that your study is able to answer all of its intended research questions and address its hypotheses.

Source: Author

TABLE 6-2 Steps in Preparing a Study

Literature review

Development of specific and measurable research questions, null, and alternative hypotheses

Development of research question matrix

Development of protocol with multidisciplinary team of investigators (multiple iterations)

Meet with community to discuss and ensure community- and cultural-appropriateness of study

Creation/adaptation of instrumentation

Pre-testing/piloting of instrumentation and study protocols

Development of quality assurance plan

Submission to institutional review boards and relevant organizational, local, state, or federal bodies for approval

Training of field staff

Study implementation

Ongoing data and study quality assurance measures

Assessment of fidelity to intervention (if applicable)

Data cleaning

Data management

Data analysis

Interpretation

Public health action as needed

Dissemination

Recommendations for future study

them. (This should not be the entirety of their training, of course, but should take place after the training and before going live with the study.) Instrumentation such as surveys and questionnaires should be practiced, too. Once the study procedures have been piloted to the point of being efficient and smooth, it may be useful to consult peer educators or CAB members to identify suitable consumers who can offer insight into a real participant experience; any issues that arise may then be addressed prior to study implementation. Supervision, training, and ongoing quality assurance are also important. This process will assure that the investigators know exactly how the study will be executed. Though painstaking, this process is crucial to systematic and high quality data collection and, in the case of any study that requires multiple visits from participants, increases follow-up and participation rates.

The steps leading to the study's development are many, but done up front, the work is worthwhile and reduces the burden of work later on, when the study begins. Once the front work is completed—the literature review based on the research question, creation of H_0 and H_A, operationalization of variables and how to measure the independent and dependent variables of interest, creation of a data analysis plan, submission to requisite committees, and trial runs and pilot exercises—the study may be implemented. In the following chapters, details of each of the study designs will be provided in more detail, giving a basic understanding of the steps required in conducting each design. When involved in research in the field, there will always be manuals detailing specifics of how to conduct the study—often called field or operations manuals. These augment the detail found in the protocol and are the rules and regulations for how the study must be conducted. They not only ensure consistency from site to site, but also make the field personnel's lives simpler, by allowing them to follow a "recipe" for conduct of the study.

transfers from the academic realm into the practical realm. These pilot exercises should run through all parts of the study using role-playing to ensure that the procedures are all smooth and that the staff is trained and well acquainted with all of

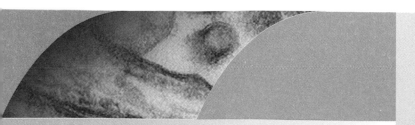

Discussion Questions

1. Identify a research question you are interested in regarding a specific infectious organism. Create the appropriate null and alternative hypotheses for this research question.

2. Create a research question matrix to accompany your research questions.

3. Imagine you were going to conduct this study. What types of multidisciplinary investigators would you want to work with you to help inform your study? What community members would be important to talk with and gain input from prior to beginning your study?

REFERENCES

1. Centers for Disease Control. Preliminary report: foodborne outbreak of *Escherichia coli* O157:H7 infections from hamburgers—western United States, 1993. *MMWR*. 1993;42:85–86.

2. Centers for Disease Control. Update: multistate outbreak of *Escherichia coli* O157:H7 infections from hamburgers—western United States, 1992–1993. *MMWR*. 1993;42(14):258–263.

3. Centers for Disease Control. Summary of notifiable diseases—United States, 2004. June 16, 2006. *MMWR*. 2004;53(53):1–80.

4. Devasia RA, Jones TF, Ward J, et al. Endemically acquired foodborne outbreak of enterotoxin-producing *Escherichia coli* serotype O169:H41. *Am J Med*. 2006;119:168.e7–168.e10.

5. Heymann DL. *Control of Communicable Diseases*. 18th edition. Washington, DC: American Public Health Association.

6. Nelson K. *Infectious Disease Epidemiology*. Gaithersburg, MD: Aspen.

CHAPTER 7

Experimental Designs as a Foundation for Observational Studies

EXPERIMENTAL DESIGNS IN BROAD STROKES

Experimental studies are designs in which the investigator decides which participants get which exposures and which are essential epidemiologic designs used to compare two or more conditions. They can test drugs, medical devices, interventions, social marketing campaigns—really, just about anything. In a nutshell, these designs allow the investigator to randomly assign individuals or communities to a condition and follow them to see what outcomes of interest occur. By doing this, instead of all our individual characteristics influencing our decisions and healthcare (or other) outcomes, a randomly assigned external factor does. This allows us to see the effect of the treatment condition under study alone, controlling for the many factors that make us do what we do and behave the way we behave. By doing this, we level the playing field for all persons or units under study.

Countless texts are available to teach you how to understand, conduct, and analyze clinical trials. Experimental designs are generally not the most commonly used methods within infectious disease epidemiology, where they are prima-

rily used in the development of drugs to treat infectious diseases, or interventions to change behavior by which infectious diseases are transmitted. Still, they are an essential step in grounding an understanding of other infectious disease epidemiologic methodologies. They set the stage for a greater understanding of the importance of methods in the study of infectious diseases that we have already used and those we will soon encounter. The purpose of this chapter is to describe randomized controlled designs so that we can refer to them in the coming chapters as a foundation for observational studies.

Let us think in broad strokes for a while. In this chapter we will jump to some conclusions that in real life—and particularly in real science—we would never jump to. In some cases, I will present the most extreme cases so that we can identify some basic principles and think things through in a vivid fashion. This will help us begin to be more comfortable with how the methodologic considerations will play a role in what we find and what it means. Note that the following scenario is simplified for the purpose of explanation.

Imagine this: You are working with a team to assess the efficacy of a new medication for HIV, an antiretroviral drug. The design is as follows: HIV-infected individuals are asked whether they want to try a new medication. If they accept, they are offered it and are followed at the HIV clinic every month; if they decline, they continue on their standard medication regimen or are offered another Food and Drug Administration (FDA)–approved drug and are followed per U.S. Public Health Service guidelines at the HIV clinic. Patients come into clinic appointments about every 3 months for follow up depending on their treatment regimen, co-morbidities, and immune status. In this example, the patients are asked what they want to take from a selection of regimens proposed by their provider based upon the patient's medical status. They are then given this prescription. Of the 500 people at your local primary HIV clinic whom you have asked to be involved in the study, we are going to think about just two. Remember, these are broad strokes to highlight the principles of randomized controlled trials; these are clearly exaggerations and hypotheticals to help imagine the individuals as people, in order to understand what their data really mean. Otherwise, it is easy—too easy—to allow the numbers that emerge from the data to take the place of the real person in one's understanding and interpretation of them. Always remember: Data should describe people; People cannot be forced to conform to data.

First, imagine the participant who requested the investigational medication. What is he like? He might be more educated than others at the clinic (for example, he may be aware of the increased potential many investigational drugs have to reduce HIV viral load, and he has read up on the drug in the literature and previous studies). He might be wealthier (for example, he might have sufficient resources such that coming to the clinic monthly and missing a day of work each time in addition to the cost of the visit is not problematic). He might have a car so that transportation is not a concern. He might be sicker than others, making him more willing to take chances on a new medication. He might be more likely than others to take the treatment on time and adhere to all of the food-related restrictions. Remember, these are certainly not "truths" about what people are like; they are imagined descriptions as we work toward a greater understanding of the myriad factors influencing any given person's actions and behavior.

Now let us imagine the participant who requested a currently FDA-approved medication. What is she like? Perhaps she is more likely to be a woman, because she may wish to become pregnant in the near future and knows her current regimen is safe for the fetus. She may not wish to come in for monthly visits because she has a new job and cannot request the time off, or she has no transportation to attend the visits. She may be healthier and does not feel she needs a new medicine. She may not be educated on the risks of the drug or fully understand clinical trials, so she may be concerned about the risks and unaware of potential benefits. She may be nonadherent to her current treatment regimen, so her medical provider may not fully and openly offer the investigational new drug due to concern about her not being adherent.

By the same token, these profiles could be completely reversed. The person who opts for the study treatment might be a female who is on public assistance and is unemployed, who can come to the clinic as often as she wants. She might be uneducated on the effects of the new drug and healthy at the moment but game to try it because she does not like to take her current medicine. She may have learned about the trials and believe the new medication offers her a better chance to stay healthy. The person who opts for the control might be affluent and educated, but fully employed at an all-consuming job, unable to take time off work. He might be so busy that adherence is difficult.

Can you imagine these descriptions? Can you imagine the people behind them? Each person will have a completely unique reason, or set of reasons, for deciding or not deciding to take the new medication. When individual choice enters the equation, there are infinite individual-level characteristics associated with the outcome of taking the medicine. Recognizing that there are no random reasons that people do what they do is an essential step toward understanding the need for randomized controlled trials.

The point is, how people behave cannot be divorced from who they are. If what people did were divorced from their underlying characteristics and behavior could be truly random, this study could work: People would assign themselves the drugs randomly. But in fact, that is not possible. Each person's characteristics influence what they decide to do. And worse, they influence how they report what they did, and how they actually end up doing with regard to the outcomes under study. For example, with the first scenario, the male who selected the investigational new drug, how do you think he would do health-wise, with regard to HIV-related indicators (e.g., lower viral load, higher CD4 count)? Irrespective of the medication selected, he might be more likely to do better than his counterpart. That would not be due to the new medication, but just due to the factors that make him himself. In each of these imagined scenarios, one can imagine in which direction their health indices might go—and all without knowing anything about the treatment under study.

So one of the most important things to do in evaluating a treatment is to remove the effects of the individual under study from the equation and make it possible to assess *only* the treatment of interest. Because people are not the same, because behavior is never random, the best thing to do is make assignment of the treatment random. This is one of the most important reasons for a randomized controlled trial: to remove individual-level factors that can drive with "self-selection" of exposures or treatments.[a]

---

[a]When we say "self-selection," it rarely implies that the subject actually selected the condition him- or herself in an open, blatant fashion. This phrase is used to differentiate it from situations in which chance or an investigator assigns treatment. When we think of self-selection, it generally means that there are forces in a person, in every person, that are interrelated. For example, a higher level of education is often associated with a higher income and a greater likelihood of having steady employment. That a person has these two latter conditions is thus a function of having had a good education. In this sense, this person did not just "turn up" at the higher paying job; he or she self-selected it by virtue of other conditions (e.g., education, family) he or she had. Again, this does not mean that he or she chose it consciously but that there are interrelated factors that everyone has that push them in one direction or another.

STEPS IN A RANDOMIZED CONTROLLED TRIAL

Now let us see how the study could be performed using an experimental approach. There are 500 people at the clinic who consented to participate in the study and were found eligible to be enrolled. In broad strokes, this is how the study might proceed:

- All eligible participants are told of the procedures, risks, benefits, and alternatives to treatment and have signed an institutional review board (IRB)–approved informed-consent form. The participants, providers, study sponsors, and the local IRB will not know which treatment, the new one or the standard of care, is better. This allows everyone to maintain equipoise[b] such that no one has knowledge or conviction that one of the treatment arms is "better" in any way. In this double-blind study, neither the participants nor any of the provider staff is aware of the treatment arm the participant is in. This study would not be ethical without equipoise, as it would mean that some participants are knowingly getting an inferior treatment. Only the research pharmacist who blinds all medications is aware of the status. This blinding means that no one's expectations or biases can come into play with regard to discussion of treatment, experience of side effects, or reporting; all effects, good and bad alike, are reported similarly, irrespective of the treatment arm.
- Following provision of consent, an extensive baseline assessment is conducted. This includes a physical exam, laboratory studies (e.g., blood tests) to confirm that the patient is healthy enough to be in the study, and collection of baseline values of HIV-related health status, such as CD4, viral load, HIV genotype, and so forth.
- The patient is then randomized into the study. Study staff use a computer program that assigns patients to one of two treatment arms:
  - the new drug plus one currently FDA-approved antiretroviral or
  - the standard of care (the control), an FDA-approved antiretroviral selected by the participant's medical provider from a list of those that can be given concomitantly.

Nothing but random assignment decides what the participant receives: not the participant, not the provider, not the nurse, not the circumstances—only chance.

- All participants are then followed forward in time every month to see if the outcomes of interest (for this study, increased CD4 count and decreased viral load) take place the same or differently depending on the treatment assigned. The safety of both drugs also is observed; safety for this study is measured by incidence of side effects and adverse events.
- At the end of 2 years, the two groups are compared. There are several different outcome options: the drugs are the same, or one drug outperforms another with regard to efficacy and/or safety. If found to be safe and effective, the new drug would continue on its journey towards FDA approval and, ultimately and hopefully, improve the health of HIV-infected persons.

Why can we say that the drug worked and not simply that the people who took the drug were more likely to improve than those who did not? Because the decision to take a given treatment was not due to individual participant-level characteristics, but instead to chance. It is not that the sicker, healthier, more or less adherent, richer or poorer participants differentially received a specific treatment: All participants had the same chance of receiving both treatments, and chance alone decided. When we look at our data before the participants received the treatments, the groups were not statistically different from one another: The only thing that might make the groups differ is chance, and in this example, they did not differ at baseline.

Here is an example of some real data from a randomized trial to assess the efficacy of a vaccine against human papilloma virus (HPV) in the prevention of persistent HPV-16 infection, which is a leading etiology of cervical cancer. When the subjects were randomized to receive either the placebo or the experimental treatment, there were no differences between the two groups, as you can see from Figure 7-1. After the participants received the treatments, however, you can see an obvious difference in Figure 7-2: There were no cases of HPV-16 in the treated group, but there were in the placebo group. Because we know that the groups were assigned purely due to chance—not because they were sicker, more or less sexually active, or chose to have the treatment—we can be sure that any difference we see at the end is due to the treatment, not due to a participant or other characteristic.

We can attribute all differences in the outcomes of interest to the drugs utilized and not to anything else because the key difference between the groups was the randomly assigned treatment. Assuming every effort was made to promote retention and adherence in both arms, and there were no systematic

---

[b]Equipoise is a basic tenet of ethical research conduct. In order for a study to be ethical, the conditions being compared must be felt to be on par with one another such that no one condition is relatively advantageous/disadvantageous compared with the others. This makes intuitive sense: In a trial of antibiotics for bacterial meningitis, it would not be ethical to compare a new broad-spectrum antibiotic with a placebo, when it is known that the placebo not only is not effective, but also puts the participant in danger. In addition to this being a violation of research subject rights, it also makes it difficult for providers to become engaged in a study. They will not want their patients to participate if they know (or feel) that one treatment is worse than the others.[1]

FIGURE 7-1 Baseline characteristics of women in the Phase III placebo-crontrolled study of the HPV vaccine

Characteristic	HPV-16 Vaccine (N=768)	Placebo (N=765)	Total (N=1533)
Age — year Mean ±SD	20.0 ± 1.63	20.0 ± 1.61	20.0 ± .62
Range	16–25*	16–23	16–25*
Race or ethnic group—no. (%)			
White	601 (78.3)	561 (73.3)	1162 (75.8)
Black	41 (5.3)	63 (8.2)	104 (6.8)
Hispanic	56 (7.3)	66 (8.6)	122 (8.0)
Asian	49 (6.4)	46 (6.0)	95 (6.2)
Other	21 (2.7)	29 (3.8)	50 (3.3
Current smoker—no. (%)	183 (23.8)	190 (24.8)	373 (24.3)
Lifetime no. of sex partners—no. (%)			
0	38 (4.9)	34 (4.4)	72 (4.7)
1	218 (28.4)	200 (26.1)	418 (27.3)
2	173 (22.5)	173 (22.6)	346 (22.6)
3	138 (18.0)	131 (17.1)	269 (17.5)
4	105 (13.7)	144 (18.8)	249 (16.2)
5	96 (12.5)	83 (10.8)	179 (11.7)
Thin-layer Papanicolaou test results on day 0—no. (%)			
Normal	666 (86.7)	656 (85.8)	1322 (86.2)
Abnormal†	84 (10.9)	96 (12.5)	180 (11.7)
ASCUS or AGUS‡	47 (6.1)	58 (7.6)	105 (6.8)
LSIL	35 (4.6)	34 (4.4)	69 (4.5)
HSIL	2 (0.3)	4 (0.5)	6 (0.4)
Unsatisfactory	18 (2.3)	13 (1.7)	31 (2.0)

*At the time the data were audited, it was found that one woman was 24 years of age, and two women were 25 years of age.

†ASCUS denotes atypical squamous cells of undetermined significance, AGUS atypical glandular cells of unknown significance, LSIL low-grade squamous intraepithelial lesion, and HSIL high-grade squamous intraepithelial lesion.

‡Only one woman had atypical glandular cells of unknown significance on her day 0 Papanicolaou test. To prevent the unblinding of this woman's treatment allocation, she was grouped with the women who had atypical squamous cells of undetermined significance.

This figure indicates that there is no significant difference between women in the placebo or the HPV-16 vaccine group at baseline. The randomization "worked," and there was random allocation to the two groups with no resulting statistical differences between them with regard to knowable and measurable characteristics (and likely unknowable and immeasurable as well). Sometimes, in the case of small sample sizes, there will be random assignment that does not evenly distribute the sample characteristics between the treatment arms. Statistical expertise is needed in this case to weight or adjust the findings appropriately. This can occur in cases of larger sample size as well—we are, of course, dealing with random events so this could happen—but is less likely.

Source: Koutsky LA, Ault KA, Wheeler C et al. A controlled trial of human papilloma virus type 16 vaccine. NEJM 2002;347:1645–51, with permission.

differences in the way participants were followed up with for outcomes, documented, or treated, our design does something important: We can have confidence that one thing that was different between the groups and controlled in that way—the treatment arm—is the thing responsible for any differences in the outcomes that are found. We do not have to worry that the healthier people took the medicine, and that is why they got better. Or that the sicker people got the standard of care and that is why they did not. The treatment was assigned by chance and so we can remove the effects of everything else.

For us to truly have confidence in our findings, however, we must analyze the data in a way that maintains the initial randomization. This is essential to our thesis here. This method is called intention to treat analysis, and it means that even if some participants stop taking the treatment to which they were assigned, we still analyze them in the arm to which they were randomized. If we analyze our data in this fashion, we will always underestimate the effect of the treatment and make the effect of the treatment look less than it actually is. (This is also known as a bias towards the null.) If we do not do this, and we instead analyze data as if the participants took the treatment they *chose themselves*, as in the non-random example at the HIV clinic where participants were able to select their own treatment, we obviate the purpose of randomizing—just what we did before by letting people choose their exposures. Use of intention to treat analysis ensures that we evaluate outcomes on all participants in association with the treatment under study, and that the effects of other predictors do not obscure the treatment effects we are trying to study.

We have randomized exposure and followed up on each participant's outcomes so that we can clearly see the effects of one exposure—beautiful, elegant, easy to understand. We carefully assigned people to a given treatment such that individual behavior and characteristics are divorced from treatment exposure, and we isolated the effect of the treatment. This enables us to have a clear understanding of the treatment effects—not the people effects. Instead of seeing a blurry picture when individuals select their own treatments, we see the effect of the treatment alone. Finally, we use intention to treat analysis so that the randomly assigned treatments were maintained throughout (randomization through analysis), and at no time did individual behaviors or characteristics obscure the view of the effects of treatment.

FIGURE 7-2 Efficacy analyses from a Phase III placebo-controlled study of the HPV vaccine

Type of Analysis	End Point	HPV-16 Vaccine				Placebo				Observed Efficacy (95% CI)*	P Value
		No. of Women	Cases of Infection	Women-Yr at Risk	Infection Rate per 100 Women-Yr at Risk %	No of Women	Cases of Infection	Women-Yr at Risk	Infection Rate per 100 Women-Yr at Risk %		
Primary per protocol efficacy analysis†	Persistent HPV-16 infection	768	0	1084.0	0	765	41	1076.9	3.8	100 (90–100)	<0.001
Efficacy analysis including women with general protocol violations‡	Persistent HPV-16 infection	800	0	1128.0	0	793	42	1109.7	3.8	100 (90–100)	—§
Secondary per-protocol efficacy analysis†	Transient or persistent HPV-16 infection	768	6	1084.0	0.6	765	68	1076.9	6.3	91.2 (80–97)	—§

*CI denotes confidence interval.

†The per-protocol population included women who received the full regimen of study vaccine and who were seronegative for HPV-16 and negative for HPV-16 DNA on day 0 and negative for HPV-16 DNA at month 7 and in any biopsy specimens obtained between day 0 and month 7; who did not engage in sexual intercourse within 48 hours before the day 0 or month 7 visit; who did not receive any nonstudy vaccine within specified time limits relative to vaccination; who did not receive courses of certain oral or parenteral immunosuppressive agents, immune globulin, or blood products; who were not enrolled in another study of an investigational agent; and who had a month 7 visit within the range considered acceptable for determining the month 7 HPV-16 status.

‡The population includes women who received the full regimen of study vaccine and who were seronegative for HPV-16 and negative for HPV-16 DNA on day 0 and negative for HPV-16 DNA at month 7 and in any biopsy specimens obtained between day 0 and month 7.

§P values were calculated only for the analysis addressing the primary hypothesis.

This figure indicates that there is a significiant association between receipt of the vaccine and having no HPV-16 infection. This is a criticial finding that has led to the recommendation of this vaccine in girls and, perhaps in the future, one day to boys as well. This vaccine has the potential to drastically reduce the morbidity and mortality due to cervical cancer, the chief cause of which is HPV.

Source: Koutsky LA, Ault KA, Wheeler C et al. A controlled trial of human papilloma virus type 16 vaccine. *NEJM* 2002;347:1645–51, with permission.

As mentioned earlier, randomization can be performed not only on the individual level as in the previous examples, but also on the level of communities, clinics, regions, schools, hospitals, or any unit of analysis that one wishes to study. The nuances become statistical and logistical in nature, but their conceptual simplicity remains the same as when individuals are randomized.[c] Although we typically think of randomized controlled trials in the context of drugs and the drug approval process, this methodology is used in a variety of settings. These include comparison of medical devices, behavioral interventions, social marketing media, ancillary services, nursing or provider practices, complementary medicine, and more. We can also assess any number of interventions in the context of group-level randomization and outcomes, clustered randomization with individual outcomes , and other designs specific to the research question under study.

---

[c]Some complications stem primarily from limitations in sample size and types of analytic methods required. Even if one has thousands or even millions of people in a study, it is the unit of analysis—the level on which the individuals are randomized—that counts. For example, imagine you are conducting a randomized controlled trial of a new infection control procedure. The study compares traditional hand-washing methods versus installation of antiseptic hand sanitizer wall mounts at 30 hospitals. Although the 30 hospitals serve over 4,000 patients in total and have hundreds of provider staff, the sample size that you will use is actually only 30. Statistical methods will be used to adjust for the clustering of the hospitals and other factors, but in the end, the sample size is not as great as it would seem on the surface. In addition, with multiple facilities or areas, the logistical issues are very different than when conducting studies on the individual level. Especially with studies that involve an intervention, study implementation and data collection must be identical from place to place to ensure that the intervention can be correctly analyzed.

Group Randomized Trials of Interventions Other Than Drugs

Malaria is a chief cause of death throughout the world, with highly endemic areas including Africa, the Southwest Pacific, parts of South America, Southeast Asia, and parts of India. The parasite, carried by mosquitoes, is responsible for over 1 million deaths each year.[2–4] Four types of malaria are found in humans: *Plasmodium falciparum, P. vivax, P. ovale*, and *P. malariae*. Of these, *P. falciparum* poses the most severe risk of morbidity and mortality. Mosquitoes are the vector responsible for malaria transmission, although it may also be spread via contaminated needles (either medically related or for illicit drug use). In areas where chloroquinine-resistant strains are widespread, methods for reduction of infectious mosquitoes and transmission are sorely needed.[3,4]

New methods to reduce exposure to infectious mosquitoes and acquisition of disease are being identified and include new drugs, insecticides new and old (e.g., DDT), and insecticide-treated bed nets[3]. One prevention—bed nets, impregnated with the insecticide permethrin—was assessed for efficacy in reducing malaria infections in Kenya. The study was performed among a cohort of 833 children that was followed from birth to 2 years. The study was conducted within a community-based group randomized controlled trial, which randomized village clusters (and the villages in the clusters, and the households in each village) to receive the permethrin-treated bed nets or not (the standard of care). Twice annually, the bed nets were retreated with the chemical to maintain effective doses. After the intervention part of the study was completed, control villages were also supplied with the nets.

Although the unit of randomization was the village, the unit of analysis was individual-level data in the form of each child's ultimate infection status. Outcomes of interest included incidence of morbidity determined at follow-up clinical visits; time to the first malaria event; and an important and unique measure called the force of infection (also known as instantaneous attack rates). This measure takes into account that in any given time interval, the subject could have cleared and acquired a new infection; usual morbidity rates do not take this into account, thus underestimating the true incidence rates.[3] Demographic, clinical, and behavioral information on village, household, family, and child were ascertained in addition to laboratory specimens. The data were analyzed using methods that account for the correlated nature of the villages.[d] The intervention was found to significantly reduce

continues

---

[d]The authors indicate that they used SUDAAN release 8 (Research Triangle Institute, Research Triangle Park, NC), Stata Version 7 (Stata Corporation, College Station, TX), and SAS 8.2 (SAS Institute, Cary, NC), all statistical programming packages that can take into account the randomized clustered nature of the design. They used a repeated measures approach in SAS, with compound symmetry covariance structure to account for the intravillage correlation—the clustering—that occurred. Although this is beyond the scope of the text, there are several basic things to think about in this sort of design: the households are clustered within the villages, and the people within the households. Statistical techniques can be used to adjust for the fact that there are fewer within-village, within-household differences than between-villages, between-households. This has an impact on the overall variance, and the resulting estimates can be biased in the event these are not taken into account. Sample size calculations in clustered designs are especially important because the overriding sample size calculation depends upon the clusters and their size, not just the individuals. For example, in this study there were 833 participants but only 19 village clusters that received the randomization.

Group Randomized Trials of Interventions Other Than Drugs—continues

the force of infection among the children, reduce time to first infection, decrease incidence of symptomatic malaria, and improve nutritional outcomes among exposed children. Importantly, the fear that a reduction in maternal exposure to malaria during pregnancy could result in worsened infection (as a result of an unknown mechanism that could, conceivably, confer protection from the parasite with exposure during gestation) was not realized. There was no evidence that this intervention was associated with worsened outcomes, making this a safe and effective potential addition to the armamentarium against malaria. This is a useful study for evaluating group randomization methods.

The current accepted means of communicating results from a randomized controlled trial involves a flowchart schema that is very helpful for viewing what took place during the study's implementation as far as recruitment, enrollment, follow-up, and analysis. This enables one to tell at a glance what was done, and even see potential biases that may be there (e.g., intention to treat analysis, proportion of loss to follow-up). Figure 7-3 shows the schema from the aforementioned study; Figure 7-4 shows the mosquito responsible for spreading many infectious diseases.

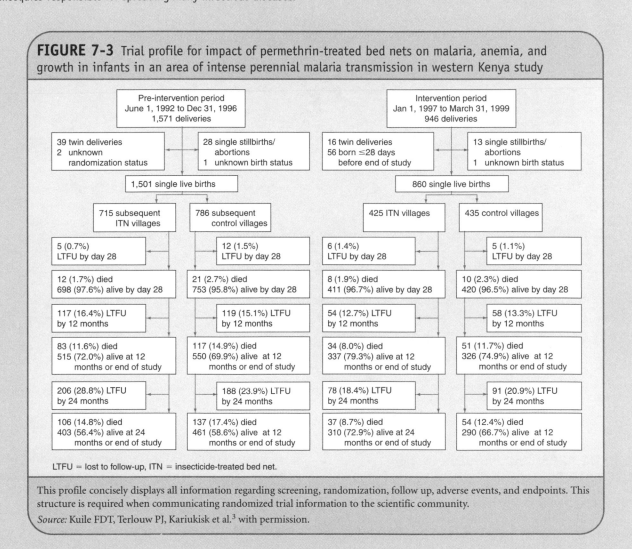

FIGURE 7-3 Trial profile for impact of permethrin-treated bed nets on malaria, anemia, and growth in infants in an area of intense perennial malaria transmission in western Kenya study

LTFU = lost to follow-up, ITN = insecticide-treated bed net.

This profile concisely displays all information regarding screening, randomization, follow up, adverse events, and endpoints. This structure is required when communicating randomized trial information to the scientific community.

Source: Kuile FDT, Terlouw PJ, Kariukisk et al.[3] with permission.

continued

Group Randomized Trials of Interventions Other Than Drugs—continued

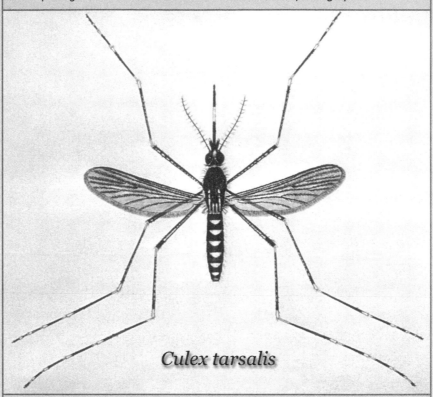

FIGURE 7-4 Female *Aedes aegypti* mosquito while she was in the process of acquiring a blood meal from her human host, the photographer

Culex tarsalis

Mosquitoes are a vector responsible for the transmission of many infectious diseases. This particular species is associated with transmission of Dengue Hemorrhagic fever, among other illnesses. Malaria is most commonly transmitted by the *Anopheles* mosquito that tends to feed at night.[2–4]

Source: CDC/ Prof. Frank Hadley Collins, Dir., Cntr. for Global Health and Infectious Diseases, Univ. of Notre Dame James Gathany Public Health Image Library, 2006.

THE DRUG APPROVAL PROCESS IN THE UNITED STATES

In the United States the government agency responsible for the approval of drugs and devices is the Food and Drug Administration. Until relatively recently, the FDA approval process that was required in order to license drugs and devices did not require randomized controlled studies to substantiate their efficacy. Legislation initiated the requirement that all drugs seeking approval and licensure need to have undergone a randomized controlled trial and meet other strict requirements for clinical evaluation. What emerged was a system of study phases that has been created to describe the approval process. In brief, this approval process (as applied to drugs here) has four phases:

- *Consent form:* Prior to any involvement in any research study, the participant will sign an IRB-approved informed consent form and be properly consented. Informed consent is more than just "signing a form"; it is a full understanding of all protocol procedures, risks, and benefits. All universities or agencies conducting research must comply with the complex and important IRB regulations that are intended to protect the rights of the participant as well as clarify the institution's role and responsibilities in the research from a legal standpoint. For animal studies, there is generally a parallel board overseeing the appropriate and ethical treatment of animals.

• *Preclinical phase:* Studies in this phase usually begin in laboratories with *in vitro* techniques and then move on to animal models. At the end of this phase, an appropriate animal model is generally identified; that is, one that is the most applicable to humans for the drug/host/ disease combination under study. This phase will usually identify a maximally tolerated dose (MTD) within the animal model, and give a hint as to what types of side effects should be monitored in subsequent studies.

• *Phase I:* Studies in this phase provide early data in a small number of participants, suggesting how well the drug will be tolerated. Phase I is intended to assess safety and tolerance of the drug under study. In general, participants in Phase I studies are either healthy volunteers or those who have tried every other available treatment and have few treatment options left. Phase I designs have several basic strategies, including the following:
  ○ *MTD:* To see how much of the drug can be given to humans before reaching unacceptable levels of toxicity
  ○ *Dose escalation strategies:* To establish pharmacokinetics and pharmacodynamics of the drug (how drugs are metabolized and circulated throughout the body)

• *Phase II:* Studies in this phase utilize all the information gained in the preclinical phase and Phase I studies. Although the correct dose of the drug under study may not have been determined precisely in the Phase I study (it sometimes can be narrowed down but not established exactly), it will be by the end of the Phase II study. In this phase, the assessment of rates of adverse events and side effects begins to be made, and level of potential biologic activity starts to be identified. Relatively few people are included, however, and many side effects and adverse events may not be observed, simply because they are so rare. This phase, like the two preceding it, is generally not randomized. There are many approaches to Phase II designs, some of which utilize a semi-randomized structure, or a two-part structure with nonrandom assignment for the first part and random assignment for the second.

• *Phase III:* Phase III studies assess the ability of the drug to do what it is intended to do. In general, for drugs that are undergoing an FDA-approval process, these will be

double-blinded, placebo-controlled randomized controlled designs, but the design depends on the available information, resources, research questions, and ethical construction of the trial. There are multiple variations on this theme, but—in its most basic framework— individuals are randomly assigned, like flipping a coin (though generally performed using a random number table or a computer program), to a treatment arm, either the drug under study or a placebo. In some cases the placebo may actually be a "sugar pill," something that has all the physical attributes of the study drug but is inactive. In other cases, where a treatment exists that works for the condition under study, the standard of care is the comparator. Prior to enrollment of the subject, he or she is assessed for eligibility to be sure it will be safe for them to participate in the study and that they meet criteria that will enable the analysts to later identify how well the drug worked. If the participant is eligible and has provided consent, the participant is enrolled in the study and randomly assigned to one of the treatment conditions: the study drug or the comparator. The individual is then followed by the research or clinical staff at regular intervals, and assessed for safety and tolerance of the drug, adverse events, side effects, and the outcomes of interest. Outcomes and endpoints are decided upon in advance. They are necessary to drive the study and determine, in a systematic manner, whether the treatment under study "worked." (For example, in testing of a new prophylaxis for PCP pneumonia, the endpoint could be development of PCP, need to switch to an alternate prophylactic regimen, or an adverse event.) Once they reach an endpoint specified by the protocol that directs the study, they either are taken off the drug, are given other treatment options, continue to be seen for follow-up, or are discontinued, as specified by the protocol. Data are analyzed by intention to treat analysis, as discussed above, and an estimate of the effectiveness of the drug is calculated.

Three types of blinding can be used:

• *Unblinded:* The providers, staff, and participant know what treatment the participant is being given. Unblinded studies are common in Phase I trials for assessment of safety and tolerance. Such studies are generally small and involve assessment of characteristics that are unlikely to be biased or biasing. For example, in a Phase I study of the pharmacokinetics of a new antibiotic, blood might be repeatedly taken at specific time points following drug administration. These samples will then be analyzed to assess the dose and the rate at which the drug is metabolized. Knowledge of which drug one is on is unlikely to influence the analysis of the specimens, or interpretation of the data. In addition, in cases of exploration of new treatments, exposure to fewer people reduces the occurrence of unknown risks that may emerge from the treatment. A blinded study would involve—and put at risk—more individuals than is required, resulting in an unethical study. Unblinded studies are also used in trials of behavioral interventions. The provider knows which intervention to provide to the participant and the participant may as well. In such cases, often the outcomes of interest are assessed by persons who are blinded to the status of the participant. For example, in a randomized trial of a group-level intervention to improve condom negotiation skills, the provider and the participant both may know to which group—program X vs. program Y—the participant was randomized. Imagine if the outcome of interest were assessment of condom negotiation skills in a role-playing situation, in addition to self-report of condom use at last sexual encounter. Though difficult to blind to the treatment assignment, one can blind the assessment of the outcome. For example, the role-playing outcome could be conducted by individuals who are unaware of the treatment assignment of each participant, and are thus less likely to be swayed or biased—consciously or subconsciously—towards assessing participant skills in one or another direction. Compare this to the participant's self-report of condom use at last sex: Which is more likely to be biased based on knowledge of treatment status? Likely the latter. Because it is not possible to blind the participant to treatment condition, knowledge of the treatment assignment may influence his or her responses to the question, which gathers the outcomes data. This is why blinding the person judging the outcome, where possible, can be extremely helpful in reducing bias that can result from an unblinded study.

- *Single-blinded:* The providers and staff know what treatment is being given but the participant does not. Single-blinded studies are often used in cases where it is not feasible or practical for the providers to be blinded. For example, in a study of a new surgical treatment for lesions from genital warts, participants might be randomized to receive either the traditional surgical approach or the new surgical approach. Given that the surgeon and providers need to know, in order to perform the procedure and care for the participants, it would not be feasible to have a double-blinded design. Clearly, the provider must know the treatment assignment. But the participants do not necessarily need to know their treatment assignment, unless it is somehow obvious from the outside or impacts their care. As in all studies, it is essential that the participants know that they are involved in a study and provide complete informed consent. Just because they are not aware of their treatment assignment, they still must know that they were part of a study, and know the risks and benefits associated with each treatment and with participating in the trial. Another example of a type of study that may be single-blinded is a Phase II study. For example, a new drug for the treatment of SARS may be in development. Phase I trials may have indicated that it is safe and tolerable, a dose has been definitively determined, and in the latter half of the Phase II trial, exploration of outcomes begins (though, as above, not to the in-depth degree that it will be in Phase III trials). In this case, it might not be feasible or advisable to blind the provider but it might be possible to blind the participants to treatment status.

- *Double-blinded:* No one knows what treatment the participant is being given. This is the standard that is required in almost all cases to approve a treatment in the United States. A double-blinded trial is the most difficult to execute, but because minimal bias enters the trial, it is the most accurate for assessing outcomes of interest, as well as safety and side effects. Double-blinding is generally reserved for Phase III studies that will determine if the treatment is effective at attaining the ends desired (e.g., reduction of symptoms, remission, cure). For example, in an early trial of highly active antiretroviral treatment (HAART) in the treatment of HIV (see Randomized Controlled Trials and Eligibility Criteria), participants were randomized to receive zidovudine and ddI or HAART. The study was double-blinded, thus only the research pharmacist handling the medications in a secure fashion knew the status of each participant. No one else—from physician to nurse to participant to data management personnel—knew the treatment being given to each person. When outcomes data, including CD4 count, viral load, development of AIDS-defining diagnoses, and lab indicators of and participant self-report of side effects and adverse events were collected, entered into the computer program, and then analyzed, no one knew to which arm each participant was randomized. This ensured that bias was minimized to the greatest extent possible. Not knowing whether they were on the new treatment, participants and providers could not perceive that the treatment was either "better" or "safer" or "worse" or "more dangerous." Not knowing whether they were on the old treatment, the standard of care at the time, participants and providers could not perceive that the treatment was "older" or "safer" or "had fewer side effects" or "was more effective." All the participants and providers could assess was the actual state of the participant with regard to side effects and clinical and laboratory outcomes. Data personnel, too, could not introduce bias into the data collection, entry, or management of the data, by unwittingly changing the existing data to fit a preconceived notion of what each participant was experiencing *in conjunction* with the treatment assignment. This results in reduction of bias and ensures, to the extent possible, that the findings truly reflect the treatment and not just what those involved expected or wanted to find about the treatment.

APPLICATION OF RANDOMIZED DESIGNS

As mentioned earlier, randomized controlled designs may also use larger units of analysis, not just individuals. The same methodology presented above is generally used, with several modifications. Blinding is usually difficult to implement, though the need for it may be lessened when dealing with group-level interventions and/or outcomes. For example, in a randomized controlled trial comparing the effects of two social marketing campaigns on use of methods to reduce exposure to mosquitoes and West Nile virus, 10 similar communities in different neighborhoods might be randomized to be exposed to each of the different campaigns. One group might be assigned to the new social marketing strategy (a new print and television media campaign plus standard public service announcements), and the other to the standard of care social marketing strategy (public service announcements alone). Data might be collected on several outcomes: individual-level report (via survey) of exposure to campaigns and use of mosquito reducing techniques (e.g., use of DEET repellent, staying indoors at dusk hours, reduction of environmental areas prone to mosquito infestation), aggregate (by neighborhood) reports of DEET purchase, and surveillance data to quantify number of West Nile virus cases during the study period. Collection of outcomes data on this type of trial may be difficult, and can suffer from the problem of the ecologic fallacy: Did the person who contracted the disease see the social marketing campaign? Did she use suggested techniques to reduce risk but were they unsuccessful? It may not be possible to link individual-level exposure and outcome data. In addition, depending on the communities selected, it may be difficult to determine how many people were exposed to the treatment arm. What about people who were exposed to the social marketing campaign while visiting friends or family? If an individual were visiting family in

a neighborhood assigned to the new social marketing strategy, but lived in a standard of care social marketing strategy area, the actions she takes (use of DEET, for example), may be affected by the alternate campaign. When her risk reduction behaviors are measured, they would be influenced not by her own neighborhood's campaign, but by her family's. Due to this crossover, the neighborhood in which she lives will appear "better" than it should. This individual will act based on the new strategy but be counted as the standard, skewing the results.

This situation is termed crossover and, although sometimes a problem in randomized controlled trials, it is particularly problematic in community designs, as in this example. Although the treatment portion of community-based designs is often more straightforward than that of individual-level designs, outcomes assessment can be very difficult. Ascertaining individual responses from within the population base exposed to the treatment can be difficult; linking exposure and outcome can be challenging, especially in the face of limited data sources for each; and the problem of crossover is hard to surmount. Still, many important studies have been conducted with this design and so it is essential to be aware of it.

Other forms of monitoring and evaluation can be used (see Chapter 13) to overcome some of these challenges. Evaluation differs from research, though the two often overlap in methodological approaches. The evaluation approach to this research question (Which social marketing campaign works better?) might be less likely to involve a randomized controlled trial comparing the two campaigns, and might be more likely to use creative application of existing data sources to answer the same question. As with most things, there are multiple ways to "skin a cat" and answer a research question. Although each epidemiologist becomes an expert in his or her own most frequently used methods, collectively, many designs are needed to answer important infectious disease research questions. This allows comparison of results and, hopefully, as time moves forward, ultimately arrival at an understanding of the research question under study.

Ethical Concerns

Randomized controlled trials, of drugs or other interventions, require the highest degree of attention to ethical concerns. Why is this attention so essential? In all other study designs, you as the investigator or research staff observe what is already happening or has happened. In experimental designs, however, you actually *make something happen*. This means that you as the researcher must be absolutely certain that the provision of the treatment and control under study—whatever they are—are safe and will be likely to improve or maintain the health status of the participants. In addition, you must be sure that those in the placebo or standard of care arm(s) of the study are not being prevented from having access to a necessary new treatment that would be better for them, and that there is no knowledge or suggestion that one treatment is better than the other. (If there is, one must of course ethically give that one.)

The realization that experimental trials create an environment requiring absolute attention to ethics and the rights of human subjects cannot be stated too firmly or frequently. Before ever embarking on any study, but particularly a clinical trial, it is essential to work with a multidisciplinary team to develop the protocol and instrumentation, and review the study's ethics. Multiple disciplines are necessary, because what a physician finds objectionable might differ from what a nutritionist, nurse, or behaviorist would. All persons who write, conduct, and work on studies should be thoroughly trained in Health Insurance Portability and Accountability Act (HIPAA) regulations, the Belmont Report, and other information guiding the protection of research subjects' rights.

HOW TO CONDUCT A RANDOMIZED CONTROLLED TRIAL

Randomized controlled trials are not something to be entered into lightly or without appropriate expertise. This section will not make you an expert in the conduct of randomized trials, but will hopefully provide you with an understanding of how they work. Many epidemiology and public health students are able to work as clinical trials coordinators or data managers, so a general understanding of the flow of clinical trials is useful. Working in clinical trials environments is a fascinating opportunity to interface with real research that has public health implications. In addition, a clear, applied understanding of clinical trials implementation will facilitate your reading of articles while grounding your understanding of other analytic epidemiologic study designs.

There are as many randomized controlled studies and specifics as there are diseases, medications, and unique populations of patients. Thus, there is no one-size-fits-all mentality when it comes to this study design. However, the usual structure is similar from study to study. Nearly all randomized designs are driven by a protocol, a comprehensive guide to the study that details all one needs to know about the study and how to conduct it. The protocol is also important because it makes implementation of the study the same across providers and sites, wherever the study is being conducted. This protocol will usually provide the following sections:

- A background literature review encompassing the new intervention under study, the comparison (control) arm(s), the design, the risks, and potential benefits.

- A rationale for the study
- A schema or summary of the design
- Detailed inclusion and exclusion criteria
- Specific details on the intervention and the control arms
- Randomization procedures, including instructions for the research pharmacists
- Step-by-step specific instructions regarding clinical, laboratory, or other examinations that must be conducted and when they are to be conducted (including, in general, an easy-to-read flow chart of the same information)
- A data analysis plan, including endpoints, stopping rules, sample size, and power calculations[e]
- Template consent documents to facilitate IRB submission and review
- A variety of appendices, tailored for the study's unique needs, including instrumentation and data collection tools, requirements for source documentation, and reporting requirements to ensure reporting of adverse events to the regulatory body responsible for the study's conduct

The nuts and bolts of conducting of a randomized controlled clinical trial are similar to those of cohort and case-control studies you will see in the next chapters and to the study planning described in the previous one. For all of these, careful attention must be paid to literature review, development of the research question, null and alternative hypotheses, variable selection and operationalization, and the data analysis plan. For randomized trials, inclusion and exclusion criteria must be especially well detailed so that all participants are subject to the same rules and there is a specific composition of the study sample. Inclusion and exclusion criteria are similar conceptually to the case definitions we developed in our outbreak investigations.

These assist in the compilation of the desired sample and, later, the study's ability to generalize its findings to the target population. The most essential difference between experimental and observational studies is the random assignment of treatment to each participant. The active role of the study in assigning treatment to subjects is what makes this design different from all others. Here there is no self-selection of exposure, no purposive provision of treatment. What treatment each person receives is entirely 1) up to chance and 2) out of everyone's control. How does this occur? Although logically simple—in essence it is no different than flipping a coin—it

---

[e]That is, how many subjects need to be enrolled and maintained on the study in order to see a difference between treatment conditions, if a difference exists.

Randomized Controlled Trials and Eligibility Criteria

Here is an example of eligibility criteria from one of the early trials of HAART in the treatment of HIV. The double-blind, placebo-controlled study compared saquinavir, zidovudine, plus zalcitabine, vs. saquinavir plus zidovudine, vs. zidovudine plus zalcitabine.[5] This is a summary of the inclusion criteria that were published with the results. Those listed in the actual protocol would contain additional detail that clarify the inclusion/exclusion criteria and facilitate field implementation of the study.

Participants were enrolled at 10 participating AIDS Clinical Trials Units sponsored by the National Institute of Allergy and Infectious Diseases.

Inclusion criteria

Participants were required to:

- Be willing and able to provide informed consent and sign an IRB-approved consent form
- Be at least 13 years old
- Have HIV infection as documented by the protocol-specified laboratory criteria
- Have one CD4+ count of 50 to 300 cells per cubic millimeter obtained within 30 days before entry into the study
- Have at least 4 months of prior zidovudine therapy
- Have the following laboratory specifications:
  - Granulocyte count of at least 1,000 cells per cubic millimeter
  - Hemoglobin level of at least 8.5 g per deciliter (5.3 mmol per liter)
  - Platelet count of at least 50,000 per cubic millimeter
  - Creatinine level not exceeding 2 times the upper limit of normal
  - Aminotransferase and alkaline phosphatase levels not exceeding 5 times the upper limit of normal
  - Bilirubin level not exceeding 2.5 times the upper limit of normal
  - Amylase level not exceeding 1.5 times the upper limit of normal

Exclusion criteria

Participants must have documented absence of:

- Lymphoma
- Visceral Kaposi's sarcoma
- Severe chronic diarrhea
- Peripheral neuropathy
- Pancreatitis, or an active untreated opportunistic infection
- Dependence on transfusions
- Pregnancy or nursing
- Taking immunomodulatory or other experimental medications

In general, though it varies somewhat from sponsor to sponsor, source documentation (copies of lab reports, physician notes, etc.) confirming the presence of each and every inclusion criterion and absence of every exclusion criterion is required. This is to ensure that the participant is in fact qualified to be in the study and—most importantly—is in the appropriate health to be safe in the study. Some clinical studies require that a person previously has tried other types of treatment whereas others require healthy volunteers or participants naïve to a given treatment. But no matter what the requirements, what the protocol says must be followed in their exact order to protect the safety of the participants and the integrity of the research.

presents logistical issues. When are participants randomized? How does it work? How is staff prevented from "choosing" treatments?

The act of randomizing is most commonly performed by use of a random number table or computer algorithms. Random number tables provide numbers without any order or system in them. They are random, assembled by chance. Using the table, one can assign each person in a list with a number, and then treatment assignment can be based on the number assigned. For example, all persons with even numbers are assigned the intervention being tested, and all persons with odd numbers are assigned the standard of care (control or placebo).

This can be laborious due to the effort required to assign individuals, but the principle is the same. Computer algorithms in general do this very same task, but simplify the process and ensure that a proper and random process is conducted each time.[f] Computer randomization can take place in a variety of ways, from simple to complex.

Getting the information regarding random assignment of the participant to the field can be the hardest part of this process. The simplest strategy is to run a list of numbers using a table or a computer and, based on these, put "assigned intervention" or "assigned control" on individual index cards. Place these index cards in opaque envelopes (so the treatment assigned cannot be seen from without the envelope). As participants are entered into the study, draw, in order, an envelope for each participant, open it, and determine their treatment assignment. This information may be written in code or kept secret as dictated by the blinding design of the study, and can then be conveyed to the pharmacist as needed. However, even if this step is taken, this method has a large degree of active involvement by the staff, so extensive safeguards are needed to protect against cheating, nonrandom allocation, or staff meddling in the process. (With use of envelopes to randomize in the field, there is the potential for violation of randomization. Often, staff will try to randomize those subjects that they perceive to be sickest/least sick to a particular treatment assignment. Envelopes are sometimes steamed open, looked at with bright lights, and even, frankly, switched to change assignments. This is then nonrandom, and makes the entire process invalid. Treatment assignments are being assigned nonrandomly, just as they were in our first example! In certain studies, however, use of an alternate procedure is not possible. In these cases, procedures should be developed to guard against tampering and check data for evidence of tampering with randomization processes on a regular basis.)

If a computer is available, it may be programmed to provide real-time random assignment to subjects; this is substantially safer than the envelope method. The computer lets the staff member overseeing randomization know a number, which corresponds to the treatment assignment and may either be given to the pharmacist by the staff or may be provided automatically by computer. In the case of a double-blind study, this coded procedure prevents all parties except the intended research pharmacist from knowing the treatment assignment. This procedure may be associated with reductions in procedural difficulty as well as tampering with treatment assignments. As indicated by technology available in the field as well as the study's needs, other procedures may involve a phone or

a faxed randomization. Irrespective of the method used, the information gleaned from the randomization process is the same: Participants are randomly assigned to a particular study arm (e.g., treatment, placebo, standard of care, new vs. old treatment), and then the treatment is provided to the participant. Once the process of randomization is complete, the participant is randomized and followed up, just the same as on cohort and case-control studies. Like these other study designs, as you will see, follow-up is imperative, so every effort may be made to identify outcomes for each and every person in the study.

Individual-level randomized controlled trials generally have multiple procedures for ensuring that individuals are healthy enough or, depending on the trial type, sick enough to participate in the study. These inclusion and exclusion criteria are important, serving two purposes. First, they ensure that the sample has the necessary characteristics to draw the desired conclusions from it. This includes having sufficient statistical power to be able to discern a difference if one exists, to generalize the findings to a particular type of target population, or to compare certain subgroups within the sample. Second, and even more importantly, inclusion and exclusion criteria are there to protect the participant. In the case of experimental designs, the investigators are actively intervening in the care of the participant. This intervention may include medications, surgeries, devices, or behavioral interventions. Ethical treatment of research subjects demands that we take good care of those volunteering to be in our studies. In the case of studies for healthy participants, Phase I studies of drugs for example, a healthy sample may be required; using a sicker sample could put already-ill individuals at unneeded risk. At the same time, "salvage" trials may use, for example, persons who have tried every available treatment for AIDS or cancer. In these studies, it is crucial to ensure that participants are sick enough to be in the study so that healthier persons who may still benefit from nonexperimental approaches have a chance to do so.

As you can see, the range of concerns with any study in which the investigator is *doing* something instead of just *observing* something is quite large. And as with all studies, experimental or observational, you need to inform the participant of potential risks and benefits, provide the specifics of each and every procedure, remind them that participation is voluntary, and explain that declining to participate in any or all parts of the study will not result in any change to the services or care to which the participant is otherwise entitled.

It is incumbent upon all persons involved with research in any capacity—from the data entry person all the way to the lead investigator—to do everything possible to conduct research ethically. No matter what role you are in, when in doubt about any facet of a study that you are working on, always

---

[f]Some computer algorithms employ a quasi-random method.

bring it to the attention of your supervisors, individuals at your institution's IRB, or office of legal counsel. Working to protect the rights and safety of research participants is everyone's job.

Strengths and Limitations

Randomized controlled trials in many ways are the "gold standard" of study designs. They allow for random assignment of treatment condition for participants, such that participants do not "choose" their exposure status. A key strength of the randomized trial is that confounders are equally distributed across arms, along with treatments, so that there is an equal distribution of the treatment condition and the arms may be compared—treatment vs. control. Structurally and methodologically, this difference is critical. When it is ethical, feasible, and logistically possible to use this design, its many strengths override its limitations.

Primary among the limitations for this study design are the following:

- Randomized controlled designs must be designed with attention paid to equipoise and ethical distribution of treatments. Because the investigator plays a central and active role in giving participants the exposure, the investigator has enormous responsibility to provide treatments and conduct the study ethically. Better to not conduct the study, or to find an alternate methodology, than to conduct an unethical trial. If everyone, from the study architects to the front line clinicians to the data entry personnel, does not feel that they are giving all participants access to an ethically appropriate treatment, then the study should be redeveloped. Failure to do so can result in a violation of the rights of the participants. In addition, it may open up the study to being conducted badly: When staff do not "buy in" to a study, they are much more likely to circumvent study procedures, including that of randomization. This can make the study that much more dangerous, and likely to violate subject rights.
- Randomized controlled trials are not free. Resources required for this design can be substantial. Studies of medical or other types of treatment have unique needs; they will require a multidisciplinary team of experts, including physician, nursing, pharmacy, instrumentation specialist, behaviorist, epidemiologic, biostatistical, and other collaborators, depending on the study's emphasis. Monitoring and institutional involvement in randomized controlled trials can be the costliest of all studies, with costs driven not only from the administration of the treatments but follow-up, safety, and monitoring. Follow-up can be expensive with reminders, incentives, longitudinal study visits, and more. It is necessary to have comprehensive follow-up for all subjects. Without follow-up on all participants, we will not have outcome data on everyone, making it difficult to analyze and interpret the data. To avoid the biases that derive from attrition, resources devoted to this end are warranted. Still, this can be a limitation depending on the type of study, and even optimal resource allocation to preventing attrition is not always successful.
- Randomized studies are not effective for outcomes that are rare. This is the same as for cohort studies, as you will learn in the next chapter. They are too short and too small to assess rare outcomes and outcomes that take place over a long period of time. Imagine that you are interested in studying an intervention to reduce death from rabies. In the United States, rabies is most frequently acquired through bats; however, overall, rabies is very rare. From 1985 to 2000, of 57 human deaths attributed to rabies, 35 resulted from exposure to bats.[4,6] Death from rabies is thus extremely rare. Perhaps you are interested in studying the use of netting over beds at camp cabins that tend to have a large population of bats therein. To do this, you conduct a randomized trial of camp cabins, randomizing half of the cabins at a summer camp to use individual bed nets and the other to have the standard, which is no nets. Your outcome is death from rabies. In view of the rarity of this outcome, you would be highly unlikely to see a difference between the bed netting arm and the standard, simply due to the fact that the outcome—death from rabies—is so small. It is rather like looking for a needle in a haystack: The probability of something taking place needs to be sufficiently large that you will expect to see it. Even looking for a difference between contracting and not contracting rabies would be difficult, because that itself is low. Outcomes that would be more possible might include bat bites, but that too is a very rare event.[g] Consider now, though, the same design used to evaluate malaria in tropical Africa. In an area endemic with malaria, this design would be feasible and useful. Sadly, one could use deaths from malaria, incidence of malaria, or mosquito bites as an appropriate outcome because not one of these is rare in that region. In the United States, however, that would not be possible.

---

[g]As humans increasingly move beyond urban boundaries, and proximity to bats increases, exposure to rabies has become more common in the last two years. Still, the rates are low—but on the rise.

Given the strengths of a randomized controlled design, you may be asking yourself why having other design approaches is so necessary. The answer is that a great many things—most things even—cannot be tested by intervention. As in the examples you saw in this chapter, treatment assignments could be dangerous, unethical, or not feasible given the construct of day-to-day life. Outcomes of interest may take place too infrequently to evaluate with this design. Or resource expenditure may be too high. Given this, analytic observational designs are required. These are the bulk of those used in infectious disease epidemiology, although drugs are, of course, tested using randomized controlled trial designs.

MOVING FROM RANDOMIZED TO OBSERVATIONAL STUDIES

Why not always do such trials to explore how different characteristics impact infectious disease? The reason is that it is simply not always possible. Epidemiologic methods largely are built upon the conceptual framework of the randomized controlled trial. What you will study in the next chapters—the cohort and case-control designs—emerged as a substitute for the randomized study in cases in which more ideal study design cannot be used. The following are a few examples of situations in which a randomized trial cannot be performed.

- We are interested in learning about the effects of malaria on hemoglobin levels of children. Can we randomize children to be exposed to infectious vectors (mosquitoes) vs no exposure, and follow them prospectively to assess their hemoglobin levels? Of course not!
- We are interested in the effect of gender on acquisition of SARS. Can we randomize fetuses to gender and follow them forward in time to assess for development of SARS? Of course not!
- We are interested in the effect of a person's specific chromosomal composition and quantity of E. coli required to cause illness. Can we randomize persons to a specific chromosomal makeup? Of course not!

Although these are outrageous examples, the point is clear: In many situations, it is impossible, unethical, or not feasible to randomize individuals to the condition we wish to study in order to compare treatment effects. In these instances, we take an observational yet analytic approach. In its simplest form, the cohort study, the approach mimics the randomized study. Individuals are classified based upon their exposure to the characteristic under study (in the previous examples, exposure to mosquitoes in a malaria-endemic location, gender, and chromosomal makeup), and followed forward in time for the outcomes of interest (in these examples, hemoglobin levels, SARS, and manifestations of E. coli). More complicated is the case-control study, which strives to overcome disease-specific characteristics that the cohort design demands. We will build on this in the next two chapters, but these include rarity (the prevalence of disease in a given population), long latent periods, and more. In addition, case-control designs and retrospective cohort (nonconcurrent cohort) designs overcome logistical and feasibility issues that sometimes arise in their prospective counterparts. Each of these in its own way builds upon the randomized controlled design in their ultimate construct. Details regarding how these studies are performed are described in Chapters 8 and 9.

Conceptually speaking, the key difference between an experimental and an observational study is that the exposures in the latter are not randomly assigned. One might argue that it does not matter because gender, for example, is hardly "self-selected," thus there can be no impact of its being nonrandom. Although this may be true (though individual characteristics of the parents or the environment in which they live or a multitude of other factors may affect an individual's gender), the characteristics that are associated with gender are certainly nonrandom; in fact, in many cases they are distinctly systematic.

As a construct to guide our understanding of observational studies, randomized trials are very useful. In the next chapters, observational designs will be presented against the conceptual backdrop of the randomized trial. As biases of special importance within infectious disease are discussed, this useful construct will continue to aid our understanding of these pivotal epidemiologic designs.

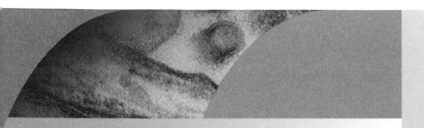

Discussion Questions

1. You are interested in evaluating the efficacy of the interventions shown in Table 7-1. Design a randomized controlled trial to assess each of them. Be sure that your design is ethical in its treatment of subjects and would be realistic to implement. For each one, operationalize both the intervention (the exposure) and the outcome (primary endpoint).

TABLE 7-1 Interventions and Primary Endpoints

Intervention	Primary endpoint
1. Group therapy	Injection drug use
2. Directly observed therapy	Adherence to HAART
3. Smoking cessation	Immunocompromise among HIV+ patients
4. Disclosure of herpes simplex virus type 2 (genital herpes) status to partner	Use of antivirals during outbreaks
5. HIV education curriculum	Use of condoms
6. Food handling preparation training	Outbreaks of common foodborne pathogens

2. Make up specific steps involved in conducting a randomized controlled trial of one of the interventions listed in Table 7-1. Be sure to create eligibility criteria and consider any ethical implications of the intervention and control arms.

3. In most of the examples in this chapter, for simplicity, we have used only two arms: a treatment arm and a control arm. Design a study for a research question of interest to you with more than two arms: What would you compare? How would you conduct the study?

4. Unanticipated consequences sometimes develop from research. For example, the control arm can result in a safer participant experience than the new treatment under study. What are other unanticipated consequences that you could imagine occurring? What research questions could be developed to follow up on your study and test the preliminary results?

REFERENCES

1. Sackett D. Why randomized controlled trials fail but needn't: 1. Failure to gain "coal-face" commitment and to use the uncertainty principle. *Can Med Assoc J.* 2000;162:1311–1134.

2. Nelson K. *Infectious Disease Epidemiology.* Gaithersburg, MD: Aspen; 2001.

3. Kuile FOT, Terlouw DJ, Kariuki SK, et al. Impact of permethrin-treated bed nets on malaria, anemia, and growth in infants in an area of intense perennial malaria transmission in western Kenya. *Am J Trop Med Hyg.* 2003;68 (4 Supp):68–77.

4. Heymann DL. *Control of Communicable Diseases.* 18th edition. Washington, DC: American Public Health Association; 2004.

5. Collier AC, Coombs RW, Schoenfeld DA, et al. Treatment of human immunodeficiency virus infection with saquinavir, zidovudine, and zalcitabine. *N Engl J Med.* 1996;334(16):1011–1018.

6. Centers for Disease Control. Summary of notifiable diseases—United States, 2004. *MMWR.* 2004;53(53):1–80.

CHAPTER 8

Cohort Studies

LEARNING OBJECTIVES

By the end of this chapter, you will be able to:

- Describe cohort designs, including prospective, retrospective, and ambidirectional.
- Delineate steps in conducting a cohort study.
- Compare and contrast internal and external control groups.
- Articulate strengths and limitations of the different types of cohort studies.

FROM THE EXPERIMENTAL STUDY TO THE COHORT STUDY

Why begin in the previous chapter with experimental studies, when observational analytic studies are more common in infectious disease epidemiology? Randomized controlled trials set the stage for a more thorough understanding of cohort and case-control studies, the primary analytic "toolkit" of observational epidemiology. Cohort studies turn randomized controlled trials on their ear. Like experimental designs, they are concerned with the relationships between the exposure and the treatment but in cohort studies, the investigator has nothing to do with who gets which treatment or exposure. Participants do what they do, are exposed to what they are exposed to, for their own reasons. Although most of the time exposure is not "chosen" intentionally to be studied, it is experienced by the participant independently and not in the control of the investigator. This is the central characteristic of the cohort paradigm that differentiates it from the experimental design: The investigator does not randomly (or otherwise) assign treatment in the cohort study; rather, the participant—

or his or her circumstances in life, health, sickness, poverty, occupation, or other situations—ultimately selects it.

How does a cohort study work? In brief, the investigator finds individuals who have been exposed to the predictor or exposure of interest and a group of similar individuals who have not been exposed, and follows all of them forward in time. No one has the out outcome of interest at the start of the study and all participants are followed forward in time to see if they develop it. That's it! It is the same structure as a randomized controlled trial; the only difference is that the investigator does not randomly assign treatment. However, this difference, although only a sentence long, makes a tremendous difference in the way we interpret results, the limitations of the study's findings, and the types of things we can study.

TYPES OF COHORT STUDIES

There are three types of cohort studies. All follow exposed and unexposed individuals, with the only difference being where the investigator stands in relation to whether the outcomes have occurred at the study's start. All start with disease-free individuals, those who have not experienced the outcome of interest.

Concurrent Cohort Studies

These studies are also called prospective cohort studies, prospective studies, incidence studies, follow-up studies, and longitudinal studies. When one hears of a cohort study without specification of type, in general, this design is being used. These studies have the exposure happening right at the study's start, and the outcomes are undetermined at that time. Participants are followed forward in time to see if they do or do not develop the outcome of interest.

For example, imagine a large group of children who were exposed to varicella (chickenpox) at a sleep-away camp in the summer of 1952. In 1953, researchers become interested in finding out the prevalence of herpes zoster (also known as shingles) among this cohort, in order to calculate the expected rates of shingles among varicella-exposed individuals. Medical records were kept on the children who developed chickenpox when at the camp, and [following institutional review board (IRB) approval and individual parental consent and participant assent] the participants and/or their parents were asked to complete a questionnaire annually regarding their

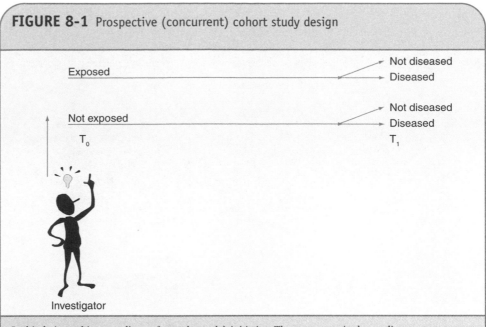

FIGURE 8-1 Prospective (concurrent) cohort study design

In this design, subjects are disease-free at the study's initiation. They are categorized according to exposure status (exposed/not exposed) and then followed forward in time to see the outcome (disease/not diseased).
Source: Author

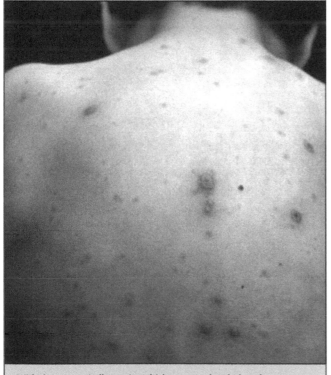

FIGURE 8-2 Pancorporeal varicella, also known as chickenpox

With the new varicella vaccine, chickenpox outbreaks have become rarer than ever before.
Source: Courtesy of CDC/Public Health Image Libray, 1995

health status. In this form, occurrence of shingles during the interval year was ascertained. Individuals who report shingles are asked to provide supporting medical documentation. Follow-up continues for 25 years, at which point the study is closed.

Nonconcurrent Cohort Studies

These studies are also known as retrospective cohort studies and are performed when information on both exposure and outcome is available at the study's start, *and* the exposure (and its documentation) took place before knowledge of the outcome of interest.

For example, imagine the same scenario as in the previous section with the varicella outbreak at sleep-away summer camp. Add the following information, however: the camp attendees are primarily repeat attendees, with families returning generation after generation. Every year, the camp sends out questionnaires and information requests to all of its families. In 1952, one of the camp nurses was very concerned about the chickenpox outbreak at camp, so she started sending out—as a part of the annual questionnaire—a health outcomes form. Shingles was included as a question, as were a variety of other ailments. Now fast-forward to 1999. One of the camp counselors, who was entering this information into a database one summer, decides it might be a rich data source for a medical school project. He starts the study in 1999, closing the database to new information after that point. When he starts the study, the exposure (varicella) and the outcome (shingles) have both taken place. The exposure precedes the outcome in temporal sequence. But for him, the information is available all at one time. He does not have to wait decades for the outcomes because they have already occurred.

Ambidirectional Cohort Studies

These studies are a hybridization of concurrent and nonconcurrent cohort studies. This study design is best described by example: Imagine the nonconcurrent cohort study we just described. Now imagine that the medical student would like to continue to obtain data between 1999 and 2006, thus giving him seven additional years of data. The camp continues to send out

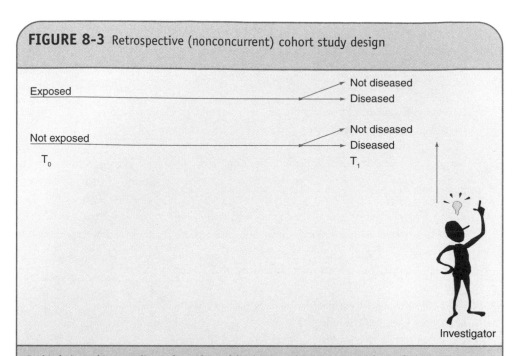

FIGURE 8-3 Retrospective (nonconcurrent) cohort study design

In this design, subjects are disease-free at the study's initiation. They are categorized according to exposure status (exposed/not exposed) and then followed forward in time to see the outcome (diseased/not diseased). The only difference between this design and the prospective (concurrent) cohort designs with regard to classification of exposure and outcomes is where the investigator stand in relation to the activities. Here the exposure and outcome have both concluded at the time of the study's start. However, at the time of the exposure, the disease had *not* yet occurred.

Source: Author

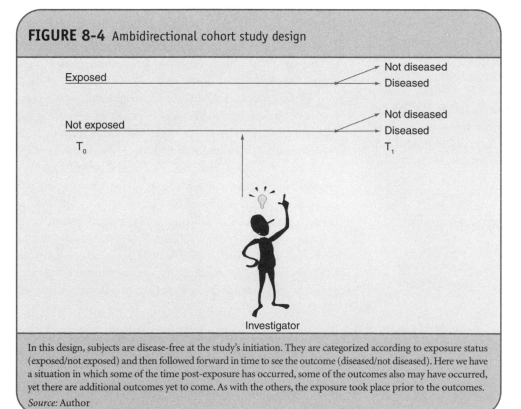

FIGURE 8-4 Ambidirectional cohort study design

In this design, subjects are disease-free at the study's initiation. They are categorized according to exposure status (exposed/not exposed) and then followed forward in time to see the outcome (diseased/not diseased). Here we have a situation in which some of the time post-exposure has occurred, some of the outcomes also may have occurred, yet there are additional outcomes yet to come. As with the others, the exposure took place prior to the outcomes.

Source: Author

the forms, and he continues to enter them. Thus for individuals who did not develop shingles by 1999, more information is prospectively collected; this is the concurrent part. For those that already had developed shingles, the database is closed; this is the nonconcurrent part. By combining these two study designs, if resources are available, the investigator maximizes the number of outcomes that are available to study as well as adding potentially important information about the longevity of the response to varicella virus. The invesitgator can also compare the differences in data obtained retrospectively and prospectively, and assess any potential for bias that is present in either subset.

Cohort Study Similarities

All of these designs have four things in common. In each:

1. The participants were categorized according to exposure.
2. All were disease free at baseline.
3. The exposure occurred first.
4. The exposure categorization—that is, exposed vs. not exposed—was documented *prior* to the outcome.

Let us break this down and apply it to our examples:

1. *The participants were categorized according to exposure:* having varicella or not having varicella at the study's start.
2. *All were disease free at baseline:* all had no shingles at baseline.
3. *The exposure occurred first:* among exposed, varicella occurred first, not the shingles.
4. *The exposure categorization—that is, exposed vs not exposed—was documented prior to the outcome.* The varicella/no varicella status was documented first, before the shingles occurred, not the other way around.

This temporal sequencing is important, because it has impact down the road when we interpret the findings of the study, particularly with regard to biases that may impact the study's internal validity. This sequence is identical to that of the randomized controlled trial. The only difference between the two with respect to the exposure is that in the randomized controlled trial study, the exposure was assigned by the investigator whereas with the cohort study it is not. With respect to the outcome, the concurrent cohort is the same as the randomized controlled trial. The non-concurrent cohort is somewhat different, however—more like looking at the results of a trial that was conducted many years ago, where the exposure and outcome data were collected but never analyzed.

COHORT STUDIES IN INFECTIOUS DISEASE RESEARCH

Cohort studies are frequently used in infectious disease research. Many examples of cohort study methodology are in the literature:

- Studies to understand the natural history of disease
- Studies to confirm the source of an outbreak
- Treatment cohorts
- Studies to assess sequelae (follow-up conditions resulting from an illness or a condition) of infectious diseases

In order to see the underlying construct of the cohort study in each of these, one must understand the concept of exposure and outcome. Build upon your learning from previous chapters:

- Other words for exposure include risk factor, predictor, and independent variable. (This is often denoted as *X*.)
- Another word for outcome is dependent variable. (This is often denoted as *Y*.)

We are interested in the association between these two things, *X* and *Y*. Independent variables are the items under investigation: We wonder whether they "cause" an illness or a problem or—alternately—whether they "prevent" an illness or a problem.[1] A few examples may make this clearer:

- If we had a research question of, "Is varicella virus exposure associated with development of chickenpox?" Varicella virus exposure is the *independent variable* and the development of chickenpox is the *dependent variable.*
- If we had a research question of, "Is varicella vaccine exposure associated with prevention of chickenpox?" Varicella vaccine exposure is the *independent variable* and the development of chickenpox is the *dependent variable.*

Going back to the randomized design as a construct, the exposure is the treatment being assessed and the outcome is the illness being investigated. I will discuss confounders and effect modifiers in Chapter 11, but these are generally considered independent variables, although they work in peculiar ways that differentiate them from the exposures or independent variables of interest.

As you have seen, cohort studies in epidemiology categorize participants with respect to the exposure of interest and follow them forward in time to assess the outcome of interest. Sometimes, the more traditional nonepidemiologic use of the word "cohort" is used in studies. This can be confusing to new epidemiologists, as the word "cohort"—with its meaning of a group of similar people based on a given characteristic—is different from the more technical use of the word "cohort" as in cohort designs. In studies of the natural history of disease, we often see large cohorts of people with the same characteristic or disease assembled and followed prospectively for the purposes of understanding the disease. Sometimes researchers

---

[1]Note that we often think of research questions in causal terms: X *causes* Y; Q *prevents* Z. But with observational designs we cannot demonstrate causality. Unlike randomized controlled trials, which, under certain conditions when executed and analyzed appropriately, can demonstrate causality; observational studies cannot. What we can say is that X *is associated with increases in* Y; Q *is associated with decreases in* Z.

may also use occupational groups (e.g., nurses, doctors, lab technicians) to study en masse. Although on the surface these studies may appear to lack categorization with respect to an exposure of interest, they actually do not. Such cohort studies have several layers of research questions underlying their construction. For example, the researchers may wish to follow a group of people simply to characterize their disease descriptively; from that, as the data begin to inform our understanding of the disease, specific research questions may emerge. Then characteristics of interest may be compared/contrasted using the more technical use of the cohort terminology.

For example, in learning about the natural history of HIV/AIDS, two large cohort studies—the Adolescent/Adult Spectrum of Disease (ASD) study and the Men's AIDS Cohort Study (MACS)[1,2]—have been instrumental in understanding the disease, its symptoms, and its characteristics. Researchers of the MACS, in particular, have published extensively on this cohort, contributing a wealth of data to inform our understanding of the HIV/AIDS. Comprehensive data are collected in both of these cohorts, so that many exposures and outcomes can be evaluated. Both of these studies have had multiple analyses, with each their own exposures and outcomes of interest. Thus, although the overall cohort may have participants who are followed before being categorized in a particular way, in the end, the criteria for a cohort study are met. The participants are categorized with respect to exposure for each particular research question of interest. They are followed forward in time for the outcomes of interest and extensive data are collected on a variety of variables. For example, an analysis of the parent cohort's data might be a comparison of people treated with antiretrovirals at low CD4 counts vs. people treated with antiretrovirals at high CD4 counts—and all followed forward in time to determine the association with treatment start time and development of an opportunistic infection. For this analysis, categorization of exposure and its documentation preceded outcome meets the criteria of a cohort study. Through this method, much has been learned about the natural history of many diseases. With the identification of HIV/AIDS, were it not for the large cohort studies such as MACS, ASD, and others, little would be known about the disease's progression, potential treatments, or how the disease affects the body. The same goes for many other diseases. Cohort studies such as these maximize the ability to study multiple exposures and outcomes while not collecting additional samples of individuals. Because comprehensive information is collected prospectively, multiple analyses may be performed based on the same people and data.

Cohort studies are sometimes also conducted following an outbreak investigation. They may often be used to confirm the existence of the relationship between the pathogen, or the pathogen's source, and the illness or with long-term effects of the infection. In most cases where a strong case may be made for the putative causal agent, public health action takes place immediately, as we saw in outbreak investigations. But then it is important to follow through and be sure the conclusion drawn was the right one. So, persons, who were exposed to the source that investigators think is responsible for the illness, are followed over time, and compared to a group of similar persons who were not exposed, to see who develops the disease.

An Example of When To Use a Cohort Study in an Infectious Disease Situation

Although randomized controlled trials are used to assess the safety and efficacy of drugs that treat infectious diseases, cohort methodology is generally used to identify treatment guidelines in situations where either it would not be ethical to randomize or more information is needed to understand uses of the treatment, side effects, or sequelae. They are also often used to assess the utilization and effects of treatment in the "real world"—that is, outside of the ideality of the clinical trials setting.

Cohort studies can also be conducted to assess sequelae to a given disease. Many infectious diseases are acute, but may become chronic or create after–effects that are lasting. Good examples of these are Lyme disease, with its acute phase and later long-term disability, and *Staphylococcus aureus*, which may result in arthritis and related joint and cardiac dysfunction over time.[3–7] A cohort study is ideal for situations where an emerging or re-emerging disease needs studying to better understand sequelae. People with the disease in its resolving state are compared to a group of similar people without the disease and followed forward in time to ascertain information on the effects of interest. In the case of a newly identified disease, where little is known about it, such studies are essential. West Nile Virus, a good example, cohort studies were performed to better understand its effects over time, and differentiate those with subacute disease from those with acute neurological manifestations.[6,8–10]

HOW TO CONDUCT A COHORT STUDY

The basic construct of a cohort study is the same for concurrent, nonconcurrent, and ambidirectional studies Like all studies, consider the following things: What is the research question you are trying to answer? What do you want to find out? What is the exposure of interest and what are the outcomes of interest? Setting up a research question matrix that contains the relevant information in a nutshell—including research questions, independent and dependent variables, potential confounders, and the like, as in Chapter 6—is very helpful for cohort studies. Consider these additional factors:

Types of Cohort Studies

Is the exposure of interest something that continues to happen or happens only once? This dictates the type of cohort to be studied. An open cohort, also known as a dynamic cohort, is one in which individuals may continuously be added or removed. A fixed cohort is one that has only a finite group of people included but people can exit the cohort, while a closed cohort is one that is closed to entry and exit.

For example, if one were looking at children exposed to vectors such as mosquitoes and ticks while camping in the mid-Atlantic region, the open cohort will increase each year with new exposures and decrease as there is attrition from the group (also known as loss to follow-up). A fixed cohort, however, could include all children exposed to ticks at a particular campsite in the mid-Atlantic region between June 1, 2000, and September 30, 2000. This group of children is finite and set: No one may enter the cohort that was not there from the beginning. However, there may be losses as attrition occurs over time. If campers were followed for Lyme disease for only a short period of time, perhaps 3 months following the summer that qualified them for the study, and no losses were permitted by study protocol and follow-up, then this would be a closed cohort.

Measures of Incidence by Cohort Type

Although cumulative incidence can be calculated for a closed cohort (because all of the people exposed are staying in the ultimate cohort being followed), incidence rates, using person-time in the denominator, must be used for open and fixed cohorts to accurately describe incidence. For example, you might opt to have all families who reserve a campsite complete informed consent when they register to camp. When they arrive at the campsite, they might be asked to have blood drawn for Lyme disease assessment, which involves a two-stage antibody assay in combination with a clinical questionnaire. Then they would complete a log regarding exposures of interest during their stay. Upon turning the log in to the office prior to departure, they could leave contact information for monthly follow-ups and contact by study staff. This would provide estimates of follow-up time, exposures, and outcomes for all participants in the study.

Internal or External Comparisons Groups

There are two types of comparison groups in cohort studies: internal and external This design choice is usually made in conjunction with the research question being studied and the specifics of the study design selected. In many studies, a group of similar individuals is assembled and followed forward in time with data collected systematically on all participants. From within this cohort, a variety of comparisons may be made to identify differences in the prevalence of the outcome between exposed and nonexposed subjects.

For example, if one took the campers described above in the fixed cohort, a research question could be, "Is campsite proximity to bushes associated with acquisition of tick-borne Lyme disease?" The campers who camped closer to the bushes could be considered exposed and those further away could be considered nonexposed. This would be an internal comparison group. Another research question within this cohort could be, "Is use of 10% DEET insect repellent associated with acquisition of tick-borne Lyme disease?" The campers who used 10% DEET spray more than once daily could be considered exposed and those who used it less frequently or not at all could be considered nonexposed. Note that individuals who were exposed for one research question would not necessarily be considered exposed in the other research question.[2]

A benefit of assembling a cohort such as this is that multiple research questions may be addressed, generally based upon the same routine instrumentation being utilized. However, it is important to remember that each individual question really represents a unique study. In each of these cases, the exposure preceded the outcome—at the start of the study, all persons were disease-free (here proven by clinical findings in combination with self-reported symptomatology), and persons were categorized based on exposure, *not* outcome. Following people forward in time is the means by which outcome data can be ascertained. Multiple outcomes associated with each exposure—here, proximity to bushes and DEET use—may be identified if data are available. (This is a benefit of cohort studies I discuss in the next section.) In addition, multiple levels of the exposures of interest may be utilized; for example, one could examine differences among low, medium, and high levels of DEET use, or close, far, farther levels of proximity to the bushes.

---

[2]This illustrates the problem of confounding, which will be covered in more depth in Chapter 11. These exposures overlap: It is likely that campers camping closer to the bushes may use insect repellant more assiduously than their counterparts. There would then be an uneven distribution of insect repellant use by proximity to bushes. This is the central characteristic of confounding, and it can blur our perception of the relationship between exposure and outcome.

Now imagine a slightly different research question: "Is camping in the mid-Atlantic region associated with Lyme disease?" For this question, we have a situation in which our internal comparison group will not work. Everyone in the cohort described previously was camping, thus there would be no source of comparison. In this situation, we need an external comparison group. This group would be composed of disease-free individuals (based on the same measures of course) who were *not* camping. We would do our very best to identify non-exposed individuals who were like the exposed individuals, except that they had not been camping. External comparison groups are typically drawn via one of three methods:

- Random samples of the general population. This can be costly and time-consuming, and may result in a comparison group that differs substantially from the exposed group)[3]
- Comparison cohorts: groups of individuals who are similar in major criteria, such as socioeconomic status, educational level, type of work, availability of data, and so on. These groups are followed as their own cohort, allowing comparison with those with the exposure of interest
- General population statistics, such as mortality from a given reportable disease.

Deciding on Length of Follow-up

Based upon the exposure and outcomes of interest, how long is appropriate for follow-up? In our Lyme disease example, incubation times range from 3 to 32 days from time of tick exposure, with an average time of 7 to 10 days. If the research question involves acquisition of Lyme disease, then it may be perfectly reasonable to use 6 months as the time frame for follow-up from this fixed cohort. This is the upper range of time in which one expects symptoms to show and diagnostic procedures to reveal positives—one should have caught all individuals exposed at the campsite. Having a longer follow-up period may cause individuals not exposed at the same time at the campsite to appear exposed and diseased, when they in fact should be counted as nondiseased. On the other hand, if the outcome of interest is Lyme-associated arthritis, a follow-up time in years may be required. Similarly, one must consider the interval at which to contact members of the cohort.

Defining Exposure and Outcome

How should the exposure and outcome variables be operationalized? This crucial question should always be considered. In order for the study's findings to be informative and meaningful, variables need to be described and data obtained on them systematically. In the case of exposure assessment for the campsite distance from bushes, contrast the following two possibilities:

- Two rangers come by campsites at 5:00 p.m. on the date of each camper's arrival. One measures the distance from the closest bush or shrub to the campers' nearest gear with a specific device dedicated to this study; the second ranger remeasures it to check for reliability. This distance is recorded on a case report form, which is then entered along with other study data into a secure data system.
- Campers report how far they thought they were to the nearest bush on a survey that is sent to them upon their arrival back at home, within 3 weeks of their visit to the campsite.

These appear different? Indeed! It is important to note that although the former is more precise and probably more valid and reliable than the latter, a study could succeed with the latter, if this is the systematic method that is *always* used. But the meaning of the study would be different. The former can actually describe the association between the outcome and the distance to the bushes; the latter can only describe the association between the outcome and the camper's self-report of the distance to the bushes. If both modes of data collection are used and they are inconsistent, then this results in an even bigger problem in interpreting the data. Similarly, for outcome assessment: If in some cases self-report is used and in others lab values are used, the results will be difficult to interpret. Instead, selecting the desired exposure and outcome variables at the beginning of the study, and articulating specifically how they are operationalized, is critical. There are many data sources for variables, and these should all be examined during the planning phase of the study. Creativity in finding good data sources is a key element in designing and conducting good studies. Training to ensure systematic, quality data collection then follows.

Once these items are addressed in the study design and the other preliminary steps have been taken, including creation and validation of instrumentation, IRB approval, training of staff, and communication with community and relevant stakeholders, the cohort study activities may begin. Instrumentation—data collection tools—a key means of collecting quality data, can make or break a study. The development of systematic tools to collect data, which have been extensively trained upon, is critical.

---

[3]We will discuss the healthy worker effect in Chapter 11. Briefly, this bias occurs when the base population at home during a workday is sicker, less healthy overall, than the healthier workers who are on the job in the middle of a day. This is a problem with case-control studies as well. When comparing cases to a sicker base population, one may find fewer differences between cases and controls than would be found with a population-based estimate of a working population.

Use of a Cohort Design to Examine Increased Risk of HIV-1 Transmission in India

India is home to a growing and serious HIV epidemic. Approaches to reducing risk factors for HIV, including behavior, are sorely needed, as are biomedical approaches. Sexually transmitted infections (STIs)—both ulcerative (e.g., syphilis), and nonulcerative (e.g., chlamydia)—have been associated with increased risk of HIV transmission and acquisition. Dubbed the HIV/STI cofactor hypothesis, it is thought that there are specific mechanisms for heightened transmission.[11–17] With ulcerative STIs, genital ulcers create a portal for entry and exit of the virus. With nonulcerative STDs, the accumulation of lymphocytes in the genital tract due to the STI means that CD4 cells—the cells that carry and also acquire HIV—are proximal to the source of infection. In addition, HIV virus shedding creates increased volumes of viral particles in the genital tract, ready for transmission.

Syphilis outbreaks have occurred recently in India, creating concern about the added risk of HIV transmission. Reynolds and colleagues conducted a prospective cohort study of STI clinic attendees to assess the relationship between acquisition of syphilis and that of HIV-1.[17] Of the 2,324 participants who were syphilis and HIV negative at baseline and returned for follow-up, 172 developed a new (incident) case of syphilis during follow-up, yielding a crude (unadjusted) rate of 5.4 cases per 100 person years.[4] The authors found that syphilis incidence was higher among those less than 20 years old compared with those over 30 years old, those lacking in formal education, and those with recent (after the start of the study) HIV infection. The primary outcome of interest was acquisition of HIV. The greatest risk of HIV was found within 6 months of syphilis infection (RR 4.44, 95% CI 2.96 to 6.65, $p < 0.001$).

What one major question does this study opens up for us? Temporality. The majority (22/27 = 81.5%) of those with HIV *and* syphilis were diagnosed at the same clinic visit. How do we know that the participant did not acquire HIV first and then, by virtue of a suppressed immune system, acquire syphilis? Given the data on those cases taken together with cases without dual diagnosis, it is difficult to tell. In this study, only those with syphilis at a visit prior to HIV acquisition help to answer this question. Time becomes a problem for us, and so we need to consider all the elements at work. Here, we have the problem of syphilis, which in its latent stage does not usually cause genital ulcers,[5,17] and HIV, tested here using and enzyme-linked immunosorbent assay (ELISA), a form of antibody testing which, is subject to a "window period" during development of antibodies. This all has to be added into the interpretation of a cohort study to evaluate this complex research question.

FIGURE 8-5 An electron photomicrograph of two spiral-shaped *Treponema pallidum* bacteria

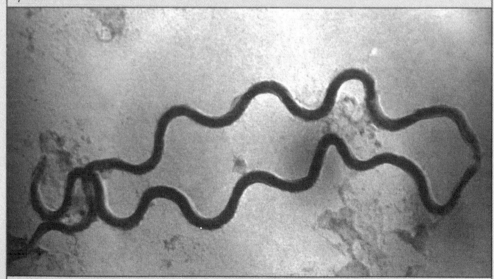

Here we see two *Treponema pallidum* bacteria scanned by an electron microscope, magnified 36,000X. *T. pallidum*, the causative agent of syphilis, contains one of the smallest prokaryotic genomes consisting of about 1000 kilobase pairs.

Source: CDC/Joyce Ayers 1969. Public Health Image Library

---

[4]After reading Chapter 5, you may wonder why we are using person-years here. Remember, it is a prospective cohort and we have individual-level data; thus, we can calculate the actual amount of time each person was under study.

STRENGTHS AND LIMITATIONS

Cohort studies approximate the design and construct of randomized trials, and this is an important design facet that drives most of its strengths. Chief among them is that exposure precedes outcome, helping the temporal relationship to be clearer and reducing biases that result when there is less clarity in what came first. Chapter 11 discusses specific biases that are found in studies. For now, though, realize that there are several methodological limitations of the cohort design:

- One of the primary limitations of cohort studies is the potential for loss to follow-up. Within this, loss to follow-up that can occur when the attrition is associated with the exposure of interest is of particular concern; this is termed differential loss to follow-up. Follow-up of participants in any study is not free. Resources, including study staff, space, overhead costs; incentives for participation, visit reminders, and more are required to keep people in studies, particularly those with long-term follow-up. Chapter 11 teaches about loss to follow-up and other biases related to follow-up, a serious problem to reckon with.
- Cohort studies are not intended for the study of rare outcomes. Imagine this: You are interested in studying rabies, using a different approach than that described in Chapter 7. As described there, to study rabies and its association with exposure to bat bites, it would be inappropriate to use a prospective design: To compare individuals exposed to bats to those not exposed, and follow them forward in time to assess death from rabies would not be feasible, due to the rarity of this outcome. One would need to follow a great number of people at great expense in order to have sufficient outcomes (death from rabies) to see whether an association exists. In other areas, however, where rabies are more common, this may be an appropriate design. However, when the prevalence of the outcome is low, it would not work with a cohort design.
- Cohorts are not efficient for outcomes that take a long time to develop. For such outcomes, the follow-up period includes a time "waiting" for the outcome to occur; this waiting time not only requires resources, but also increases the risk of attrition from the study due to death or loss to follow-up.

- In the case of nonconcurrent cohort studies, data on exposures, outcomes, or confounders may be missing. If they are present, they may be inadequately documented to allow in-depth analysis of the exposure-outcome relationship. This is generally because the data are collected for a nonstudy purpose, and they therefore reflect the underlying needs of the initial data collection impetus rather than study of the research question at hand.

These limitations notwithstanding, the cohort design has numerous strengths:

- It does approximate the randomized controlled design, by ensuring that the exposure precedes the outcome. Especially in concurrent cohort designs, where data collection instruments are developed to collect all necessary exposure, outcome, and confounder data, information collected can effectively describe the relationship between the exposure and the outcome, and clarify (though not prove) the temporal relationship between the two.
- Cohort studies are very good for studying multiple outcomes. In the case of general cohorts, where multiple research questions can be asked of the data, many different outcomes can be assessed. Thus if the exposure is camping, for example, a variety of outcomes associated with camping can be evaluated if the instrumentation is designed to collect data on them.
- Cohort studies, like randomized controlled trials, provide an actual measure of risk of the outcome of interest. We can extract incidence. This is because we are following people forward in time in two groups—exposed and unexposed—and we are able to see how many in each group develop the outcome. The beauty of this is that the exposed and unexposed groups are the whole "universe" of exposed in our sample; this then gives us a denominator that we can use to see how many of the exposed did and did not have the outcome, and how many of the unexposed did and did not have the outcome. This is unlike the case-control and cross-sectional designs introduced in the following chapters, in which we generally find cases first and see how many of them were exposed.

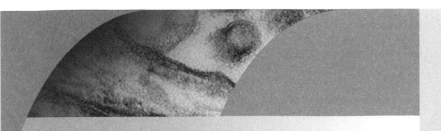

Discussion Questions

You are interested in assessing the sequelae (late effects) of exposure to rotavirus among infants in a day care center.

1. Design three cohort studies: one each for prospective, retrospective, and ambidirectional.

2. What are the relative benefits/limitations of each?

3. What are potential data sources for each study?

4. How will you operationalize your exposure and your outcome? Do these differ depending on which design you are using?

REFERENCES

1. Blair J, Hanson D, Jones JL, et al. Trends in pregnancy rates among women with human immunodeficiency virus. *Obstet Gynecol.* 2004;103(4): 663–668.

2. Cain LE, Cole SR, Chmiel JS, et al. Effect of highly active antiretroviral therapy on multiple AIDS-defining illnesses among male HIV seroconverters. *Am J Epidemiol.* 2005;163(4):160–165.

3. Centers for Disease Control. Lyme disease. *MMWR.* 1982;31(27): 367–368.

4. Carnicer-Pont D, Bailey KA, Mason BW, et al. Risk factors for hospital-acquired methicillin-resistant Staphylococcus aureus bacteraemia: a case-control study. *Epidemiol Infect.* 2006;134:1167–1173.

5. Heymann DL. *Control of Communicable Diseases.* 18th ed. 2004 Washington, DC: American Public Health Association.

6. Nelson K. *Infectious Disease Epidemiology.* Gaithersburg, MD: Aspen.

7. Centers for Disease Control. Notice to readers: caution regarding testing for Lyme disease. *MMWR.* 2005;54(5):125.

8. Centers for Disease Control. Outbreak of West Nile-like viral encephalitis—New York, 1999. *MMWR.* 1999;48(38):845–849.

9. Centers for Disease Control. Assessing capacity for surveillance, prevention, control of West Nile Virus infection—United States 1999 and 2004. *MMWR.* 2006;55(6):150–153.

10. Centers for Disease Control. West Nile Virus activity—United States, January 1 to November 7, 2006. *MMWR.* 2006;55(44):1204–1205.

11. Laga M, Manoka A, Kivuvu M, et al. Non-ulcerative sexually transmitted diseases as risk factors for HIV-1 transmission in women: results from a cohort study. *AIDS.* 1993;7:95–102.

12. Grosskurth H, Gray R,et al. Control of sexually transmitted diseases for HIV-1 prevention: understanding the implications of the Mwanza and Rakai trials. *Lancet.* 2000;355:1981–1987.

13. Grosskurth H, Mosha F, Todd J, et al. Impact of improved treatment of sexually transmitted diseases on HIV infection in rural Tanzania: randomised controlled trial. *Lancet.* 1995;346:530–536.

14. Ghys P, Fransen K, Diallo MO, et al. The associations between cervicovaginal HIV shedding, sexually transmitted diseases and immunosuppression in female sex workers in Abidjan, Cote d'Ivoire. *AIDS.* 1997;11: F85–F93.

15. Ghys PD, Dialloa MO, Ettiegne-Traore V, et al. Increase in condom use and decline in HIV and sexually transmitted diseases among female sex workers in Abidjan, Cote d'Ivoire, 1991 to 1998. *AIDS.* 2002;16:251–258.

16. Wawer M, Sewankambo N, Serwadda D, et al. Control of sexually transmitted diseases for AIDS prevention in Uganda: a randomised community trial. Rakai Project Study Group. *Lancet.* 1999;353:525–535.

17. Reynolds SJ, Risbud AR, Shepherd ME, et al. High rates of syphilis among STI patients are contributing to the spread of HIV-1 in India. *Sex Transm Infect.* 2006;82:121–126.

CHAPTER 9

Case-Control and Cross-Sectional Studies

LEARNING OBJECTIVES

By the end of this chapter, you will be able to:

- Define case-control epidemiologic designs, including the variants of case-cohort study and nested case-control studies.
- Define cross-sectional epidemiologic studies.
- Delineate the steps for conducting a case-control study.
- Delineate the steps for conducting a cross-sectional study.
- Identify at least two types of controls.
- Identify methods for ascertaining control data.
- Articulate the strengths and limitations of case-control studies.
- Articulate the strengths and limitations of cross-sectional studies.

FROM THE COHORT STUDY TO THE CASE-CONTROL STUDY AND CROSS-SECTIONAL STUDY

The case-control study is a unique design that further inverts the paradigm derived from experimental studies. This study design is very useful in infectious disease epidemiology and used perhaps more frequently than other analytic designs. Cross-sectional studies are yet another epidemiologic study design based on the same conceptual framework. Together, case-control and cross-sectional studies comprise a large proportion of the epidemiologic work conducted in the field in the arena of infectious disease.

As you learned in previous chapters, experimental and cohort studies share an important characteristic: The exposure comes first, then the outcome. There are two groups, exposed and unexposed, and they are followed forward in time to observe the outcome, the disease or condition of interest. Even in nonconcurrent cohort studies this is the case; the only difference is that both the exposure and the outcome have oc-

curred at the time the investigator initiates the study. In that cohort study variation, at the time the exposure took place, all persons were disease free. There were no outcomes at the time the study was initiated. As you saw, however, that design has distinct limitations. Case-control studies were developed in large part to overcome the limitation of cohort studies with respect to rare outcomes. How can one study rare outcomes, when prospective designs simply will not work well?

The answer to this very logical question is that one must first look for the outcomes of interest and then check back in time to see the antecedent exposures (exposures that took place prior to the outcome). Then diseased persons can be compared to nondiseased with respect to the exposure of interest. So case-control studies work in the same way as cohort studies and randomized controlled trials—but in reverse! Instead of looking at disease among the exposed and nonexposed, we are now looking at exposures among the diseased and nondiseased. This elegant study design overcomes the problem cohort studies have of being able to only look at diseases without long induction periods, rare outcomes, and costly expenditure of resources while waiting for outcomes to occur. With case-control studies we find people who are diseased, find similar counterparts who are not diseased, and look backward in time to see if they were exposed or unexposed to the exposure of interest.

Case-Control Studies

In some ways, the answer to the question of how to conduct this type of study could be phrased as, "Easier said than done." Conceptually, it is not difficult. Find cases (the diseased individuals), and find similar controls (nondiseased individuals) who are so similar that if they were cases they would have been found in your study as cases, and compare their exposure status.

But what does this assume?

1. There is a good way to find cases.
2. There is a good way to find controls. In addition, these controls must be those that *would have* been identified as cases in your study. This means that the controls are a subset of your population that actually gives rise to your cases.
3. All the exposure information required was systematically maintained at the time the exposure under study took place, and these data are of sufficient detail to describe the exposure.

Many times, these assumptions are met and important case-control studies can be conducted. But the trick is to be careful in designing case-control studies in order to minimize the problems that result when these assumptions are not met.

There are many excellent resources that provide detailed instruction on how to conduct case-control studies. The purpose of this text is not to recreate those, but rather to discuss how various designs are used in infectious disease epidemiology, and to provide the introductory reader with enough information to understand other available resources. As it happens, case-control studies are a frequently used approach within outbreak investigations, because the data required are retrospective, meaning that there is little or no waiting time for information to accrue. That means that public health action can generally be implemented earlier rather than later, an important facet of study design selection when urgent public health problems exist. Figure 9-1 shows an example of a straightforward subject for a case-control study. For this example, we will consider a design that might be conducted to assess the risk factors for hospital-acquired methicillin-resistant *Staphylococcus aureus* (MRSA).

Suppose there is an outbreak of MRSA at a local hospital, a very serious infection because it is not susceptible to the usual antibiotics, including front line antibiotics such as penicillin G all the way to methicillin, antibiotics that are administered in the hospital. CDC surveillance data from 2006 indicate that there was one case of vancomycin-resistant *S. aureus* that year. Vancomycin may be the only drug left that can be effective against certain resistant strains of bacteria; that we have even one case of this notifiable disease is extremely serious. This is a case where we have "helped" dangerous bacteria; those previously held in check with our arsenal of antibiotics, develop resistance. The hospital's infection con-

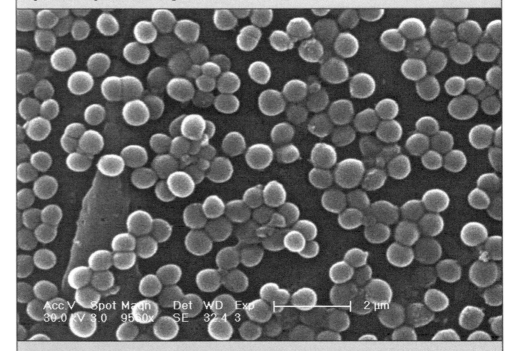

FIGURE 9-1 This 2005 scanning electron micrograph (SEM) depicted numerous clumps of methicillin-resistant *Staphylococcus aureus* bacteria, commonly referred to by the acronym, MRSA; magnified 9560x.

Methicillin-resistant *Staphylococcus aureus* infections, (e.g., bloodstream, pneumonia, bone infections) occur most frequently among persons in hospitals and healthcare facilities, including nursing homes, and dialysis centers. Those who acquire a MRSA infection usually have a weakened immune system. However, the manifestation of MRSA infections that are acquired by otherwise healthy individuals, who have not been recently hospitalized, or had a medical procedure such as dialysis, or surgery, first began to emerge in the mid- to late-1990's. These infections in the community—dubbed community-acquired MRSA or CA-MRSA—are usually manifested as minor skin infections such as pimples and boils but also can manifest as the more severe diseases such as sepsis and pneumonia. Transmission of CA-MRSA has been reported most frequently in certain populations (e.g., children, sports participants, or jail inmates).

Source: CDC/Janice Carr/ Jeff Hageman, M.H.S. 2005. Public Health Image Library.

trol department is concerned about an increase in MRSA infections in the ICU, and needs a study done to identify potential causes of it. A description of the cases is developed, and a small outbreak investigation is performed. The preliminary data suggest that the problem, perhaps, stems from the cleaning of the IV pole equipment, but it is difficult to be sure that this is the problem, or to be sure there are not other problems as well. A case-control study is initiated to expand the findings of the outbreak investigation.

Why not select an alternate method? Our options are somewhat limited. We could use an experimental approach, but that is most useful if we want to observe the effects of an intervention to reduce infections, for example. It is less useful in the exploration of root causes of the increased incidence. A cohort study could be conducted, where patients are classified as either exposed or unexposed based on exposure to a characteristic in the environment. This would be difficult however; what should be considered the exposure? Without a clear picture of the etiology we might have to gather substantially more information than in other designs. We would then need to follow exposed and nonexposed forward in time to assess the proportion developing MSRA in each. As people are generally not tested for this disease at all possible anatomic sites, it would require excess testing, which would be expensive and burdensome to the patient. This leaves only one design that can help us beyond the outbreak investigation: the case-control design.

The first thing to do is to define who we want as our cases; then we identify suitable controls. After that, we can develop means of exposure assessment. In studies such as this example, where the time from exposure (in ICU) to outcome (diagnosis of MRSA) is brief, and records are available, it is relatively easy to do this. However, in other studies, when the exposure may be years or even decades prior to the initiation of the study, exposure assessment will be considerably more difficult than in this example.

As with the outbreak investigation methodology, use of strict case definitions is very important. We saw a similar importance in cohort studies and randomized controlled trials with inclusion and exclusion criteria, paralleling the use of a case definition. Whether they cast a wide or narrow net, being deliberate about who is considered diseased or not and exposed or not, we are able to be sure that we are always comparing apples with apples—or not—as we intend. Failure to know what types of persons are in the study makes it difficult to make comparisons, makes analysis difficult, and makes it hard to know how to generalize findings or how to develop appropriate interventions to reduce risk in the target population.

So, whom do we consider a case? For this example, we will consider as a case anyone who comes back with MRSA diagnosed in a laboratory. Specimens must have been collected from a site that otherwise should have been sterile using the protocol specific to assessing MRSA isolates.

Salmonella Outbreak: Case-Control Example

Recall the example on the salmonella outbreak in alfalfa sprouts discussed in Chapter 4. This is a useful example for case-control studies as well. From 1988 to 1998, there was an outbreak of a particular strain of salmonella, the Mbandaka strain, which increased acutely, and an outbreak investigation was launched. Because of the uniqueness of the strain, a case-control approach was utilized to see whether the disinfection process worked. Cases were operationalized as those with the Mbandaka infection that was laboratory-confirmed taking place between January 1, 1999, and April 15, 1999. Age-matched, population-based controls were identified through telephone numbers similar to case numbers; cases and controls were systematically asked about their sprout consumption and consumption of other foods known to have salmonella during the prior week.[a] Cases who did eat alfalfa sprouts had their food traced back to the source in order to identify the specific sprouts and lot that were consumed. (This is called a trace-back and trace-forward investigation.) Because of the rarity of the strain, it was possible to genetically identify the specific strains. The comparison of cases and controls suggests that the disinfection process was, in fact, effective in reducing disease caused by salmonella. This is a good example of the use of case-control methodology in conjunction with laboratory techniques, outbreak and descriptive epidemiologic methods, and good old-fashioned detective work.

---

[a]The authors indicate that their research from FoodNet showed that approximately 10% of the population in Oregon, where the study was conducted, consumed alfalfa sprouts weekly. If the frequency of consumption was too low, it would have been difficult to compare disinfected sprouts to nondisinfected sprouts: the comparison of interest. In that case, however, it would have been possible to compare sprout consumption vs. no consumption, but that was not the research question of interest.

In this example, these would be incident (new) cases although for other disease processes the use of prevalent (existing) cases might be the only feasible approach. Using incident cases provides a degree of matching with respect to time of development of disease as well as reduction of biases that can emerge from use of prevalent cases. This sort of time matching is important: Secular trends that may have taken place will be controlled for in the design such that they are less likely to confound the study's findings. Use of prevalent cases—particularly for diseases with long induction periods or asymptomatic periods—may cloud our understanding of the relationship between the exposures and outcomes of interest. This usually takes place because prevalent cases that were just diagnosed and those who have had the disease for a length of time. Who should be controls? It is crucial that the control group is selected from among people who *would* have been cases had they (the controls) developed the disease. This means that we are clear about who is in the study sample, and we ensure that the controls are sufficiently similar to the cases. With case-control designs, this is particularly important, even more so than with other designs. Where randomized designs provide that treated and untreated are similar by virtue of chance, and cohort studies provide that both exposed and unexposed need to be followed similarly to see who among all the subjects develop the disease (ideally), case-control studies rely upon design to make the controls similar to cases, except for their disease status; this allows a valid comparison to be made. In this example, a possible control group would be patients with *S. aureus* but without MRSA.[b] This would be useful for two key reasons:

1. These patients all have been worked up for *S. aureus* infection in a similar fashion, and would all have had the same laboratory diagnostic activities conducted.
2. The controls, those who ultimately had non-resistant *S. aureus*, are those who give rise to the cases. That is, they were worked up the same, asked to have the same diagnostic testing, and likely had similar referral patterns into the hospital, comparably serious health conditions, similar insurance payors, and so on. In some cases, it will be important to match cases to controls on the basis of age, gender, race, disease type, or date of diagnosis. Matching is a means of controlling for confounding and helping to hone in on the differences that are associated with cases being cases. Depending on design, though, matching can be detrimental. It can make cases appear too much like controls ("overmatching")—so much so,

that there are no obvious differences between them, and the controls look like the cases even when they are, in fact, very different with regard to their exposure distributions. Matching also makes it impossible to assess the variable on which you have matched, in association with the outcome of interest. This makes sense: if you match cases and controls on, for example, gender, all the cases and all the controls will be in sets based on gender. This will mean that looking for differences in the distribution of disease by gender will not be possible. Specific types of analysis (such as conditional logistic regression) are needed in order to analyze matched case-control studies. Although this is not necessarily a limitation, it is something to be mindful of when planning one's study (and one of the many important reasons why involving a biostatistician during the study design process is vital). Matching with respect to time does not present quite the same issues, and is a useful technique in many cases.

Control selection is often much more complicated than development of a suitable case definition and case selection. Controls may derive from several sources, each with its own strengths and limitations.

Population-Based Controls

Population-based controls are those that are drawn not from existing comparison groups, or the study base itself, but are drawn from the healthy population at large. Population-based controls may be identified through a variety of sampling schemes, including population-based lists. These lists include things such as voter registration lists, drivers license listings, telephone directories, and others—with the key being that the sampling frame (the list from which the controls are selected) must be the same population that gave rise to the cases in the study. This is important. If cases derive from a national sample, and controls are from only a county-wide listing, then the cases would not be reflective of the controls. Once a sampling frame is selected, a random sampling procedure most suitable to the population source is selected, and information from each member of the sample of that population contacted is ascertained.

One method that is very common for sampling the population as controls is random-digit dialing, but door-to-door interviewing and mailed interviews are other potential methods. One strength of the population-based control is that if done properly, it may be most likely to truly represent the underlying population base that gave rise to the cases, though it takes a great deal of work to develop a population-based con-

---

[b]The referent needs to change with the research question. For example, if we were comparing hospital-acquired MRSA to community-acquired MRSA, then the latter could be the control group.

trol that does this. This is because of the inherent limitations in any sampling frame—not necessarily in the design itself. For example, with telephone sample strategies, many people may not have telephones, introducing bias into the control group selection. Cell phones present another problem, as more and more individuals have cell phones and not landlines. Cell phones are difficult because people frequently move without changing their cell phone number, thus the number may seem to reflect one geographic area when in fact it is another, or the number itself may have changed hands. Phone numbers may also be disconnected or belong to businesses instead of individuals. Although there are sophisticated methods available to overcome these problems, they create limitations in the random-digit dialing approach.

Another problem with the population-based control is the problem of the healthy worker effect. Because people at home are more likely than others to be unhealthy—people who work tend to be healthier than those who do not—this bias can result in the unfortunate finding that the "sick" people (the cases) are actually healthier than the controls. This bias is an important one that can make studies with population-based controls a little more difficult to interpret at times.

Finally, obtaining accurate exposure, outcome, and confounder histories from persons in the population can be difficult. Especially when people are not sick, it is hard for them to remember what they were exposed to or experienced. This is the flip side of recall bias: when people are healthy, their ability to recall exposures is logically reduced. They feel healthy; so why would they recall exposures when nothing is anchoring them to the time in the same way that something may be for cases? What makes them inclined to participate in data collection?

These are some of the limitations in this approach, though population-based sampling for controls has an important role in case-control research.

Hospital- or Clinic-Based Controls

Hospital-based controls are selected from the hospitals where the cases are most common. Sometimes they may be selected from a consortium of hospitals depending on the research question under study and referral patterns underlying the hospitals. This type of control overcomes many, though not all, of the limitations seen in the population-based controls while adding its own limitations. Here we find controls that are similar to the cases—at the same facility, maybe there for a disease or procedure similar to the cases—in their overall characteristics. Controls may resemble cases with regard to many characteristics; but the point is to classify them with respect to disease and then to assess what each subject had as an exposure

or exposures. Individuals seen at the same facility and who are similarly unhealthy generally derive from the same source population (demographic, behavioral, and clinical characteristics) as the cases. Most importantly, these are the individuals *who made it to care*—like the cases.[c] This levels the playing field as far as circumstances that lead up to seeking/being able to seek care, making the controls similar to the cases. Because they are at the facility for a health-related concern or procedure, they are more like cases with regard to their ability to remember exposures of interest when compared to a population-based control. This type of control is easy to identify and takes fewer resources to collect data on than other types of controls.

Hospital- and clinic-based control groups represent the tip of the iceberg, as do cases in a case control study: they are the individuals who can and do access care, making them different from individuals who cannot and do not access care. In addition, people seen in hospitals and clinics are necessarily different from those who are not (this is called Berkson's bias, and will be discussed in Chapter 11e), which may make results more difficult to generalize.

Friend or Family Controls and Dead Controls

Friend, family, and dead controls are when individuals closest to the cases (but obviously without the disease or condition of interest) are used as the controls. In general, these types of control groups are fraught with hazards. Use of family members or friends of cases can sometimes be useful if the characteristics of the cases make them especially hard to find a suitable control. However, such controls may be *too* similar to that of cases, obscuring identification of exposures that differ between them. In addition, especially in areas of sensitive research such as drug use, STDs, HIV, and others, this type of control may be unwilling to disclose exposures for fear of stigma or loss of social and family support. Use of dead controls usually entails interviewing surviving relatives to find out exposure information.

Limitations of this type of control are chiefly that people cannot usually answer very accurately for someone else, even if they were close. Crucial information may not be known by

---

[c]The problem of the tertiary referral center can sometimes present itself. As multiple types of care delivery systems are becoming more common, this problem has increased. For example, imagine a hospital that has an internal medicine practice that serves primarily the neighborhood, but a renowned burn unit that is used throughout the region. In a case-control study of cutaneous infections following burns, the use of controls from the internal medicine practice would not be perfect. The patients in the burn unit, the cases, are being referred from all over the region, so the controls do not represent the base population from which the cases were derived. Patients being seen in the neighborhood clinic are from the neighborhood, and likely have different insurance payors than those in the burn unit. The referral source for these two populations is very different. In this case, bias can result.

the proxy or, for a multitude of reasons including social desirability, may not be disclosed. In addition, this sort of control is not thought to be from the same base population that gave rise to the cases. This makes sense: for whatever reason the case may have died. He or she is clearly very different from another case that survived. These types of control groups are not usually used in infectious disease epidemiology.

How to Conduct a Case-Control Study

Once the cases and controls are identified, and informed consent is obtained, the status of cases must be confirmed using the case definition and inclusion/exclusion criteria developed for the study. Figure 9-2 shows a graphic representation of what is going to happen. The steps learned with all other study designs discussed so far—development of case definitions, inclusion/exclusion criteria, interfacing with the IRB, obtaining consent, and so forth—are all operational with this design as well.

For example, if *E. coli* is the outcome of interest, lab diagnostic identification needs to be conducted on specimens to substantiate that that is the correct diagnosis. It is also possible to use symptom-based case definitions; these may be used with good success, if they are well-operationalized and strictly adhered to. Still, biomarkers, pathology, laboratory, and objective diagnostic testing are best for in defining case status. Then data on antecedent exposures (exposures that predate the outcomes) of interest and potential confounders are collected. Like all epidemiologic studies, systematic data collection is crucial. Case report forms need to be developed to ensure that study staff collect information from data sources in a systematic fashion or ask participants about their experiences systematically. Like every part of science and epidemiology, the methods count! If information is collected haphazardly, it will not be useful in identifying the associations between exposures and outcomes.

By sheer influence of the interviewers or abstractors the resulting bias may lead to incorrect conclusions. Use of a systematic process for collecting data on exposures, outcomes, and confounders—for all study designs—is necessary.

One way to reduce bias in case-control studies is the use of blinding. Interviewers and data abstractors should be blinded to disease and exposure status whenever possible. This may not always be feasible, particularly with a small staff or limited resources. Still, one may be able to be creative in pursuit of this goal. For example, imagine a case-control study following an outbreak investigation. If only two field workers are available to assess the exposure status of patients who were exposed to foods at a buffet, it may be possible for one person to conduct the interview with the participant regarding disease and one regarding exposure (food line item assessment). This would reduce the impact of the interviewer's knowledge of the participant's disease status on the assessment of the exposure. Because the exposure and disease determinations are being collected simultaneously, it is even more important to reduce bias in case-control studies than in cohort studies. Why? In the case-control studies, we are collecting information on both axes at approximately the same time. In the cohort studies, we are collecting information about the exposure *prior to* the occurrence of the outcome. This temporal difference makes it more likely in case-control than cohort studies that the field worker's or participant's perception of one axis could influence that of the other. Although it is always important to reduce bias, this type of bias is more common in case-control studies than in the previously mentioned designs.

Strengths and Limitations

Case-control studies offer an enormous amount of "bang for one's buck." But they are not without limitations. Case-control studies are more prone than other designs to recall bias (to be discussed in depth in Chapter 11). Recall bias is when people who are cases are more likely to remember their exposures than those who are noncases. This is usually because the fact of being ill creates a heightened awareness of exposure either at the time of the exposure or later on, when one is recalling exposures as they are being asked. Another limitation in case-control studies is identifying a suitable control population from which to sample, as well as overcoming the specific limitations of each control type. For infectious disease

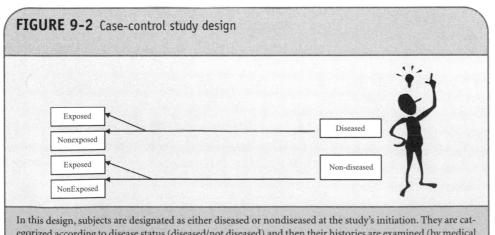

FIGURE 9-2 Case-control study design

In this design, subjects are designated as either diseased or nondiseased at the study's initiation. They are categorized according to disease status (diseased/not diseased) and then their histories are examined (by medical record, self-report, or sometimes laboratory-based or other tests) to identify antecedent exposures (exposed/not exposed).

epidemiology, case-control studies are frequently a useful adjunct to outbreak investigations, because they provide an analytic "look" at the data, and an analysis comparing cases and controls with regard to the distribution of exposures in each. But the strengths of this design are compelling. Case-control studies are generally the best design for assessing rare outcomes. For any given outcome, multiple exposures can be explored, making this design efficient. By using cases that are identified already, there is no need to follow a large cohort only to find a few cases of the disease of interest. Case-control studies are generally conducted using information that is already available, though the information can be collected in real-time, making them more resource-friendly than their long-term cohort counterparts. When little is known about a given disease—for example, an emerging infectious disease—case-control methods can be ideal. They are similarly useful when evaluating diseases with long induction and latent periods, such as HIV/AIDS or cancers with infectious etiologies, and those diseases whose exposure-disease relationships we do not understand very well.

CROSS-SECTIONAL STUDIES

Cross-sectional studies cover a range of territory, and represent an important method for epidemiologists. This design includes one most people are already fairly familiar, taken most often in the form of surveys. Figure 9-3 shows a graphic representation of what is going to happen.

Have you even been approached in the market to complete a questionnaire regarding satisfaction with the store's offerings? Have you ever been asked about your political opinion in a phone survey? These are both examples of cross-sectional studies in which the key instrumentation is a questionnaire. Cross-sectional studies, however, are often much more complex than this, and can be helpful by collecting large amounts of data that can be described with regard to person, place, and

Thinking Outside the Box: Using Case-Control Studies to Identify Risk Factors Following an Outbreak

We usually think of hepatitis B as a sexually transmitted disease, and one associated with injection drug use. Residents of nursing homes are not the "usual suspects" when it comes to hepatitis B virus (HBV). But just because we do not think of it as a prime suspect, does not mean that it should not be on our radar. With infectious diseases, one must be ready to think outside the box and examine evidence in order to draw conclusions that can result in positive public health impact.

At a nursing facility in Germany,[2] an outbreak of hepatitis B resulted from the process of routine glucose (sugar) monitoring. Not knowing the cause, however, a case-control study was undertaken using the 17 cases with a genetically linked virus. All of the 188 residents of the facility were systematically tested serologically for hepatitis B in order to identify the 17 selected as cases due to their similarity in viral identity. Controls were those individuals who were without any sign of acute or past infection, who were neither confirmed nor probable cases, and who were susceptible for HBV infection. All subjects had to live in a particular ward of the nursing home during a particular window of time. Cases and controls were sampled in an approximately 2:1 (controls:cases) fashion, but with only 26 individuals meeting control criteria.

There were two types of cases, confirmed and probable. Confirmed cases were those positive for hepatitis B surface antigen (HbsAg) and with a DNA sequence indistinguishable from the implicated HBV strain. Probable cases were those residents negative for HBsAg, but positive for a marker of recent infection (anti-HBc-IgM), and without HBV DNA sequence data.

This study indicated that after adjusting for diabetes status and practitioner taking sample, there was an odds ratio (OR) of 8.5 (95% CI 1.49–49.71, $p = 0.017$). As you will learn in Chapter 10, this suggests the following: after taking into account the diabetes status of the patient and the practitioner who took the specimen, given a resident had hepatitis B, he or she was 8.5 times as likely as a resident without hepatitis B to have been exposed to blood glucose monitoring on a specific day.[d] As a result of this study, more attention was paid to the glucose monitoring procedures at the nursing home. The multi-use alcohol dispenser that was shared by all patients during glucose monitoring was reevaluated, only people truly needing glucose monitoring were screened, and more attention was paid to infection control methods including use of disposable gloves.

---

[d]The 95% CI indicates that if similar repeated samples were taken of the same population, the population estimate of the OR would fall in the range from 1.49 to 49.17; this one may or may not. This finding was statistically significant, as indicated by the CI not crossing the null value, 1.0, and also the p-value is less than the stated level of alpha, 0.05.One may wonder why the CI is so big: from 1.49 to 49.71 is a very large range. This suggests that the sample size was very small. Still, having reached statistical significance, power is not an issue here. Power is only an issue when there is no significant finding. Power is the ability to see a difference if one exists. Here we achieved statistical significance and we see that a difference does exist, though the magnitude of that difference is not well discerned. Future studies could use this information to generate sample size calculations, should they be required.

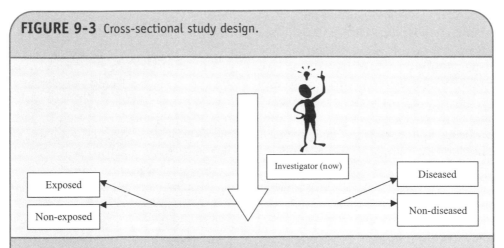

FIGURE 9-3 Cross-sectional study design.

In this design, subjects are designated either diseased or nondiseased all at one exact moment. They are categorized according to disease status (diseased/not diseased) and then their histories are examined (by medical record, self-report, or sometimes laboratory-based or other tests) to identify antecedent exposures (exposed/not exposed) if the researcher opts for the case-control approach. A cohort approach may also be taken, looking at the proportion of diseased among exposed vs. not-exposed.

Measuring Disease Trends Over Time Using Prevalence Estimates and Serial Cross-Sectional Studies

The bacterial disease *Chlamydia trachomatis* is a sexually transmitted infection, the most common nonviral sexually transmitted infection in the United States.[3–7] Chlamydia has been associated with pelvic inflammatory disease, infertility, and ectopic pregnancy among women, with sequelae increasing with repeat infections. The disease is especially common among adolescent women. Unfortunately, the prevalence of repeat infections is very high,[3,5–8] particularly among women, due to their frequently asymptomatic state. A reportable disease, surveillance is essential to monitor trends in disease throughout the country. However, surveillance for this disease is often passive, and may not be able to accurately identify smaller trends in disease. So how can we assess changes over time?

One way is to examine the prevalence in similar populations over a period of time, using serial cross-sectional studies of prevalence. Although prevalence is generally a less informative measure than incidence, when taken using the same methodology over repeated periods of time, it can be very useful.

For example, one study compared baseline screenings for chlamydial infection for women entering the National Job Training Program from 1998 to 2004.[6] Because all women were screened for chlamydia in a consistent fashion upon entry into the program, and the women were only screened once each for entry, estimates from this serial cross-sectional are very informative. Data from this study demonstrated a statistically significant decrease in the disease's prevalence among women 16 to 24 years of age entering the program: From 1998 to 2003 there was a decrease from 11.7% to 10.0% prevalence at baseline, followed by a slight increase in 2004 to 10.3%.

A similar approach was used by Ghys and colleagues to evaluate the effectiveness of an intervention to reduce sex workers' risk of HIV.[9,10] The purpose of this study was to assess behavioral and demographic characteristics in a clinic-based sample of female sex workers in Abidjan, Cote d'Ivoire. The intervention was designed to improve condom use and ultimately reduce transmission of HIV. To evaluate behavioral characteristics associated with the intervention, a serial cross-sectional approach was used. Between 1991 and 1998, community-based surveys were conducted to assess self-reported condom use. Although the women being tested in the clinic for HIV and other STDs were not necessarily the same as those being interviewed, the study provides insight into a population-based estimate of condom use over time, and trends possibly associated with the campaign. This study conceptually links the independent variable (the program) and the outcome (HIV prevalence), though because it compares aggregate values and not individual-level data (i.e., independent and dependent in the same person), it is difficult to link the two; the ecologic fallacy comes into play here. Still, this is an excellent example of how to use serial cross-sectional data to inform ourselves about trends over time.

time, and by generating hypotheses or conducting analytic studies on them to clarify relationships between exposures and outcomes.

The hallmark of a cross-sectional study is that the exposure and outcome data are collected at one time point. There is not more than one time point collected in a cross-sectional study, even though information about the past may be queried. This is often referred to as a "snapshot" study, offering one cross-section in time rather than multiple timepoints. Cross-sectional studies can be surveys, secondary data analyses of existing datasets, primary data collection of medical data, or other methods to investigate a research question at one point in time.

The most detailed cross-sectional studies can look quite different from their relaxed cross-sectional cousin, the non-random convenience sample. Take, for example, the National Health and Nutrition Examination Survey (NHANES).[11] This study uses a sophisticated random sampling technique such that it is representative of the U.S. population. Participants spend a number of hours having an extensive physical examination, with in-person measurements; extensive behavioral questionnaires; dental, visual, blood, and cardiovascular tests; food recall; and other examinations. It offers one of the most comprehensive evaluations of the heath of the U.S. population. This is very different from, say a convenience sample. A convenience sample is one composed of individuals who are in a specific location at the time of sampling; it is a nonrepresentative sampling approach. Still, this approach is valuable when observing behaviors or utilization of care services. Another way they can be used is to assess individuals about their knowledge, attitudes, and perceptions, or any types of behavior or other self-report mechanisms, risk categories, based in a clinician's office. They are different in their depth and their ability to answer public health questions. However, both are very useful, even if they serve different functions. A detailed study with precise measurements and sampling such as NHANES provides important information about the population. An attitude assessment based on a convenience sample can help generate hypotheses and help researchers understand more about the clinic population that is sampled. Both are important adjuncts to public health as well as to developing hypotheses for future studies.

How to Conduct a Cross-Sectional Study

It is difficult to summarize a generic method required to conduct a cross-sectional study because they vary quite dramatically with the specific aims of the study and the methods selected. For all types, however, the basic tenets discussed prevail: use solid case definitions, well-justified sampling schemes, systematic data collection, and blinding of study staff where appropriate and feasible. For all studies, it is necessary to collect detailed information on confounders, and potential confounders, at the point of primary data collection. This is even more important in cross-sectional than in other designs (though it is, of course, also important there) because it is unlikely if not impossible to have a second chance to ask the participant to provide data on confounders of interest. One must get all the information at the point of contact with the client or the data source; otherwise, it will be missing data and important questions and relationships may be missed.

Strengths and Limitations

Despite their limitations, cross-sectional studies make a highly valuable contribution to epidemiologic research. In infectious disease epidemiology, they can help us understand a variety of issues as well as generate hypotheses to stimulate future research. One of this design's strengths is that cross-sectional studies can be analyzed like the cohort study—in which the proportion of diseased among the exposed is compared to the proportion of diseased among the nonexposed—or like the case-control, in which the proportion of exposed among the diseased is compared to the proportion of exposed among the nondiseased. But unlike the experimental, cohort, and case-control designs, it is generally very difficult, if not impossible, to assess incident cases in a cross-sectional study. Because they are a snapshot in time, usually only prevalent cases may be assessed. In addition, it is very hard to establish temporal sequencing between exposure and disease, because information is being gathered at the very same snapshot. Accurate recollection of exposure and disease information may be very difficult for participants taking surveys, which may create a weighting towards accurate exposure and outcome classification among those more recently exposed or more recently ill. Finally, although cross-sectional studies can be inexpensive (and for the most part are less expensive when compared to case-control studies, and certainly cohorts and randomized controlled trials), that does not mean they are cheap. Conducting any study demands resources—field staff, data managers and analysts, supervisors, paper for instrumentation, telephone banks, and so on. Nonetheless, this is a useful and accessible methodology for answering questions about infectious diseases, including risk factors, etiologies, knowledge, attitudes, and behaviors.

This chapter provided the nuts and bolts, as well as conceptual underpinnings for two of the cornerstone epidemiologic designs as applied to infectious disease. As we have seen, these are directly based upon randomized controlled trials and, in turn, cohort studies. The broad strokes as shown in this chapter applied to an infectious disease context will hopefully increase your ability to read studies and later, using your newly developed intuitive understanding of design, participate in them.

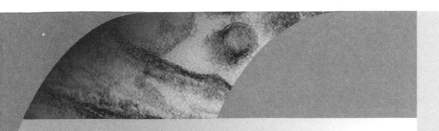

Discussion Questions

1. Imagine you have a case-control study and a cross-sectional study both designed to assess the association between ectopic pregnancy and *Chlamydia trachomatis*.
   a. Compare and contrast the study designs.
   b. Which would be the preferable study design, and why?
   c. What are the relative strengths and limitations of each of these designs in studying this association?

2. You would like to conduct a case-control study of people exposed to *S. aureus* enterotoxin after a food-borne outbreak following a large political function that was catered.
   a. Design the study.
   b. What is your control group? What are its relative strengths and limitations?
   c. Now design this as a cohort study. What would you need in order to be able to do that? Which design do you think would be stronger in its ability to assess the association between the exposure and gastrointestinal symptoms, and why?

REFERENCES

1. Gill C, Keene W, Mohle-Boetani JE, et al. Alfalfa seed decontamination in a salmonella outbreak. *Emerg Infect Dis.* 2003;9(4). Available at: www.cdc.gov/nicdod/EID/vol9no4/02-0519.htm. Accessed December 25, 2006.

2. Dreesnab JM, Baillot A, Hamschmidt L, et al. Outbreak of hepatitis B in a nursing home associated with capillary blood sampling. *Epidemiol Infect.* 2003;134:1102–1113.

3. Fortenberry J, Brizendine E, Katz B. Subsequent sexually transmitted infections among adolescent women with genital infection due to Chlamydia trachomatis, Neisseria gonorrhoeae, or Trichomonas vaginalis. *Sex Transm Dis.* 1999;26:26–32.

4. Magnus M, Clark R, Myers L, et al. Trichomonas vaginalis among HIV-infected women: are immune status or protease inhibitor use associated with subsequent T. vaginalis positivity? *Sex Transm Dis.* 2003;30(11):839–843.

5. Schillinger J, Kissinger P, Calvet H, et al. Patient-delivered partner treatment with azithromycin to prevent repeated Chlamydia trachomatis infection among women: a randomized, controlled trial. *Sex Transm Dis.* 2003;30:49–56.

6. Joesoef MR, Mosure DJ. Prevalence trends in chlamydial infections among young women entering the national job training program, 1998–2004. *Sex Transm Dis.* 2006;33(9):571–575.

7. Magnus M, Schillinger JA, Fortenberry JD, et al. Partner age not associated with recurrent Chlamydia trachomatis infection, condom use, or partner treatment and referral among adolescent women. *J Adolesc Health.* 2006;39(3):396–403.

8. Centers for Disease Control/Department of Health and Human Services. *Sexually Transmitted Disease Surveillance, 2002.* 2003;Atlanta, GA.

9. Ghys P, Fransen K, Diallo MO, et al. The associations between cervicovaginal HIV shedding, sexually transmitted diseases and immunosuppression in female sex workers in Abidjan, Cote d'Ivoire. *AIDS.* 1997;11:F85–F93.

10. Ghys PD, Dialloa MO, Ettiegne-Traore V, et al. Increase in condom use and decline in HIV and sexually transmitted diseases among female sex workers in Abidjan, Cote d'Ivoire, 1991 to 1998. *AIDS.* 2002;16:251–258.

11. National Center for Health Statistics. *National Health and Nutrition Examination Survey (NHANES).* Available at: www.cdc.gov/nchs. Accessed December 1, 2006.

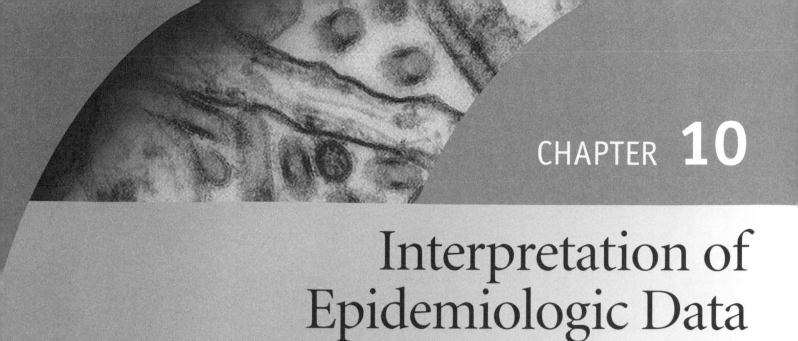

Interpretation of Epidemiologic Data

The purpose of this chapter is to give you a framework for understanding the basic analyses that can be conducted with data from analytic epidemiologic studies and that is useful for the reading of scientific literature. This chapter will not make you a statistician or provide advanced techniques for analyzing epidemiologic data. There are many, many excellent resources—from epidemiologic to biostatistical texts—available to assist the reader in learning how to analyze epidemiologic data. This is an introduction to facilitate your ability to understand how information is extracted from the study design methods discussed. Additional study is recommended in order to be able to fully analyze and interpret data.

Before moving on, I want to make sure you have the basic study designs down and that you can identify each one if you see it (as well as be able to create one appropriately if asked to do so). Table 10-1 is a study design, "cheat sheet," designed to make it easier for you to identify the correct study design and measure of association when you are presented with a specific study.

Decide three things and then follow the row across to lead you to the correct design and measure to use. The three questions are:

1. How is the study categorized? Is it categorized based on exposure or outcome? Because these two are mutually exclusive, it can be only one choice, and this simplifies this step.
2. How do participants come to choose one treatment or condition over another: Is it by design as in a process or randomization? Or do they self-select it in some fashion?[a]
3. In which direction is the study conducted? Where do you as the investigator stand in relation to the exposure and the outcome?

MEET THE 2×2 TABLE

The first order of business is to introduce you to the 2×2 table. Using this basic tool—this simplest of constructions—we are able to convey a wealth of information about our data. As you have no doubt already recognized, most of what we are talking about concerns categorical data, items that must be catego-

[a] Again, it is not that an individual would wish to self-select anything harmful. This term refers to the ability of multiple factors to come into play for each moment, exposure, and outcome. Because things are so interrelated, it is very difficult to look at an exposure as independent from other features, and this is what the statement means. Thus a person's educational level is generally a reflection of many forces (family, income, living area, awareness, past family members in college, etc.). This term is used to differentiate it from the randomization process, which is conducted based on chance alone, without any individual- or provider-level characteristics entering the decision-making process.

TABLE 10-1 Study Designs at a Glance

Categorization based on:	Exposure of interest is:	Direction	Design type	Measure of association*
Exposure	Randomly assigned by study	Prospective; follow forward in time for outcomes of interest.	Randomized controlled trial	Relative risk (RR)
Exposure	Self-selected by participant	Prospective; follow forward in time for outcomes of interset.	Concurrent cohort (aka prospective cohort)	Relative risk (RR)
Exposure	Self-selected by participant	Retrospective; both exposures *and* outcomes have occurred at the time the study starts; however, at the time of the exposure, the outcome has NOT yet occurred.	Non-concurrent cohort (aka retrospective cohort)	Relative risk (RR)
Disease	Self-selected by participant	Retrospective; both exposures *and* outcomes have occurred at the time the study starts; in almost every case, at the time of the exposure assessment, the outcome HAS already occurred.	Case-control	Odds ratio (OR)
Disease	Self-selected by participant	Snapshot; data on exposure and outcome collected simultaneously. Exposure assessment may inquire about temporal sequence, but no additional timepoint data are available.	Cross-sectional	Prevalence odds ratio (POR)
Exposure	Self-selected by participant	Snapshot; data on exposure and outcome collected simultaneously. Exposure assessment can inquire about temporal sequence, but no additional timepoint data are available.	Cross-sectional	Prevalence Ratio (PR)

Depending on analysis, other measures may also be used. These come from the 2×2 table, however.

rized. We have not talked much about continuous data, information for which there is always a number in between to be considered. For example, with heights, one could be 48 inches or 49 inches, or any fraction of an inch in between: 48.1, 48.15, 48.155, and so forth. This is opposed to categorical data. With the basic epidemiologic toolkit, we are involved most heartily with questions whose answers fall soundly in one category or another; that is categorical data: diseased/not diseased, exposed/not exposed, smoker/nonsmoker, male/female, high/medium/low exposure. We have not talked much about continuous data, like ages, weights, exposure gradients, or biomarkers like blood levels of a substance. All of these are, of course, perfectly valid ways of investigating infectious etiologies, and as you advance in the field you will begin using both categorical and continuous data in different ways, to refine your understanding of relationships between etiologies and disease. It just happens that for the purposes of the epidemiologic designs covered here we focus on categorical data, and so that is where we begin as well. We create categories even out of continuous data when there are natural cut points to help us understand phenomena. There are limitations to this approach at times, but they are more detailed than this discussion warrants.

The 2×2 table, also known as a contingency table, is simply a depiction of information in a specific format that facilitates analysis and understanding. To create one, you take the line listings that you often will have available from raw data and turn them into counts. Once counted, the numbers go in the appropriate cells. For example, imagine you are conducting a cohort study of persons living with TB-positive partners. Your exposure of interest is whether the partners were adherent to recommended prophylaxis regimens, and the outcome is a reactive PPD (pure protein derivative, a TB screening test) of >5 mm induration within one year of diagnosis of partner's TB. All of this information may be summarized within the powerful 2×2 table, by taking the individual lines of data, counting them, and turning them into the cell counts. If you have 200 partners, 100 exposed and 100 not exposed to prophylaxis, their line item data for the exposure and the outcomes might take any one of the combinations shown in Table 10-2.

Participant 001 was neither exposed nor reactive, participant 002 was not exposed but was reactive, participant 003 was exposed but not reactive, and participant 004 was both exposed and reactive. This sort of line item could go on to describe all 200 participants in the study. More likely the database might look like Table 10-3, with additional information collected on confounders and other predictors of interest. This information, when counted, could be inserted into our 2×2 table, as shown in Table 10-4.

In this one nice, neat box we describe the total experiences with regard to exposure and outcome for 200 study participants. Powerful! Note that this will not work for continuous data; other statistical tests and methods of data presentation are required for that. In addition, this does not tell the whole story. Additional analyses that are beyond the scope of this text would be necessary to assess the independent contribution of predictors and confounders to the outcome when adjusting for all other effects or to look at confounding or interaction (effect modification), which are fundamental to evaluate and understand.

Another example: if we took John Snow's cholera outbreak from London, and put the information in a 2×2 table, we would have what's in Table 10-5. All of this information may be made more general and applied to other studies using the notation shown in Table 10-6.

The following measures of association will enable you to analyze basic infectious disease epidemiology data yourself and to understand literature when you read it. They also form the conceptual underpinnings for those who opt to go further in their studies of epidemiology.

THE RELATIVE RISK

The relative risk (RR) is one of the most intuitive measures in epidemiology. It is used to describe outcomes associated with predictors (exposures) evaluated in randomized controlled trials and cohort studies (both retrospective and prospective). Think of the 2×2 table again but instead of seeing notation, see what each cell represents conceptually, as in Table 10-7.

To see the whole scenario, first we develop our research question, our null and alternative hypotheses, and then calculate and interpret the measure of association for this study.

The two-sided research question is, are partners of TB-positive persons who take TB prophylaxis as likely to have a reactive PPD within one year of the partner's diagnosis as those who do not?

The two-sided null hypothesis is,

H_o: There is no association between receipt of TB prophylaxis among partners of TB-positive individuals and development of a reactive PPD within one year of the partner's diagnosis

---

TABLE 10-2 Sample Data Listing

ID number	Prophylaxis 0=no; 1=yes	Reactive PPD (>5 mm)[1] 0=no; 1=yes
001	0	0
002	0	1
003	1	0
004	1	1
...	...	...
200	1	0

[1]Data would also be maintained on the size of the induration, as that would be useful as well. However, positivity is being operationalized as >5 mm in this study.

TABLE 10-3 Sample Data Listing, with More Variables Listed

ID number	Prophylaxis 0=no; 1=yes	Reactive PPD 0=no; 1=yes	Smoker 0=no; 1=yes	HIV status 0=-; 1=+	Gender 0=M; 1=F	Age Continuous
001	0	0	0	0	1	29
002	0	1	0	1	1	23
003	1	0	0	0	0	54
004	1	1	1	0	1	35
...	...	...	...	...	...	...
200	1	0	0	1	0	43

Or

the rate of reactive PPDs among partners who take TB prophylaxis = the rate of reactive PPDs among partners who do not take TB prophylaxis.

H_A: There is an association between receipt of TB prophylaxis among partners of TB-positive individuals and development of a reactive PPD within one year of the partner's diagnosis

TABLE 10-4 2×2 Table Portraying These Data

	Reactive PPD	Non-reactive PPD	Total
Prophylaxis	22	78	100
No prophylaxis	45	55	100
Total	67	133	200

or

the rate of reactive PPDs among partners who take TB prophylaxis ≠ the rate of reactive PPDs among partners who do not take TB prophylaxis.

The one-sided research question is, are partners of TB-positive persons who take TB prophylaxis less likely to have a reactive PPD within one year of the partner's diagnosis than those do are not?

The one-sided null hypothesis is,

H_o: TB prophylaxis among partners of TB-positive individuals is associated with equal or increased development of a reactive PPD within one year of the partner's diagnosis

or

the rate of reactive PPDs among partners who take TB prophylaxis are equal to or greater the rate of reactive PPDs among partners who do not take TB prophylaxis, within one year of the partner's diagnosis.

H_a: TB prophylaxis among partners of TB-positive individuals is associated with lower rates of development of a reactive PPD within one year of the partner's diagnosis

TABLE 10-5 Example of the 2×2 Table Snow Conceptualized

	Cholera	No cholera
Southwark and Vauxhall Company (exposed)	Diseased and not exposed	Not diseased and not exposed
Lambeth Company (not exposed)	Diseased and exposed	Not diseased and not exposed

Table 10-6 General 2×2 Table Notation

	Diseased	Not diseased	Total
Exposed	a	b	a+b
Not exposed	c	d	c+d
Total	a+c	b+d	a+b+c+d

TABLE 10-7 Relative Risk 2×2 Table

	Reactive PPD	Non-reactive PPD	Total
Prophylaxis	The people who took the medicine and had a reactive PPD	The people who took the medicine and had a non-reactive PPD	Of the total, the people who were exposed to the medicine
No prophylaxis	The people who did not take the medicine and had a reactive PPD	The people who did not take the medicine and had a non-reactive PPD	Of the total, the people who were not exposed to the medicine
Total	Of the total, the people who had a reactive PPD	Of the total, the people who had a non-reactive PPD	All of the participants

or

the rate of reactive PPDs among partners who take TB prophylaxis are less than the rate of reactive PPDs among partners who do not take TB prophylaxis, within one year of the partner's diagnosis.

What we are hoping to do now is to compare the proportion of exposed participants who became reactive to the proportion of nonexposed participants who became reactive. This will give us the full picture about how the exposure is associated with the outcome. Note that I did *not* say "causes" the reactive PPD. The only information that we are able to determine from an observational study is whether characteristics are associated with each other, and whether this association is likely to be due to a true association or observed due to chance. We do not know from this type of study design whether one thing is responsible for the occurrence of another; most of the time it may be difficult even to determine what happened first. To

do this using our 2×2 table is now intuitive. We just need to take the steps shown in Table 10-8 and then compare these two groups, exposed and nonexposed, to see how they differ with respect to development of disease. So what do we have? We have our relative risk (RR). (This makes sense, because it looks at risk in one group as compared to that in another. It is not an absolute risk, but a relative one.)

$$\text{Relative risk (RR)} = \frac{\text{the people who took the medicine and had a reactive PPD} \div \text{the total number of people who were exposed to the medicine}}{\text{the people who did not take the medicine and had a reactive PPD} \div \text{the total number of people who were not exposed to the medicine}}$$

This may be generalized more simply to:

$$RR = [a/(a + b)] / [c/(c + d)]$$

TABLE 10-8 Relative Risk 2×2 Table—Conceptual

	Reactive PPD	Non-reactive PPD	Total
Prophylaxis	The people who took the medicine and had a reactive PPD	⟹	As a proportion of the total, the people who were exposed to the medicine
No prophylaxis	The people who did not take the medicine and had a reactive PPD	⟹	As a proportion of the total, the people who were not exposed to the medicine

TABLE 10-9 Relative Risk 2×2 Table—Reversed

	Reactive PPD	Non-reactive PPD	Total
No Prophylaxis	The people who did not take the medicine and had a reactive PPD.	⟹	As a proportion of the total, the people who were not exposed to the medicine.
Prophylaxis	The people who took the medicine and had a reactive PPD.	⟹	As a proportion of the total, the people who were exposed to the medicine.

This measure may be, as its name implies, interpreted as a risk. It still may not be interpreted as a cause of the outcome, but it can assess risk, unlike the odds ratio (OR) that we will visit in a moment. In this example:

$$RR = [a/(a + b)] / [c/(c + d)]$$
$$= (22/100) / (45/100)$$
$$= 0.22/0.45$$
$$= 0.489$$

What does this tell us? It continues to be intuitive. The data suggest that the risk of developing a reactive PPD test is less if the partner takes the TB prophylaxis. How do we know that this information tells us that development of TB is less, and not more? All you need to know is that if the RR is less than 1.0, then the exposure of interest is associated with a reduced risk of the outcome. If the RR is greater than 1.0, then the exposure of interest is associated with an increased risk of the outcome. We can say that persons taking medications are 0.489 times *as* likely (almost half again as likely) to become reactive than those not taking them. Another way of looking at it is to consider it as a percentage: 100% without medications −48.9% = 51.1%.[b] Thus, we can say that there is a 51.1% reduction in risk of a partner of a TB-positive individual developing a reactive PPD in the year *relative to* someone who is not on medications.

One of the beautiful things about the 2×2 table is that it allows us to look at things from two different perspectives, what is called counterfactual. If taking medications is associated with reductions in risk, then *not* taking them is associated with increases in risk. So to that end, if this is the case, we

see a reversal in the numbers though no change in their essence (see Table 10-9).

Note that each cell is still referring to the same thing, exposed/diseased. The difference is that now the exposure is considered absence of medication. This makes sense: if you are considering vitamins or vaccinations, the absence of something can be very detrimental, even if there were no other problems.

Now we see this:

$$RR = [a/(a + b)] / [c/(c + d)]$$
$$= (45/100) / (22/100)$$
$$= 0.45/0.22$$
$$= 2.045$$

What does this tell us? The data suggest that the risk of *not* taking prophylaxis is associated with an increased risk of reactivity 2.045 times that of people who do. There are two ways one could calculate this number. One could do the same thing all over, $[a/(a + b)] / [c/(c + d)]$ with the exposure now considered not taking the medicines and the RR indicating, instead, the risk of *not* taking the medications. This is the easiest conceptually. But once you are familiar with the approach, you may do a trick that is mathematically correct and also simple: You find the reciprocal of the value you obtained as your RR. That value is your new RR. In other words:

$$RR = 1/2.045 = 0.489$$

which is exactly what we say when we think about the number of people who took the medications.

This works simply because our exposed/nonexposed categories are the reverse of one another. If you were working with more than two categories, for example low, medium, and high categories, this would not work. It only works when the categories are mutually exclusive and there are only two to

[b]This is not to say that the risk of the positive PPD is 100% in the absence of medications, just that this is the referent group, the one to which we are comparing taking medications. The 100% is arbitrary and indicates that we are comparing taking medications to not taking them.

work with. Then this works well while illustrating the counter-factual property.

When is the RR used? In general, the RR may be used any time there are data that follow exposed and unexposed persons forward in time to assess for the outcomes of interest. This includes randomized controlled trials and cohort studies, both prospective and retrospective.

THE ODDS RATIO

The odds ratio (OR) is the measure used to describe associations demonstrated by case-control studies. It uses the same notation within the 2×2 table to describe it, as shown in Table 10-10.

Note that the construction of the table is the same irrespective of the study design. It is a construct used to describe counts of data. How the data are collected is crucial to their analysis and interpretation, but they may be displayed in exactly the same types of grids.

However, to use an example that is set up as a cohort study does not make much sense. Measures and designs are integrally related, and it is not correct to change one without changing the other. So let us change it ever so slightly so that you may meet the OR. Imagine we have a new study design to work with. Now the design is as follows: Persons with reactive PPDs one year after their primary partner was diagnosed with TB were compared to controls (those without reactive PPDs) who sought care at the same ID clinics as the cases. The exposure of interest remains whether or not they took the prophylaxis medications.

Here we have:

$$\text{Odds ratio} = \text{OR} = \frac{\begin{array}{l}\text{the people who did take the medicine}\\ \text{given they had a reactive PPD} \div \text{the}\\ \text{people who not did take the medicine}\\ \text{given they had a reactive PPD}\end{array}}{\begin{array}{l}\text{the people who did take the medicine}\\ \text{given they had a nonreactive PPD} \div\\ \text{the people who not did take the medi-}\\ \text{cine given they had a nonreactive PPD}\end{array}}$$

This may be generalized more simply to:

$$OR = (a/c) / (b/d)$$

This reduces to (using your algebra!):

$$OR = ad / bc$$

What is different about a case-control study versus a cohort study or randomized controlled trial is that the totals (a + c, b + c) are fixed. They are determined by the investigator. We no longer allow the proportion of the sample that is made up of cases to float, as we do in the cohort and randomized controlled designs. Because these are now fixed, we need to look at the odds that a person had an exposure given he or she was diseased, instead of the risk that a person will get the disease.

Let us consider that we had the counts shown in Table 10-11. We still have 200 subjects, only they are half reactive and half nonreactive on their PPDs. For this reason, we know that it would not be a correct statement to say that half of the sample became reactive because half of the subjects are ill and half are not. That would be drawing the wrong conclusion from the data. If you are ever in doubt about how to remember this, try this memory trick: Case-controls are designed for rare diseases, generally less than 5% of the population. If the disease being studied is rare, would half of the sample have it? No! That does not make sense. In a case-control study we "fixed" the case and control sample sizes by virtue of our study design. Thus, you will be able to remember how to interpret findings from case-control studies. What you can say is that 0.22 of the participants who had a reactive PPD had taken their medications, whereas 0.12 of the nonreactive PPD had. All told, this works out to an OR as follows:

$$\begin{aligned}OR &= ad / bc\\ &= (22 \times 88) / (12 \times 78)\\ &= 1936/936\\ &= 2.07\end{aligned}$$

TABLE 10-10 General 2×2 Table Notation

	Diseased	Not diseased	Total
Exposed	a	b	a+b
Not exposed	c	d	c+d
Total	a+c	b+d	a+b+c+d

TABLE 10-11 Odds Ratio Example

	Reactive PPD	Non-reactive PPD	Total
Prophylaxis	22	12	34
No prophylaxis	78	88	166
Total	100	100	200

What does this tell us? That given an individual had a reactive PPD, he or she was 2.07 times as likely to have not taken medications than someone who had a nonreactive PPD. Note that this is not stated as a risk, as the RR is. The RR actually provides a basis for estimating risk, because the exposed and unexposed populations are considered base populations, and the development of the outcome of interest is allowed to "float". Here, in the case-control situation, the number developing the disease is 100% fixed by the design and the selection of the cases and controls. If there were a 1:1 ratio of cases:controls, then 50% of the sample developed the disease. If there were a 1:4 ratio of cases:controls, then 20% of the sample developed the disease. In this case, it would be wholly inappropriate to consider the OR an estimate of risk. We do not know the population of exposed people that go onto become diseased, since we have intentionally picked out the number of diseased in relation to nondiseased. It is therefore fixed. But what it does do, is, under certain circumstances, provide a fairly good estimate of the RR. This is very helpful, especially because, in many cases, it is not possible to conduct a cohort study, and there are situations in which even if it were possible it would not be an appropriate disease process for doing so (e.g., rare diseases). When the OR approximates, the RR is a source of great discussion, to be abbreviated considerably here. There are many good resources for investigating this question for those who are interested. For now, however, suffice it to say that the following are conditions in which the OR is a good estimate of the RR:

- Controls are representative of individuals in the base population.
- Cases are representative of all individuals in the base population with the disease of interest.
- The disease is relatively rare (generally < 5% of the base population).

What does it mean if these assumptions are not met? It suggests that the association being measured in a prospective study design, the risk, may not be the same as what you are finding in your case-control study. Your OR may be biased, either towards or away from the null hypothesis. (This is another way of saying either towards the null value, 1.0, or away from it, less than or greater than 1.0.) The difficult part of this is that you will never be able to know the direction or extent of the bias, because there is seldom a "true" value to compare your OR to. So we do the best we can, estimate the associations, and try to understand the limitations surrounding each individual measure of association. When possible, we conduct adjunct analyses to try to determine, or at least suggest, the direction and extent of the bias or make adjustments to remove it where possible.

THE PREVALENCE RATIO

Cousin to the RR is the prevalence ratio (PR). This measure is used when conducting cross-sectional studies. It is extremely useful because it does not give the reader any false impressions about it: It is not estimating risk like the RR; it only takes one cross-section and includes only prevalent cases (or possibly incident ones, though it is impossible to distinguish the two). Imagine we have a study where we are again investigating the relationship between adherence to medications and reactivity on the PPD test. This time, though, we take a random sample of a TB clinic population (see Figure 10-1).

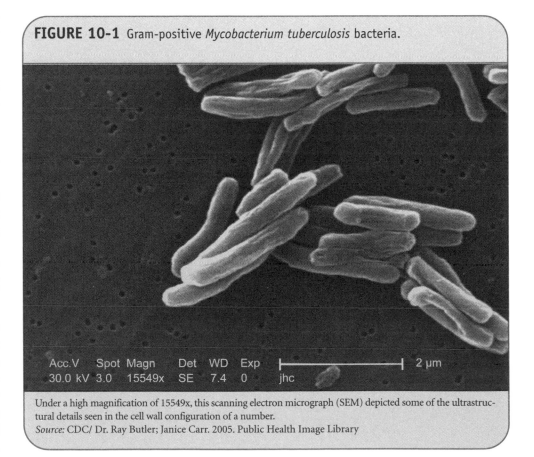

FIGURE 10-1 Gram-positive *Mycobacterium tuberculosis* bacteria.

Under a high magnification of 15549x, this scanning electron micrograph (SEM) depicted some of the ultrastructural details seen in the cell wall configuration of a number.
Source: CDC/ Dr. Ray Butler; Janice Carr. 2005. Public Health Image Library

Each of the participants is asked to be in the study; if interested, they sign an institution review board (IRB)-approved informed consent form, and sign an IRB-approved Health Insurance Portability and Accountability Act (HIPAA) or other consent form that gives study personnel the ability to see each participant's medical record so that measurements from client self-report are standardized. Cross-sectional information is abstracted systematically from the medical record and from the participant self-report, and—as we saw before—placed in the 2×2 table. The calculation of the PR is identical to that of the RR. Thus,

$$\text{Prevalence Raio (PR)} = [a / (a + b)] / [c / (c + d)]$$
$$= (45/100) / (22/100)$$
$$= 0.45/0.22$$
$$= 2.045$$

The interpretation here is the same as for the RR, helping to quantitate the association between the exposure and the outcome. The null value is 1.0, as we have seen before. The PR, though, is clear on the fact that we are looking only at *prevalence*. We are not able to infer much about temporality because all the data were collected at one point in time, at our snapshot or cross-section. The PR measure reminds us of the limitations of the underlying design.

THE PREVALENCE ODDS RATIO

Cousin to the OR is the prevalence odds ratio (POR), in a neat parallel to the relationship between the RR and the PR. The POR is calculated exactly the same as the OR, and as does the PR, the POR reminds us we are looking only at prevalence. This prevents us from being casual about temporality in the absence of any data suggesting relationship in time; it keeps us from what might be wishful thinking, if we wish we had incident cases but only have those prevalent cases presented in cross-sectional data. Our POR is then calculated like this:

$$\text{Prevalence Odds (POR)} = ad/bc$$
$$\text{Ratio} = (22×88) / (12×78)$$
$$= 1936/936$$
$$= 2.07$$

While these measures are not mathematically different from the RR (for the PR) or the OR (for the POR), they are important—and useful for analyzing and interpreting cross-sectional data analysis.

INTERPRETING THE MEASURES

Interpretation of these four measures of association is important. Though it might seem that epidemiologists can sometimes be "splitting hairs" or paying too much attention to syntax and grammar, it is crucial that you understand the basis

for these measures of association and express what they mean carefully and correctly. The difference is important: finding an association between a potential etiologic agent and an infectious disease is very different than saying that the agent "caused" the disease. Since it is so very different, as epidemiologists, we must be very careful when communicating our findings to others in the public health, scientific, or journalistic communities with which we interact.

As you have seen, the RR (and the PR) provide a comparison between the proportion of people exposed who end up diseased and the proportion of people not exposed who end up diseased. This is a different thing entirely than the OR (and POR), which provide a comparison between the proportion of people who were exposed given that they were diseased to the proportion of people who were exposed given they were not diseased. The RR and PR give an estimate of risk of developing the disease of interest; the OR and POR give an estimate of the odds that one was exposed given they were diseased. The methods matter—and they dictate how we must interpret and communicate our results. By nature of the design we have a very different measure of association, and a different meaning.

Each of the measures we have discussed has a different way of being expressed—but the same statement of no difference. Fortunately, this is very straightforward. The RR (and PR) and OR (and POR) are, respectively, looking at a ratio of risks and of odds. If our study shows that the two conditions—of risks or of odds—are the same, then the top will equal the bottom of our equation. And we will have a measure of association equal to 1.0.

For example, imagine we are calculating an RR. Among those exposed, 45.6% of the participants developed the outcome of interest, and among those nonexposed, 44.9% did. The numerator would be the former, the denominator the latter, and we would see the following RR:

$$\text{RR} = 45.6\% / 44.9\% = 0.99 \sim 1.00$$

This is because the conditions, diseased among the exposed and not exposed, are nearly equal. The statement of no difference is 1.0. In this case, there is no difference in the proportion of exposed who became ill when compared to the proportion of nonexposed. Does this mean that the illness or the exposure is not of concern? Does this mean that the healthcare providers in the area need not prepare healthcare resources to treat the ill? Of course not. This only provides one estimate of the relationship between the exposure and the disease and compares it to another category of people, those people who were not exposed. The term *relative risk* means just that—it provides an estimate of the risk of one category relative to that of another category—it does not explore absolute risk at any point.

Similarly we have the OR. Imagine among diseased, 5.6% of the participants were exposed and among nondiseased, 5.5% were. The numerator would be the former, the denominator the latter, and we would see the RR as follows:

$$RR = 5.6\% / 5.5\% = 1.02 \sim 1.00$$

This is because the exposure distribution between the diseased and not diseased are nearly equal. Thus, the statement of no difference is 1.0. Here, too, we are not making any suggestion about the importance or needs of persons with the disease or the exposure. We are only estimating the odds of being exposed given a person was diseased compared to those given if a person was not. Here, too, we are dealing with a situation of relativism, not absolutism.

Sometimes, people get confused thinking that the statement of no difference should be 0. This makes sense in a way, because when we think of differences, the statement of no difference is, in fact, 0.

For example, if you are interested in comparing hepatitis viral loads between two groups, the null hypothesis would be H_o: $mean_{group\ 1} = mean_{group\ 2}$ which, algebraically (remember: subtract one side of the equal sign from the other sign; here we take $mean_{group\ 2}$ and subtract it from the left-hand side of the equality) converts to H_o: $mean_{group\ 1} - mean_{group\ 2} = 0$. This is why understanding what the measures really mean can be helpful in remembering what the null hypotheses should be. If there is no difference in the proportion of diseased among the exposed (for the RR or PR) or in the proportion of exposed among the diseased (for the OR or POR), then the measure of association will be 1.0.

What is different about how we interpret our measures of association for the RR and the OR? It goes back to what they mean and what the 2×2 table tells us.

The best way to discuss how to correctly communicate a measure of association is to give an example. Imagine you have just conducted a study of the relationship between a newly identified virus and a syndrome. This is early research, and you are searching for etiologic agents. You conduct a case-control study. Laboratory, ecologic, and cross-sectional studies have already been performed, and you have just completed the first case-control study of it. Your OR is 1.64. This suggests that, given one was diseased, the odds of having been exposed to the infectious agent is 1.64 times that of one who was not diseased. Or you could say that the odds of being exposed given one was diseased were 64% higher. This measure compares the odds of having been exposed in each of the two groups, diseased and nondiseased.

Now let us imagine that you go back and conduct a cohort study, basing your design on previous research into this asso-

ciation. The RR is 1.75. This suggests that the risk of becoming diseased given one was exposed is 1.75 times that of one who was not exposed. Or you could say that the risk of becoming diseased is 75% greater among exposed than not exposed. This measure compares the probability of becoming diseased in each of the two groups, exposed and nonexposed.

What can you not say in both cases? You cannot say that the infectious agent "caused" the disease, "created" the disease, "made" the disease happen, "is responsible" for the disease, "increased" the disease—or any other phrases suggesting or implying causality. We just do not know enough from observational studies to be able to support these statements. If your estimates were less than 1.0, thus the exposures were associated with reduced outcomes or exposures, what can you not say? You cannot say that the infectious agent "prevented" the disease, "reduced" the disease, "fixed" the disease, "lessened" the disease—or any other similar statement implying causality. All we can say is that we demonstrated an association between two variables, the infectious agent and the disease of interest. Begin noticing when you read articles in journals or even those in the lay papers how relationships are presented. Are words suggesting causal relationships used in observational studies? They should not be! Only randomized controlled trials, which have very specific assumptions met during their conduct and analysis, should ever have causal terminology linked to their findings. Even then, caution should be used.

A BRIEF EXPLORATION OF THE ROLE OF CHANCE

Before leaving this chapter, let us briefly visit the role of chance in basic epidemiologic studies used in infectious disease. Statistics takes up the explication of the role of chance in research (and other) realms. Most readers will have had some prior exposure to the subject matter in other texts, or will be reading such texts concurrently. But a reminder of how to interpret the data that are derived from 2×2 tables and other sources is necessary to ensure that everyone is on a level playing field while reading the remainder of the text. Other references are readily available for those requiring additional information.

Imagine you are researching viral loads for a newly identified lentivirus in a population of 1,000 patients in an emerging infectious disease registry.[c] You take a group of four patients, and measure their viral load. The mean viral load is 350 with a standard deviation of 36.1 and a range 160–466 for this group. Is this high? Is this low? How sure are you that you did not just get this number by chance? Out of all the many,

---

[c]This example is fictitious.

many thousands of groups of four, is it possible that you could have gotten this particular one by chance? Perhaps the true mean viral load is actually 832 instead; how would you know?

So you begin the process of taking more samples of four. You get one that is 420, another that is 550, another that is 224, and so on and so forth. The mean of these means is 386. Now what do you say? Does it seem more or less likely that your first sample was due to chance alone? At what point do you stop and feel pretty confident that the sample you first got was not an aberration, that it was fairly on target describing the mean of the group and not just a chance fluke?

When we are looking at the role of chance in assessing numbers, this is part of what we are looking at. Each time we have a sample for a study, it is taken from an underlying population base. It is unfortunate yet true that in general, we have only a conceptual framework for the population base: We do not know its exact characteristics because we cannot. We sample smaller batches from the underlying population to try to draw conclusions about the population in the absence of census data that would describe it more precisely.

We use two primary ways of calculating the role of chance in relation to numbers gained from epidemiologic studies. They are essentially the same information communicated in different ways: the p-value and the confidence interval (CI). Each of these provides a numeric description of how likely something you found in your data happened by chance alone. There are two outcomes possible: both are based on the data we have, and related to the research question and the H_a and H_o we developed and on which we structured our study. If the probability that what you found is very unlikely to have happened by chance alone, then you are likely to reject your null hypothesis under study. This means that the relationship you proposed in your alternative hypothesis may be accepted.

If, on the other hand, it is highly likely that what you found in your study happened by chance alone, then you fail to reject the null hypothesis. This does not mean that it is false—or that you accept your null hypothesis—just that given the information you have and the data that are available, you have insufficient information to reject the null. What does this mean? It means that our data do not support us saying that the H_o is not correct; and therefore we cannot conclude that the H_a is correct. Of course, we only had one question in play; if we fail to reject the null, it means only that—we could not reject the null and accept the alternative. It does not mean that the null is true, as that would be a different question all together. The whole process looks at each H_o at a time, and assesses whether we can reject it (in which case we can conclude the H_a is correct) or not (in which case we only can say we fail to reject the null).

Factors that go into deciding what role chance plays include two primary items: the sample size and the variability of the measure under study. The sample size is how many people (or units of analysis) are in your study; the variability of the measure is how much it changes between or within people or between time points (e.g., standard deviation). As the sample size increases and the variability decreases, we are able to focus in on the relationship; chance is less likely to be as strong a factor in what is found in the study. To determine power of the study the difference you wish to detect is also required. In the earlier examples, if you had just several groups of two from your population, it would probably take more for you to believe that the numbers you found as your means were representative of the "true" population means. However, if you had groups of 30 taken from the same population 100 times, you would be more likely to believe your findings. And if you had groups of 1000 taken 1000 times, you would be far more likely to believe your findings still.

As the name implies, hypothesis testing—assessment of the role of chance or random error in your findings—involves the use of your carefully constructed null and alternative hypotheses. These hypothesize two distributions, one the null and one the alternative. Your data will better reflect one of the distributions than the other, and understanding the role of chance tells you how likely you are to have gotten what you got because it is real or because you got "lucky". p-values articulate the probability that you obtained a value as or more extreme as the one you did if the null hypothesis were true. Another way of saying this: you are trying to determine whether the null hypothesis or the alternative hypothesis is correct, given the data you have. If the question is, "How likely were we to find this same information if it is not true under the alternative hypothesis, or due to the role of chance alone?" then the p-value tells you the answer. If the p-value is small, chances are this is unlikely; you are unlikely to have found the answer you did if it were just by chance alone. If the p-value is large, however, chances are better that this is more likely.

Let us see how this looks. In the Table 10-12, information is given about rates and also about measures of associations found describing data. Each row has a p-value associated with it, describing how likely—based on the information available including sample size and variability that went into the numbers—we were to have found the values we found, or those more extreme, by chance alone, meaning that they may not really reflect the true underlying population base. Typically, a cutoff of 5% will be selected to suggest significance, or the state in which chance has little role. This means that we are willing to tolerate a 5% risk of there being an intrinsic error on this assessment; that we could reject the null when, in fact, we should not have. Maybe we are wrong! When this is our

TABLE 10-12 Examples in Assessing the Role of Chance in Interpreting Your Data

Measure	Estimate(s)	*p-value*	*Comment*
Prevalence of a new infection among a sample of HIV+ persons with CD4<200 vs. ≥ 200	1.01% vs. 0.99%	0.92	Based on the study from which these data were derived, it is very likely that a finding this or more extreme would have happened. We do not reject the null.
Mean HIV viral load at clinic A vs. clinic B	10,012 vs. 422 RNA copies/mL	0.02	Based on the study from which these data were derived, it is not very likely that a finding this or more extreme would have happened by chance alone. We reject the null. There is only a 2% chance that we have rejected the null when it should not have been.
Case-control study of *M. listeriosis* in relation to exposure to cocktail hotdogs	OR=5.03	0.001	Based on the study from which these data were derived, it is not very likely that a finding this or more extreme would have happened by chance alone. We reject the null. There is only a 2% chance that we have rejected the null when it should not have been.

cutoff—and it is a common though arbitrary one but by no means the only one—we are stating that we are willing to be incorrect about what we assume the underlying population is like 5% of the time. This is called α (alpha) = 0.05.

But would you like any more information? We now have enough information to decide whether we reject or fail to reject our null hypothesis. It is sort of like a fork in the road: if we decide to go one way, then we have decided *not* to go the other way. The decision-making process underlying hypothesis testing is that (if we construct our null and alternative hypotheses correctly), when we ask one thing of our data, it will either be true or not true. And that "truth" corresponds to only one "fork" in the road. The *p*-value is the metric by which we decide which road to take and where to go from there.

The *p*-value is a yes or no phenomenon: because up front (*a priori*) we use our α level to set how much chance we are

willing to accept. For example, look at Table 10-13. It does not give a deeper understanding of the data that gave rise to the test statistic or the *p*-value.

Confidence intervals (CI) do, however. The CI emerges from calculations that include the number of people (or units of analysis), the variability in the measure, and other characteristics under study. The CI is related intrinsically to the *p*-value. It includes all of the same ingredients required to construct it as does the *p*-value (which you will learn in your statistics courses). A wide CI may mean that the sample size is too small or the variability is too great to be able to be able to focus in on what was identified, leading us to fail to reject the null hypothesis on which we are working. The tighter the CI, the more precise our estimate is. This may result, as before, from too small a sample size, too small a difference to be detected, or too high a variability. How do you interpret a CI? Simple. Let us return to our example of the OR from the above table. Imagine we now have the information in Table 10-14.

Based on this information, we can say that if we took similar repeated samples of the target population again and again and did exactly the same thing to each of these samples to ob-

TABLE 10-13 When Do We Reject the Null Hypothesis?

If α=	And our *p*-value =	Then we:
0.05	0.04	Reject the null hypothesis.
0.01	0.04	Fail to reject the null hypothesis.
0.10	0.06	Reject the null hypothesis.

TABLE 10-14 Example of Data From a Case-Control Study of *M. listeriosis*

Measure	Estimate	95% CI and p-value
Case-control study of *M. listeriosis* in relation to exposure to cocktail hotdogs	OR = 5.03	95% CI 4.35–5.67, $p < 0.01$

tain estimates of the OR, 95% of the time the true population estimate of the OR would be in the range 4.35 to 5.67; this one may or may not be. Another way of saying this is to say that 95% of the time the true population estimate of the OR will be from 4.35 to 5.67. We are very unlikely to have found an estimate this or more extreme by chance alone.

Note three things here:

1. The null value (1.0) is not contained within the corresponding CI when the *p*-value is significant.
2. The *p*-value and the CI agree (i.e., one does not reject and one fail to reject; they must reach the same conclusion).
3. The estimate of the OR is contained within the CI.

These things are necessarily true and follow from the way the *p*-value and confidence interval are generated. In fact, they are so true that if you ever find these three things not to hold, then you know there is an error (usually just mathematical) going on somewhere.

Let us try another example. This time we have one cohort study, with two outcomes being investigated (see Table 10-15).

TABLE 10-15 Interpreting Confidence Intervals

Measure	Estimate	95% CI and p-value
Prospective cohort study of women exposed to tampons and toxic shock syndrome (TSS)	RR = 8.03	95% CI 7.05–9.77, $p < 0.01$
Prospective cohort study of women exposed to tampons and bacterial sinusitis	RR = 0.93	95% CI 0.76–5.77, $p = 0.85$

What do we have in the first example? Exposure to tampons is associated with an increased risk of toxic shock syndrome (TSS), with women exposed being more than eight times as likely to develop TSS than those not exposed, and this estimate is statistically significant, $p < 0.01$. If we took similar repeated samples from this base population and studied them, 95% of the time our true population estimate would fall between 7.05 and 9.77; this one may or may not. So we can say that the risk of TSS among tampon-exposed women is between these two estimates, and feel confident that we found this association because it is real and not because of random error. Our three things hold: the null value is not contained in our CI, our corresponding CI and *p*-value conclusions match, and our OR is within the CI.

Now take the second example. Here our estimate suggests a protective relationship, whereby women who are exposed to tampons are less likely to develop bacterial sinusitis than those who are not. Our *p*-value is very large, and so we expect to see that our CI *does* include the null value, 1.0—and it does. The conclusions drawn by these two items agree: We fail to reject the null here. In addition, the width of the CI—not just that it crosses 1.0 but how widely it does so—tells us that we do not have a precise estimate here, perhaps due to a small sample size or a large variability.

When the CI reveals a relationship between exposure and outcome that is not significant, it is really a bit more than just noticing that 1.0 is in the CI. If we put it in the context of what the interpretation of the CI is, it makes more sense. It is like saying if we took similar repeated samples from this base population and studied them, 95% of the time our true population estimate would fall between 0.76 and 5.77; thus in some populations it would be preferable to be exposed and could confer health and, in others, illness. The estimate we received this time, where RR = 0.93 is on one side of the null value, does not mean much because it could just as easily have been on the other due to chance alone!

Let us now put this all together: interpretation, working with null and alternative hypotheses, and assessing statistical significance. To do this, let us revisit the example regarding the new infectious agent and newly discovered disease that we covered in the previous section to make this a bit clearer. Imagine we have the following for our prospective cohort study:

H_o: There is no association between the infectious agent and diagnosis of the new disease.

H_A: There is an association between the infectious agent and diagnosis of the new disease.

Our RR is 1.75 (95% CI 1.54-1.87, $p < 0.05$). What does this mean? It means that we have sufficient evidence to reject our null hypothesis: what we found suggests that it is very unlikely that this information would occur by chance alone. There does appear to be an association between the infectious agent and the new disease.

Now imagine we found something different. Our new RR is 1.35 (95% CI 0.87-1.43, $p > 0.05$). What does this mean? It means that we have insufficient evidence to reject our null hypothesis. Our data are not sufficient to reject the idea that there is no relationship; there may, in fact, be no relationship. However, this may have occurred for many reasons: it may be that our sample size was too small. It may be that there was too much variability in the sample. It may be that the difference between the exposed and unexposed groups that we were trying to examine was too small (it is harder to see small differences than big ones). It does not mean there is no relationship between the two, only that we do not have enough information to support that there is one, and that what we found could have occurred by chance alone. This is why people do not say that "we accept the null." We cannot accept that there is no relationship based on our study; all we can say is that we cannot reject the null hypothesis.

There is so much more to the exploration of our measures of association and the role of chance in interpreting epidemiologic results. But this will be left for experts in that realm and students of that course. For now, we will use this as a stepping stone to move from what methods are supposed to be to the "real world" and begin to see methods at use in the field. It is here where the story becomes interesting. We will step into the world of bias, where problems emerge from systematic flaws in the methods instead of the simpler to handle role of chance. Not perfect, often ugly, here we see the methodological problems that exist and can suggest means to overcome them. Let the fun begin!

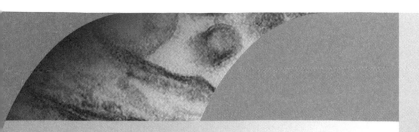

Discussion Questions

1. You have just conducted a case-control study on the relationship between meat products at a specific plant and *M. listeriosis.* Several results are below. Which ones are statistically significant at $\alpha = 0.05$? Which ones are statistically significant at $\alpha = 0.01$? Which ones are impossible? Which ones demonstrate an association that is protective in nature? For each of the results that are possible, write an interpretation of the measure of association found.

   a.   OR 2.05 (95% CI 1.41-3.01), $p < 0.0001$
   b.   OR 1.07 (95% CI 0.69-1.64), $p = 0.77$
   c.   OR 0.51 (95% CI 0.30-0.86), $p < 0.008$
   d.   OR 4.51 (95% CI 0.32-0.96), $p < 0.01$
   e.   OR 0.59 (95% CI 0.36-0.98), p $= 0.032$

2. You are the investigator overseeing a large concurrent cohort study evaluating the association between drinking alcohol and likelihood of contracting an STD over the course of a year. [Note: these numbers are hypothetical.] After data collection is complete, your 2 × 2 table looks like this:

	STD	No STD	
Alcohol	295	2116	2411
No alcohol	160	3929	4,089
	455	6045	6,500

a. What is the appropriate measure to describe the association between alcohol consumption and STDs?
   A. OR
   C. RR
   D. Incidence density
   E. Prevalence
   F. Proportionate morbidity

b. What is the measure of association between alcohol consumption and stroke?
c. How would you communicate the findings of your study if the *p*-value describing this measure of association was 0.01?
d. How would you communicate the findings of your study if the *p*-value describing this measure of association was 0.21?

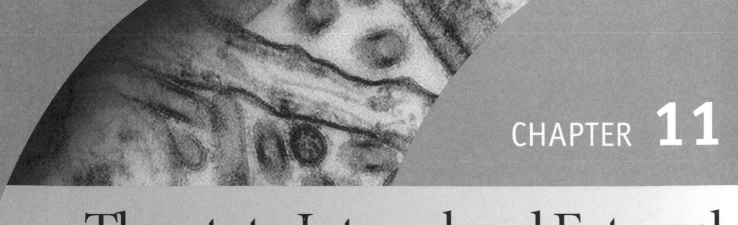

CHAPTER 11

Threats to Internal and External Validity in the Study of Infectious Disease Epidemiology

LEARNING OBJECTIVES

By the end of this chapter, you will be able to:

- Define bias, misclassification, and confounding.
- Differentiate bias from random error.
- Identify primary means of reducing bias in epidemiologic study designs.
- Describe types of bias of particular importance in infectious disease epidemiology.

FROM IDEAL STUDY STRUCTURE TO PRACTICAL REALITIES: REAL ISSUES IN STUDY IMPLEMENTATION

Epidemiology is intrinsically creative. Our set of tools, our methods, the most crucial of which you have already learned, provides us a structure by which we can answer important public health, and in our case, infectious disease, questions. When these tools are applied in the field, however, we often are struck by the barriers to the "perfect" study. In fact, there is no such thing. We need to use creativity to ensure that we are designing the best study that we can. How we define best includes incorporation of our independent and dependent variables of interest, ethics, resources (including time and expertise), and overall acceptability to the target population, public health, and scientific communities. Even when we think everything through, however, and make the best study design we can within the resource and other constraints that we have, there will necessarily be methodological issues that arise and

influence the meaning of the data we collect. Often these create biases that need to be considered and addressed after the study. It is best when we can recognize and reduce sources of bias in design; when this takes place, potential sources of bias are considered up front, and a more solid design is implemented—lending us increased confidence in our findings. As you learned in the previous chapter, the role of chance is important in assessing how likely we are to have found what we found for a reason rather than through chance. Although that involves statistics and calculations, in reality that is the easy part. More difficult is reducing the problems that derive from systematic and nonrandom phenomena. Primarily design effects and human behavior create these. Unfortunately, these cannot be statistically adjusted away or forgotten. We need to do as much as we can to reduce bias from the start of the study design and eliminate it from the study's structure. If we do not, we must live with its consequences—which often means taking a study's conclusions differently than we otherwise would.

BIAS

Bias is the systematic, nonrandom inclusion of error into a study. This error distorts the appearance of the relationship between the exposure and the disease of interest, generally by putting too many or too few individuals in one or more of the four cells in the 2×2 table. Bias means that the estimate obtained to describe the exposure-disease relationship is invalid, whether it occurs in design or in the way the information is collected, analyzed, or disseminated. The "noise" that random error introduces into a study can obscure the relationship between independent and dependent variables, making it harder for us to learn about or describe the relationship we are trying to understand. Variability, or "noise", makes the margin for error larger, so we have difficulty focusing in on the relationship of interest. But even in the presence of most variability, this random error has just as much tendency to err on the side of + as of −. What bias does is much more sinister. Because it can take place at any point in a study, from development to publication (or even post publication, if included in a meta-analysis), and because it can take nearly any form, it can create relationships that are not there; it also can attenuate or remove relationships that are there. Bias can create a situation in which the result is in the opposite direction than it should be, stronger or weaker.

The methodological approach taken by this text is designed to assist the reader to understand the epidemiological toolkit and create studies that are the best they can be. Part of this is knowing which biases most frequently occur, where, and how they can be removed in the design phase rather than after the fact. If they cannot be removed, then the trick becomes how to try to interpret the data correctly in spite of invalid estimates. This generally means understanding and articulating strengths and limitations, and knowing where findings may be generalized and where they may not be.

Epidemiologic texts are no stranger to bias; they cover it extensively and well. Articles, too, are available that catalogue the types of bias and primary situations in which we expect to see bias. Rather than re-create these exceptional resources (see the Reference list at the end of the chapter and Appendix 1), this section will describe the basic categories of bias, where they are commonly found in infectious disease epidemiologic studies, and how they may be reduced or eliminated. This is not a comprehensive treatment of this essential element of study design; rather, it is intended to provide you with a solid framework with which to add detail in the future, and a foundation for a greater insight into this important topic.

Types of Bias

There are two basic types of bias:

- Information
- Selection

Information bias has to do with whether one correctly classifies a participant's exposure and disease status, once they are in the study. This type of bias (sometimes also called observer bias) generally leads to misrepresentation, or misclassification, in which case a subject falls into the wrong cell (e.g., instead of falling into A, she falls into D in the 2×2 table). This

can happen in a vast number of ways, many surprising, and can wreak havoc on your study. Systematic inaccuracy is always a problem, irrespective of design or variable type. When we are dealing with dichotomous choices (yes/no) for both the exposure of interest and for the disease, however, the problem becomes amplified when compared to a continuous outcome or exposure.

For example, imagine you are studying CD4 counts among 1,000 HIV-negative adolescents in order to compare them to HIV-positive adolescents. If there were a systematic flaw in your laboratory analytic methods, it might result in there being a misstatement of CD4 counts: 450 might be 452, 900 might be 903, and so forth. Say in this example they were always within +/− 5. In this instance this would be a relatively minor problem because the deviations are fairly small and they are sometimes over and sometimes under, and they are not systematic based on the disease status of the adolescent. Although it is possible for there to be a typo or other data entry error, the likelihood that the flow cytometry lab in this example would report that a true CD4 count of 200 was actually 938 or a 2 was 1,003—huge differences—would be slim. Imagine the cutoff indicating "low" CD4 count is 200 cells/mm^3 and the lab report incorrectly indicates that one patient's CD4 is 203 cells/mm^3 when it is in fact 199 cells/mm.[3] Even though the difference on a continuous scale is so small, it ends up placing the outcome variable in the cell for high CD4 opposed to where it should rightly belong in the low CD4 cell. You can easily see here that biases that lead to misclassifying the data can be disastrous. When we have a dichotomous independent variable and a dichotomous dependent variable, if we are wrong in our assessment, there is only one other place for the answer to go: to the other cell. At the end of the chapter, we will discuss differential and nondifferential misclassification. In differential misclassification, the error occurs on one axis in relation to the other. For example, if the CD4 count was always misspecified for HIV+ adolescents but never for HIV− (perhaps they were done at different labs), the problem would be exacerbated considerably.

In this case the results can be especially damaging: those people who actually were diseased may be—systematically and in conjunction with the exposure of interest—considered to be not diseased! This would allow us to arrive upon the exact opposite conclusion than we should have. Thus, in studies like many epidemiologic ones where we have only a correct classification of exposure and outcome and a wrong one; systematic errors in their classification are a primary concern.

Selection bias has to do with a systematic difference between who gets into the study and who does not. Selection bias makes it very difficult to be confident in the information we obtain and whether or not we can apply that information to people who are not in our study. This is one of the more intuitive forms of bias, because it is easy to see how people who, for example, volunteer for a study are very different from those who do not. The reason to conduct research (and not just internal evaluations) is to generalize our findings to other populations. If we have decreased ability to do that because of our study design and any resulting bias, the study becomes far less meaningful.

For example, if you have a study to look at predictors of tuberculosis (TB) among family members, you may be concerned because people who are willing to participate in your study may not be representative of all the individuals with or exposed to TB. When you analyze your data and wish to understand how to reduce risk of TB among families with one member who has the disease, it may be very difficult to generalize to families who did not participate in the study.

In general, it is wise to consider first the internal validity—how free your study is from information bias and misclassification—prior to addressing external validity. External validity is how readily you may apply your findings to the target population (also known as generalizability)—how free your study is from selection bias. If, at the end of your study, you can say that your study is internally valid, free (or as free as possible) from bias with regard to the ascertainment of exposure, disease, or other variables, *then* you can explore it with regard to selection bias. If there is a minimum of bias in your design and the ultimate implementation of the study, then you will be able to generalize your findings relatively easily. On the other hand, if your study lacks internal va-

lidity and there is bias that cannot be ignored, measured, or sufficiently addressed, then the issue of whether it is externally valid becomes moot.

In both types of bias, it is crucial to remember that the issue is not solely error, but *systematic error*—error where the mistake in the estimation of the exposure or disease consistently occurs in the same direction and, worse, if the error on one axis (e.g., exposure) is related to that on the other axis (e.g., disease). For example, imagine the study of characteristics associated with contraction of TB from a family member, as above. Imagine the mother of an infant were fearful of disclosing that she did not give her child medication for TB. Now imagine this fear of disclosure is associated with the knowledge that her other child tested positive for TB (e.g., maybe

---

FIGURE 11-1 Misclassification and the 2×2 table

The "truth"

	Resistant	Non-resistant	
Exposed	a	b	a+b
Non-Exposed	c	d	c+d
	a+c	b+d	N

In the event of misclassification, misidenitfied participants will automatically be considered the opposite of their truer categorization on either one or both axes (i.e., outcome and/or predictor).

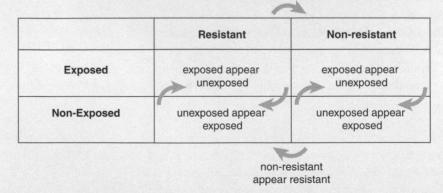

resistant appear
non-resistant

	Resistant	Non-resistant
Exposed	exposed appear unexposed	exposed appear unexposed
Non-Exposed	unexposed appear exposed	unexposed appear exposed

non-resistant
appear resistant

In the event of misclassification, there is only one other place for the client (and his or her information) to go: to the incorrect cell.
Source: Author

she felt that she "gave" her child TB and does not want to reveal to the interviewer her true behavior), bias could result. If she does not disclose her true behavior—not giving the medication—she will appear adherent and misclassification will have taken place. Description of the exposure to medication—the independent variable—is associated with the dependent variable. Unfortunately, here, it is not accurate. There is something about the design of the study that may be "creating" a situation in which incorrect information about the independent variable is being drawn from the participant, and the direction of the information depends on whether the outcome of TB in another child is present or absent.

This may be contrasted with random error, the "noise", which will usually obscure the observation of relationships. Variability will blur our understanding of relationships, biasing towards the null, and making a strong relationship in either direction look weaker.[a] Systematic error can either bias your estimates towards or away from the null, and it will be impossible to determine neither the direction of the bias nor the magnitude.

Of the more than 100 biases that have been identified and articulated, most can occur in infectious disease research. There is sometimes the sense that bias cannot occur, or always occurs less frequently, in prospective studies and those with short follow-up times. This is hardly the case. Each study design and individual study is prone to specific types of bias depending upon the research questions being addressed; broad sweeping statements or assumptions about what types of bias "can" be in a given study are usually false. It is necessary to critically evaluate the literature and one's own study to identify where there is or may be bias, how it may impact the study's findings, and how it can be reduced through design, at least in future studies.

In the arena of sensitive research, such as that on sexually transmitted diseases, sometimes the collection of the critical element of the study—for example, prevention behaviors can be woefully difficult to ascertain. Bias may be rampant, with inaccurate findings for exposure almost always associated with the outcome of interest, making it difficult to determine true relationships of interest. Even for less sensitive infectious disease topics, such as what one ate at a party or where there may have been exposure to food poisoning, memories may be poor, obscured by time or intoxicants, making ascertainment of information that would provide clues to the source difficult.

First we will learn about some key information biases, then selection biases, and then discuss the means of overcoming or reducing these biases.

Essential Information Biases

The following are some of the essential information biases. Remember, information bias has to do with whether one correctly classifies a participant's exposure and disease status, once they are in the study and related to internal validity of the study:

Reporting bias

Just as interviewers can influence the data that ultimately get into the system, things that the participants do or say also can get into the system. Reporting bias is when something about how the participant provides information is incorrect. There are multiple types of reporting bias; here are two of the most relevant to infectious disease studies:

- *Social desirability bias or unacceptable disease bias:* Incorrect reporting of information may occur because the participant does not feel confident in his or her ability to describe the truth, because the nature of the question is sensitive or because the answer may appear (or be felt to appear) socially undesirable in some respect. For example, if asked the number of new sexual partners acquired in the last three months, a respondent might say 5 when it is in fact 10. Not reporting missing a dose of medication is another good example of social desirability bias.
- *Prevarication bias:* People may lie, which is distinguished from social desirability bias by virtue of its conscious state. For example, in the case of social undesirability bias, when asked about the number of new sexual partners in the last 3 months, the respondent may have had 10 but, out of embarrassment, may only remember 5 and then report this. In the case of prevarication bias, the participant may know that he had 9 new sexual partners in the last 3 months, but consciously decide not to disclose 8 of them for personal reasons. As with other biases, this clearly alters the way in which the data are assigned to cells in our 2×2 table.

Detection bias

This type of bias can be particularly important when dealing with individuals enrolled in longitudinal studies or clinical trials. In this bias, a circular relationship evolves between the fact of being treated and/or screened and making the diagnosis of the disease. This type of bias can result in identifying a relation-

---

[a] In extreme cases of nondifferential misclassification, it is possible for the bias to be away from the null. But this is the exceptiton and not the rule, happening in only very rare and unusual cases.

ship that is there but disproportionate in one group (exposed, diseased); alternately, it can cause the appearance of an artifactual relationship. For example, imagine a prospective cohort study that is evaluating HIV-positive women on hormone replacement therapy to assess the risk of cancer. HIV-positive women in general are at high risk of developing cervical cancer, and it is an AIDS-defining opportunistic process. Women on hormone replacement therapy (HRT) often have an increased risk of abnormal vaginal bleeding. If this bleeding is followed up (as it should be) with a Pap smear and other diagnostic testing, women in the exposed group may be more likely to be diagnosed with cancer, simply because they are having symptoms that are related to HRT but not necessarily because HRT is associated with increased cancer. Yet this is how it could appear.

Poor recall

It is hard to remember things that we know about and think about. It is harder still to remember things that we do not know are happening or that are not in our sphere of understanding. Often, a study may ask about exposures or behaviors that the participant may know nothing about. This makes it very difficult for the participant in a study to be accurate. For example, in an outbreak investigation, someone may have a difficult time remembering what he or she ate at the meal in question. Often, poor recall is general and results in misclassification that is nondifferential; that means that it is not happening in the same direction with respect to the two axes; people with the outcome are just as likely as those without to remember, or not remember, their exposure. When it is differential we see again the situation in which people with the exposure (or the outcome) are more or less likely to recall the exposure about which they are being asked. This is no longer just "noise" or random error; now it is systematic and can alter the estimates that derive from the study.

Recall bias

Recall bias differs from the issue of poor recall raised above. Recall bias is an all too common bias in case-control studies. It is when the recollection of the exposure is affected by the disease status of the participant. It works like this: Imagine that you wake one morning with a dreadful cold. You cannot go to school or to work, and you are quite miserable. While in your sickbed, you mull over your primary questions: When on earth did I contract this cold? Who could have given it to me? You arrive upon your class last week, where out of about 10 students, you remember that the woman next to you had a terrible cold, not unlike the one you have at this very moment. Your mind races to the culprit: "She gave it to me!" Now imagine this: The same woman is in class, with the same cold. You, however, do not get a cold. Do you remember her nearly as well? Unlikely. The fact of your being sick with the cold heightened your memory for things that might be (or at least might seem) causally linked. Without that fact of your illness, the woman who was ill may not have stuck out in your memory at all. This phenomenon makes this one of the most common biases in case-control studies: people with diseases tend to recall exposures disproportionately when compared to people without diseases, biasing our estimate of the OR.

Interviewer bias

Interviewer training is the topic of many manuals and field guides, most of which are written to train interviewers to conduct their work in a fashion that introduces as little bias as is humanly possible. The interviewer plays a key role in how information is collected. The person collecting the data is in the "hot seat": she or he is the person who takes the information given by a participant in a study, hears and interprets it, and writes it down to turn it into coded data. Interviewer bias occurs when there is systematic error in how information is collected during an interview with a participant, how the information is understood, or how it is written down. This type of bias may occur in any study in which persons are collecting data from or about participants. In our example about TB, you may be able to imagine multiple ways that interviewer bias could sneak into the interaction between interviewer and participant. For example, the interviewer may feel—subconsciously or consciously—that a mother who is not 100% adherent to the medication regimen is a bad parent. Even if this feeling is never voiced, without training, the *feeling* of the interviewer's belief may end up revealing itself on the interviewer's tongue, even if she or he does not wish it to. It can reveal itself in body language, gesture, tonality. Even a minor difference in tone can affect the accuracy of the participant's response. If a participant perceives that their true behavior is not acceptable to the interviewer, they may not disclose the truth and this may result in bias and ultimate misclassification. This systematic difference between interviewers can result in misclassification where women who were not adherent with their child's medication are less likely to disclose this fact to one of the interviewers. All the worse if this occurs more frequently among women with other children with a diagnosis of TB. If that is the case then our determination of exposure is differential with respect to another variable of interest.

Essential Selection Biases

On the surface, understanding selection bias is intuitive. It makes sense that people who are selected or who select themselves to be in a study are different than those who are do not

Asking About Sensitive Information, Part I

Think about the following phrase:

> In the period of October 1980 to May 1981, 5 young men, all active homosexuals, were treated for biopsy-confirmed *Pneumocystis carinii* pneumonia at 3 different hospitals in Los Angeles, California. Two of the patients died.[7]

With these words in 1981, the era of HIV/AIDS was introduced—a new epidemic, a new pandemic, a new impact on individual and public health.

We have learned a lot about behavior since then, and the phrase "all active homosexuals" reminds us of one thing we have learned about people's behavior in the 25 years since the importance of sexual behavior has become even greater. Sexual behavior and orientation are generally considered two separate axes now in most behavioral research. It would be relatively rare—in the context of assessing HIV or STD risk now—to think about these five cases as only homosexual. The question is: With whom did they have sex? Sexual behavior is what a person does and when studying risks of sexual behavior, HIV transmission for example, the issue is who the person is having sex with and their sexual practices. Sexual orientation is important for many reasons, but it in and of itself is not a risk factor for disease. The behavior-related questions include: Does a man have sex with women? Sex with men? Sex with both? Are condoms correctly used at each encounter? And so forth. People may (and many do) have sex with people of the same sex and yet consider themselves heterosexual, may be married, and never would consider themselves gay. Other people would consider themselves bisexual in terms of orientation but only have sex with people of the opposite sex. For the purposes of risk behavior, it is preferable to ask about what people do rather than just their orientation. In general, now we speak in terms of sexual behavior *and* orientation, not just sexual orientation.

But how to ask about all this and obtain unbiased—or as unbiased as possible—answers? People do not necessarily like to disclose the most intimate characteristics of their lives. (And if they like to disclose it *too* much, that in itself can introduce bias.) Almost all of the time, it is not possible to observe behaviors that are sensitive. This can include things like:

- Sexual practices
- Sexual desires
- Gender identity and related behavior
- Use of condoms
- Illicit drug use
- Poor eating/nutritional habits
- Adherence to medications
- Excessive use of legal drugs (e.g., prescription, alcohol, cigarettes)
- Criminal activity

This list can also include other things that, to the interviewer, may not seem sensitive but to the interviewee are. What can one do to reduce the bias that may creep into one's study when asking about sensitive topics? The answer cannot be, and is not, "Only stick to topics that are not sensitive." This would render us unable to learn about some of the most important risk behaviors throughout public health. So a great deal of study has been done to try to improve the way we design surveys to ask sensitive questions in order to get more valid answers.

In sexual behavior research, some of the ways to reduce sources of error in survey design are as follows:[8-17,b]

- Extensively pretest all instrumentation to ensure that the questions are in a conversational tone that is speakable by the interviewer. Changes in wording are thought to occur as much as 90% of the time,[13,14] and this can result in a different questionnaire being given to each person and, obviously, substantial bias. Especially with sensitive topics, all question stems and response sets should be extensively tested in advance of field use.

---

[b] One primary problem with increased variability—due to the variables under study or due to error and misclassification—is that it reduces our statistical power to detect a difference if there is one. Recall in Chapter 10 when we discussed that power is generally the result of three things: the sample size, the variability of the variables under study, and the difference we are trying to detect. Extensive nondifferential misclassification affects the variability.

- Sampling strategies should be carefully thought out. In cases of STD or HIV risk behavior, it may be that only a relatively small portion of the population is engaging in the behavior; this may result in too small of a sample being drawn to address the research questions. Consult a biostatistician before sampling to be sure that the strategy is appropriately developed and the calculations are correct. If oversampling is necessary to ensure adequate power for a given research question or small subpopulation, work with the biostatistician to develop weights that are correct.

- Whatever sampling strategy is selected—simple random sampling, multistage cluster design, respondent-driven sampling, purposive sampling, convenience sampling, or other strategy, you must be well aware of its relative strengths and limitations. For example, if you opt for a random digit dial telephone sampling strategy, you must be aware of the specific parameters in the community under study: How many people have telephones? How many are cell vs. land phones? The sampling strategy needs to be matched to the study design and target population as well. Adolescents, for example, are unlikely to have land lines of their own but are very likely to have cell phones. Only certain strategies allow for cell phone usage, and this needs to be carefully considered. Not to mention the fact that sensitive data collection via a cell phone (while the respondent is perhaps out and about) may introduce bias (i.e., disclosure of sensitive data while in public is not likely ideal). If you use volunteers, especially for studies involving sexual behavior, finding ways to assess differences between them and the general population are important. Other studies have shown that volunteers may be more likely to differ from general population estimates regarding sexual experience and sensation seeking, and may be generally more unconventional.[18] Knowing all you can before embarking on a study will help; even if there are more limitations than strengths, being able to articulate and quantify them improves the likelihood of the study yielding useful data.

- Consider using audio or video computer-assisted self-interview (ACASI or VCASI) methods to reduce bias that may result from concerns regarding social desirability. These techniques have been shown to be useful in attaining data that are more valid where sensitive topics are concerned. If used, though, pilot them extensively, and use qualitative methods to conduct formative evaluation in advance of the study's implementation. Some subpopulations may find using computers difficult (though this has not been shown to be too much of a problem to date) or may fear disclosure of their information "through the Internet". Working with people before deciding on a tool is a good idea in case some of these problems arise.

- Use survey methods appropriate to the literacy level of your target population. If you have a population that is only functionally literate, use of an interviewer-administered survey or ACASI or VCASI might be preferable to a self-administered one.

- Be clear in defining what you are asking. Not all people define "sex" the same way. For example, adolescent women in the 1990s were frequently having unprotected anal sex to avoid pregnancy—and many did not refer to it as sex. Thus, we have a situation ripe for misclassification and bias. If the question is, "In the last three months, have you had sex?" and the answer is "No," a person would be misclassified had she had anal sex in the study interval. Better to ask about each type of behavior separately and clearly, and to define in lay or street terms what is meant. Another option is to have the respondent state what terminology he or she would prefer for the questions in the survey, and then for the interviewer to customize the interview for that specific participant. The skip patterns of the survey should be developed such that one incorrect answer at the top of the question "tree" will not prevent exposure to additional questions. For example, if there is a skip pattern such that the first question is, "In the last three months, have you had sex?" and a "No" response will skip the participant to the next question, then there may be unnecessarily missing data: One incorrect answer here precludes all the other answers. Here it would be preferable to ask a series of specific questions, such as "In the last three months, have you had oral sex?" then "In the last three months, have you had vaginal sex?" and so forth (adding codified and specific probes and definitions for interviewer use).

- Use or adapt previously validated instrumentation when possible. When using tools that have already been shown to be reliable and valid, researchers are relieved of a great deal of work. Norms may have been set and much of the pretest footwork has been done. Still, even if no changes are to be made, the researchers would be wise to assess the instrument in their own target population to be sure it is acceptable, culturally competent, and likely to collect valid and reliable information from participants. If changes are to be made to adapt the tool to the target population, they should be made with attention paid to the pretest data and pilot information; once the instrument is changed at all, it becomes an entirely different tool, and the established norms usually do not apply.

- Know the specific biases that may be at work in your study. In a study of sexual partners, heterosexual male participants may be more likely to overestimate the number of sexual partners whereas heterosexual female participants may underestimate the number of sexual partners. Males who have sex with men tend to underestimate their sexual partners who may put them at risk

continued

Asking About Sensitive Information, Part I—continued

for HIV, whereas male heterosexuals tend to do the opposite.[19] When possible, use design elements to try to reduce these biases. For example, a normalizing statement in advance of certain questions can be helpful in reducing social desirability bias: "Many people have sex with more than one person at a time; have you ever had sex with more than one person at a time?" (Be careful not to normalize too much, though, or you will get the opposite problem: People feel it is *so* normal to engage in certain behaviors that they go in the opposite direction, disclosing behavior they did not have.)

- Nonparticipation, either overall or for specific questions (item nonresponse) can be hazardous to the information to be gained from your study. If people do not participate in the study (and no one must ever be coerced), their data are not able to help develop conclusions about the target population. Sometimes nonresponse can be very high and this can be problematic. Item nonresponse is equally problematic. Extensive interviewer training regarding systematic probes, rereading the sentence, and slowing down tend to be useful techniques to reduce this problem, but other population-specific techniques may be necessary.
- There should be as little ambiguity as possible in the question stems and the response sets. Generalities should be avoided, as should vague time frames. Note the differences among the following questions:
  - ○ "In general, do you use condoms?" (yes/no)
  - ○ "Did you or your partner use a condom the last time you had vaginal sex?" (yes/no)
  - ○ "In the last three months, how many times did you have vaginal sex?" (number) "Of these times, for how many did you or your partner use a condom?" (number)

Although all of these questions strive to understand condom use, you can see that they differ quite a lot. The utility of asking about the last time someone did something is that it is very concrete: the respondent is being asked to remember something highly specific and anchored in time and memory. The limitation of this approach is that you may miss the "usual" case—that is, the last time may have been unusual in that the respondent used a condom when he or she usually does not. This may be overcome through use of a second question, along the lines of, "Is that usual for you?" Anchoring in time is also important. Behavior can change rapidly, and so making windows of time about which the instrument is asking is important. Depending on information obtained during the formative phase, you may decide to break these down into smaller or aggregate into larger time blocks. It may also be useful to have participants think of their own landmarks before starting the study, and then use their landmarks in the narrative. For example, ask the participant what he or she was doing 3 and 6 months ago. Then incorporate the answers into the questionnaire. For example, "Since you graduated high school, how many times did you have vaginal sex?" (number) "Of these times, for how many did you or your partner use a condom?" (number)

Extensive research has been published on ascertaining valid and reproducible data on sensitive topics. When you are about to embark on designing a survey to address sexual or other sensitive behavior, being well-versed is this body of research is advisable.

Asking About Sensitive Information, Part II

Getting information can be difficult on many topics, because few behaviors are validly and reliably observable. For example, adherence to study medication for participants in a clinical trial usually relies upon participant self-report: "Did you take your last dose of medicine?" may be the only way to assess adherence to the study medication. Although in some studies, technology and resources are available to facilitate use of biomarkers (for example, a blood level of the study drug in question), this is not always possible. Even when it is possible, natural variability in the pharmacokinetics and pharmacodynamics within and between individuals may make these results less than perfect, the cost may be prohibitive, or the use not generalizable to usual clinical practice. Monitoring a patient while in the hospital to assess adherence is neither feasible nor useful, because participant behavior will be influenced by the fact that they are being monitored. Other behaviors are even more difficult to measure: condom use, disclosure of HIV status to sexual partners, illegal activities, mental illness, substance use, and abuse. Even seemingly benign questions such as, "Do you have a library card?" may be sensitive. (Respondents might think: "Maybe they think I can't read" or "Maybe they think I don't have enough money for books.") Other questions are clearly sensitive ("When was the last time you injected heroin?"). How can we best measure these things? If unbiased measurement is necessary in order to conduct our study, a means of obtaining an outcome is crucial. The methods come into clear focus when assessing outcomes about sensitive issues.

Techniques, for making public health interventions in the field as well as participants in studies more comfortable in answering uncomfortable questions honestly, increasingly have been developed and researched over the last decade. Anonymous questionnaires, culturally sensitive and appropriate interviewers, tools that are visually demonstrated to the participant to be completely confidential, creative techniques such as audio or video computer-assisted self-interviewing techniques (ACASI or VCASI) are helping people to answer questions more truthfully. For example, in the field, in order to screen for risk factors for HIV, hepatitis, and other infectious diseases that would be hazardous to the blood supply, screening methods have been developed for blood banks. Upon screening for blood donations, confidential screening interviews are conducted. Potential donors answer questions about their risk factors, physical state, and symptoms they might have. This information is factored together to suggest their level of risk and whether the blood will be used. (All blood still undergoes screening; this process is a predonation screening that can further screen out those individuals at increased risk of communicable illnesses.) However, most donors are allowed to donate (if they are deemed healthy enough to do so), even those who have suggestive risk factors. Why? Because many people donate in semi-social situations, such as a blood drive at work or school. If people knew that they would be publicly dismissed as a donor, they might not be willing to tell the truth about their personal risk factors, to prevent embarrassment or inadvertent disclosure. Allowing them to donate with the others encourages frank disclosure of risk factors to the blood supply, and may in turn make it safer.

Other methods of obtaining sensitive data with reduced bias have used computers to help. Metzger and his colleagues compared rates of socially unacceptable behavior (e.g., unsafe sexual behavior, HIV testing out of study, illicit drug use) in the context of a large HIV vaccine using ACASI.[20] This study suggested that such behavior was more likely to be reported using ACASI than traditional face-to-face interview. Kissinger and her colleagues studied ACASI in the context of a randomized trial of patient-delivered partner treatment for *Chlamydia trachomatis* (an STD).[15] The outcomes under study included number of sexual partners, getting new sexual partners, pregnancy, condom use, having symptoms of STDs, and douching. Participants were randomized to have an ACASI interview first or a face-to-face interview first, but everyone got *both* types of surveys, which contained the same questions so they could be compared. Compared to the ACASI, participants were more likely to report having done more socially desirable behavior (e.g., condom use) and less socially undesirable behavior (e.g., gaining a new sex partner) in the face-to-face interview; conversely, in the ACASI they were more likely to report more socially undesirable behavior and less socially desirable behavior than in the face-to-face. No difference in the data collection modalities was seen in neutral topics, such as pregnancy. This study suggested that ACASI might be a useful tool to get at more "truth" in responses than traditional face-to-face interviews, especially in the area of social desirability bias.

Kurth[17] and her colleagues conducted a similar study, comparing responses on ACASI to the clinician's documented report in the medical record, finding that men and women differed in the types of information discrepancies between clinician history and ACASI. Women were more likely to report more same-sex behavior, oral sex, drug (amphetamine) use, and sex in exchange for goods or assistance on ACASI than to the clinician (although the authors note that it is difficult to confirm the questions were asked the same way by all clinicians). Men were also more likely to report same-sex behavior on ACASI. As in other studies, both men and women found the ACASI process acceptable.

Through research and the scientific process, we are collectively improving our ability to obtain increasingly accurate measures of sexual behavior and other behaviors that may be considered sensitive. Use of technology in both training and survey administration has much to offer, as does the use of research to identify what works, and what does not.

select themselves to be in a study. This is the central issue in selection bias. But there is a wrinkle to it that makes it a bit harder to understand. In order for there to actually be selection bias in a study, there has to be a disproportionate entry of individuals into the study, causing it to be different from the true proportion of individuals found in the base population. Another way of saying this is that the entry of cases and controls into the

study matches that in the population from which they are selected, there is not selection bias—even if cases enter the study at different rates than the controls. For example, if cases are more likely than controls to have been exposed, and this is what holds for the population as well as for our sample, then there is not selection bias in the sample in the study. However, if this proportion entered into each 2×2 cell of our study for reasons other than the true composition of the base population, then we have a problem: our sample no longer is in sync with the population, and we have selection bias.

There are several types of selection bias that are important for those with an interest in infectious disease epidemiology:

Loss to follow-up

This bias works just the way it sounds. People stop participating in studies for a variety of reasons. They may become too ill, they may move, they may decide that they no longer wish to participate, they may have died, they may not have transportation to the study visits but be too embarrassed by this fact to inform the study staff, or any other factor that intentionally or unintentionally keeps the participant from being followed up for the duration of the study. Loss to follow-up is a primary concern in any prospective study, and for studies that require more than one visit to obtain endpoint information for the study. This includes retrospective studies as well if more than one visit was required to gather the required data. In infectious disease epidemiology, this could be virtually any type of study in which the disease is being viewed over a long period of time.

Ascertainment bias

This bias occurs when data are differentially ascertained based upon the alternate axis, either exposure or disease. Imagine you are conducting a case-control study of the association between being hospitalized at the time of death and having an infectious disease. You sit with a stack of death certificates before you, systematically abstracting data. Cases are defined as those who died from an infectious disease; controls as those who died from another (noninfectious) cause. When you get to a control that was not in the hospital at the time of death, you add this information to your data extraction form and move on. This person is considered nondiseased and nonexposed. Next you get to a case that was in the hospital at the time of death and died of an infectious process. You add this information to your data extraction form and move on. Then you get to a case that was not in the hospital at the time of death. You decide to go to the local hospital and query their medical records, just to be sure that the physician completing the death certificate was correct. In fact, this patient had been hospitalized at the time of death. You code him as diseased and exposed. You continue to seek medical records only for those at the hospital with the combination diseased and nonexposed. In this sense, you have differentially ascertained information: you sought medical records only on persons who were diseased and nonexposed, creating a severe bias. All study procedures must be applied in the exact same manner irrespective of diseased/nondiseased and exposed/

nonexposed status—and any combination thereof. While it seems like this is an issue of misclassification and information bias (which some consider it to be), it can be categorized appropriately as a selection bias. Ascertainment bias has to do with who gets into the study and which information gets into the study. The information is not altered, it is differentially ascertained.

Incidence-prevalence bias (also known as Neyman's bias)

As discussed in the study design chapters, use of incident cases is preferable to use of prevalent cases. New cases have several benefits: they have not been around a long time, they have not tried treatments for their disease, and they may be younger than existing cases. Prevalent cases usually have had additional experiences with medication, treatment approaches, and other life events when compared with incident cases. Even more, they are typically sicker or with more progressed disease than their counterparts. In diseases that are acute and short-lived (due to death or to cure), this is less of a problem than when there is a long induction period. For diseases that are of a long duration, such as TB or HIV, use of both incident and prevalent cases together in the same study can obscure your understanding of the independent and dependent variables, creating substantial bias. The key problem in incidence-prevalence bias is that when a group of individuals has survived to the point of being able to enter a study, the predictors or exposures of interest may be associated with whether or not they have the opportunity to enter the study. For example, the healthier people survive to the point of being able to enter a study, and the sickest individuals have died. This gives us a distorted perspective on the frequency of exposure among the diseased. Another way of looking at this is as if we are mixing two sub-populations taken from the same base population. If you can imagine that there were hypothetical case definitions in place, or inclusion or exclusion criteria, the prevalent cases would have a different set than would the incident cases.

Time-related selection biases

- *Prevalent-cohort bias:* In cohorts of participants where the disease process has already begun, people often are included without knowing their infection status. This may be the case, for example, with HIV, due to the difficulty in identifying when transmission occurred, the window period prior to the appearance of antibodies, seroconversion, and multiple risk factors. This is a problem because participants enter the study and appear to be disease free at baseline, but are actually not. This creates a cohort that is rife with incidence-prevalence bias.
- *Differential length-biased sampling:* This is a type of prevalence-incidence bias, which results from survivor-

ship differences between study participants. It is similar to survivor treatment selection bias (below), but instead of referring only to treatment, it is for any disease or survival. What it means is that the most rapidly progressing diseased persons will not enter because either they are too ill or they die prior to being able to enter the cohort. If the covariate of interest is associated with the extent of length-based truncation, bias will enter the estimate of the association and result in a bias towards the null (estimate ~1.0).

- Survivor treatment selection bias: Survivor treatment selection bias is very similar to the differential length-biased sampling; in this case, it occurs when the healthier individuals survive to the point of being able to access superior treatments. As a result, it appears that the cohort is healthier and the treatments more effective than they would be among a cohort of sicker individuals. This is a very abstract bias with few means of reducing it, except for controlling who enters the study. By making a more homogenous study sample through use of case definitions and adherence to carefully constructed inclusion and exclusion criteria, this can be reduced to the extent possible. By including large cohorts of patients, such as that in statewide healthcare systems, large health maintenance organization databases, or public assistance programs—and following all of them over long periods of time—this bias can be somewhat measured and reduced in studies. Still, it is impossible to know if people that survive their illness to the point of getting any treatment and who enter our cohorts are different from those who do not. Why? We only can study those who enter our study; we cannot study those who do not.

- *Volunteer bias:* People who volunteer for studies are generally quite different than those who do not. Use of volunteers can introduce bias into your study, especially when behavior is a part of your research question. If motivation to be treated, to help others, or to be adherent to the study are associated with or are the outcomes of interest, then use of volunteers can be problematic.

- *Berkson's bias:* People who are hospitalized are different than those who are not. They differ in their basic demographics (e.g., socioeconomic status), clinical state (e.g., sicker than nonhospitalized patients), and so forth. Comparing hospitalized with nonhospitalized persons can be inappropriate, and likely to give biased estimates of the relationship under study.

More about time-related selection biases

The biases that relate to time of diagnosis, survivorship, and entry into the cohort are complicated. They require an understanding of an abstract world where everyone *would* have entered the study because everyone became diseased at the same time. Of course, this never happens: people get sick before others, they die before some and after others, they access treatments at different times, and so forth. Here is an example to make one of these—differential length-biased sampling—more intuitive. Because the biases are similar, this may help clarify this complex yet important bias.

Imagine this: You are interested in learning about the association between HIV-positive women with cervical cancer *in situ* and its relationship with *Trichomonas vaginalis*—an STD. You are interested in whether there is an association with cervical cancer and *T. vaginalis* as there is with HPV, so you conduct a retrospective cohort study.

Imagine you begin your study with a hypothetical group of HIV-positive women at baseline, T_0. If all of the women with the STD did in fact develop cancer and then die, it could be that by $T_{0 + 5 \text{ years}}$, all the women in the cohort who were most exemplary of the relationship between *T. vaginalis* and cancer would be drained from the cohort.

Now imagine the real world. You start your study at some time after that point, $T_{0 + 5 \text{ years}}$. You find that there is no association between the exposure, *T. vaginalis*, and the disease, cervical cancer. You had sufficient statistical power to find a difference if there was one, and there was not. What could have happened? In this hypothetical example, differential length-biased sampling drained your cohort of those with the most extreme display of the relationship under study. They are no longer in the cohort, because the people with the exposure died already of cancer—it being the strongest relationship among those that died. Unwittingly to you, as you were not able to access the full cohort because you began your study at a later point—and you cannot measure that relationship because it never was evaluated, because of this bias. Thus, your estimate is biased towards the null: it looks as if there is no, or an attenuated, relationship between the two. Sadly, because there is no one complete cohort, this may be happening but it is impossible to measure. One way to reduce the impact of this bias is to place strict entry criteria on your study, in an effort to make participants similar with regard to disease, incidence, and prevalence.

MEANS OF REDUCING OR ELIMINATING INFORMATION BIAS

Despite the wealth of valuable computers we have today, data analysis simply cannot remove the effects of bias from a study after the fact. We can adjust our data to assess things as sophisticated as the independent contribution of each variable into predicting the outcome's status, but if we have collected our data in a biased fashion, then there is no undoing it. The second most important thing to do (after protecting participant risks of course, which is always *the* most important) is to think through all elements of data collection analysis, interpretation, and dissemination prior to beginning data collection. Doing so will reduce bias substantially and ensure that you are obtaining the most internally valid data that is possible. There are several different ways to reduce bias, and they all involve work from the foundation of the study's development:

- Sometimes the best way to reduce human error in interviewing may be to eliminate the human element altogether. If a study contains sensitive questions, the study is long, a variety of interviewers are conducting the study, or there is more than one site, enlisting the help of a computer-assisted survey instrument can be very helpful. These ACASI or VCASI, or handheld computer interviewing devices, ensure that the questions are read or stated identically throughout the entire study. All participants are given precisely the same interview, without any risk of the interviewer changing words, deleting responses, inadvertently introducing a judgmental or overly sympathetic interviewer, or so forth. This type of computer-assisted interviewing also is useful because many respondents answer more honestly because they do not feel pressure to be "perfect" while talking with the interviewer.
- Piloting the study protocols and practicing interviewing and all elements of the study's implementation are good steps towards training and reducing to the extent possible imperfect survey administration. Extensive preimplementation work also helps to pilot the study with members of the target population. Piloting and working with the community early in the process is beneficial. This not only allows you to ensure that scientific needs of the study are met and that it is conducted well, but also that the community has the opportunity to provide input into how the study is done.
- Blinding is an excellent low-tech approach to reducing bias. It reduces the chance that knowing about the exposure, for example, will alter the collection of data about the disease. This can happen by accident, because it is

very difficult to not be influenced by what you experience. Having two (or more) different people work on data abstraction, interviewing, analysis, or other study related tasks—to keep individuals as far away as they can from potential biasing knowledge of disease or exposure status—can be very useful.

- Comprehensive training on the study instruments and all field technology can reduce bias substantially. Obviously, training is critical in every way. Good training and field practice may be the single most important step one can take to reduce bias. Practice, discussions about bias, role-playing regarding field worker responses in difficult situations, and rigorous supervision can make the difference between a study with lots of bias and a study with very little of it. Field workers should not only know intellectually how to reduce bias in the way they conduct the interview and comport themselves, but also have extensive training and role-playing experience using the survey in order to become facile with the instrumentation. This type of training will make it much easier to stay true to the words of the instrument, even if—as are all surveys—the interview text is not perfect. Even when this is the case, it is essential to read the questions and response sets exactly as written. This is no time for creative adaptation, which makes the training, practicing, and role-playing so important. For medical or other record abstraction, training is equally important.
- Quality assurance mechanisms including extensive supervision of interviewers, data collection and entry procedures should be developed from the beginning. The study staff should understand that quality assurance and supervision are a part of the overall team effort, striving for the best-possible study implementation. Finding an error is not a negative, but instead an opportunity for training and team-building. All study staff should be trained to regard the quality assurance and supervision protocols as an integral part of the study's conduct.

MISSING INFORMATION

On the surface, it would seem that missing data are not such a big problem: The data are not there, so they cannot and should not be worried about. *Cannot* is somewhat true—if data are missing, there are precious few approaches to dealing with the problem. *Should not* is a different story, however. Just as we must be concerned with how data are collected, we must be equally concerned with data that we try to collect but that for one reason or another cannot be collected. Bias can result in situations with missing data because the "truth" is not ascertainable if there is no information to go on. If the data are missing completely at random, and their being missing is not associated with any predictor, outcome, or confounder, it causes less of a problem. However, this is seldom the case. Usually data are missing for some reason intrinsic to the study or to the participant, and the fact that the data are missing is hardly random. Each situation is different, and the types of bias created by each type of missing data are different. Missing predictor data, outcome data, and confounder data are all important. Although the specifics of dealing with missing data can fill textbooks as well as entire courses, we are going to think about missing data here in the context of how it causes bias and why it is important to do everything we can to reduce missing data.

The purpose of studies, research, evaluation, and surveillance is to obtain information. Yet, no matter how hard we try, there will be times that we cannot get all the information that we want. Think about your own experiences: have you ever been given a survey and answered most of the questions, but refused to answer some? On those that you do not wish to answer, you are creating a situation of missing data for the researchers. (Mind you, this is absolutely okay: that is the reason for informed consent, to let us know that we do not have to participate or answer anything we do not wish to answer.) Or imagine that you are at a doctor's appointment. The physician checks your reflexes and yet neglects to document what they were. Or imagine that you are at a buffet where there is a foodborne outbreak the next day. When asked if you ate the quiche that night, you genuinely do not remember. Or finally, you are in a study to evaluate the efficacy of a vaccine to prevent HIV but you move to a different state to attend college, prior to the last follow-up visit of the study.

Each of these is an example of missing data; there are countless more. In all of these situations, problems can arise when we try to make inferences about our data from incomplete datasets. And this is because we simply lack information on which to base our conclusions. What data we have may be perfect, but the data we do not have tell their own story, a story we do not have access to. In the examples above, imagine that the people who did not wish to answer a certain type of question, say a question regarding drug use, were more likely to have hepatitis C than the other respondents; if the people who could not recall whether they ate the quiche at the buffet were less likely to have food poisoning; if the people who moved to different states to attend college and thus never were tested to see if they had HIV were more likely to have multiple sex partners than others. . . . Each of these could lead to a situation in which there are consistent and systematic patterns creating gaps in the information and missing data that would results. Besides the obvious—active follow-up, incentives, protocols, resources, and creative and innovative methods to keep clients

involved in the study—there is often nothing to do to remove missing data. And because we cannot know the answers to each of the questions we are seeking, we cannot know how to place each of these answers in our contingency table. And thus our conclusions are generated on only those people for whom we do *not* have missing data—and this creates, or can create, a false conclusion about whatever it is we happen to be studying. As we have in this situation, the missing data, as they usually are, are systematic in nature: not missing at random, but rather missing data that are associated with either independent, dependent, or confounding variables.

There are some ways to use the information that is available, to do one's best to address missing data. One can impute values (use existing data and information to develop good "guesses" to take the place of missing data). One can use actual data from the patients with missing visits; for example, if a patient was missing his or her last visit for that study, the investigator could take the visit before the last one missed—because that would be the closest in time to becoming missed—and use that information instead. Finally, one could ignore the problem altogether—assume that people missing information are the same as those not missing information, and that the missing information would not have helped to illuminate the question under study. Although the former two choices replace missing information with a surrogate (the average of other subjects or visits), or assume the last data point available is a good enough proxy for the data point that is missing, the latter can be a somewhat hazardous assumption. It is seldom realistic to assume that people with missing data are the same as those without. And yet, this sometimes is the only thing that can be done in the real world of research. At times, one must just analyze the available information and go from there.

MISCLASSIFICATION

The problem of missing data sets the stage solidly for that of misclassification—something we have touched upon already in this chapter. Missing data are relatively easy to understand: the data are missing, thus we cannot know what the outcome would have been had we known them. It is clear that this will create bias in our estimates of the relationship under study. But what happens when the information is present, appears to be correct but is actually wrong? This is the problem of misclassification, and introduces a very different problem, one that is harder to handle and yet crucial to attempt to control.

Misclassification is the result of the biases mentioned above. Misclassification is when study subjects are incorrectly classified with respect to exposure or disease status. That may happen because of the multiple biases discussed above during data collection, entry, or management; because of inaccurate and random

Using Surveys to Collect Information During an Outbreak—Nonresponse

Pertussis, also known as whooping cough in honor of the severe whoop-like cough it creates, is caused by a bacterium, *Bordetella pertussis*.[4,21,22]

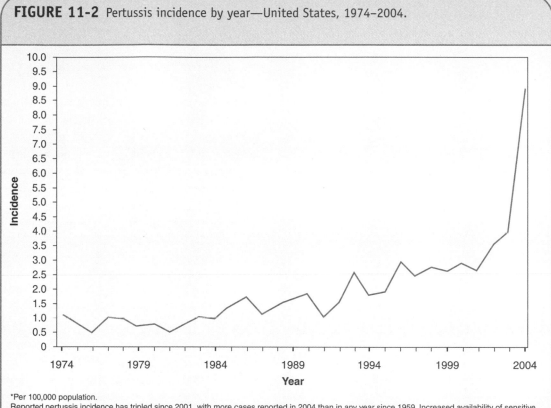

FIGURE 11-2 Pertussis incidence by year—United States, 1974–2004.

*Per 100,000 population.
Reported pertussis incidence has tripled since 2001, with more cases reported in 2004 than in any year since 1959. Increased availability of sensitive diagnostic test and improved case recognition and reporting account for an unknown fraction of this increase.

Over the past three decades, despite availability of an effective vaccine to prevent pertussis, cases have risen sharply. Much of this is due to vaccine-related behavior.

Source: Summary of Notifiable Diseases. United States, 2004. (2006). *MMWR* 53(53): 1–80.

This disease has been vaccine-preventable for decades, and current immunization recommendations include a three-shot series to infants and a booster for adolescents and adults.[23] Of all vaccine-preventable diseases, pertussis is one that has experienced increases in recent years, primarily due to two reasons:[21,22] lack of vaccination among children, and when immunity wanes from the vaccine after approximately 5 to 10 years, adults become susceptible and can get the disease themselves and/or pass the disease on to children.

In 2005, there was an outbreak of pertussis among an Amish community in Delaware. Although this religion does not prohibit vaccination, vaccination rates remain low, in part due to its insularity; previous outbreaks of other vaccine-preventable diseases (i.e., rubella and Haemophilus influenzae) have taken place in Amish communities.[21,22] In order to assess individuals having symptoms of pertussis, treatment and diagnosis, and previous vaccination, a self-administered survey was given to religious leaders, and then given one per household to all community members. Just over half (57%) of households returned the survey, with 19% of the people represented by the surveys having symptoms consistent with pertussis. Households with possible cases were contacted and a total of 274 confirmed and probable cases were identified in 96 houses.

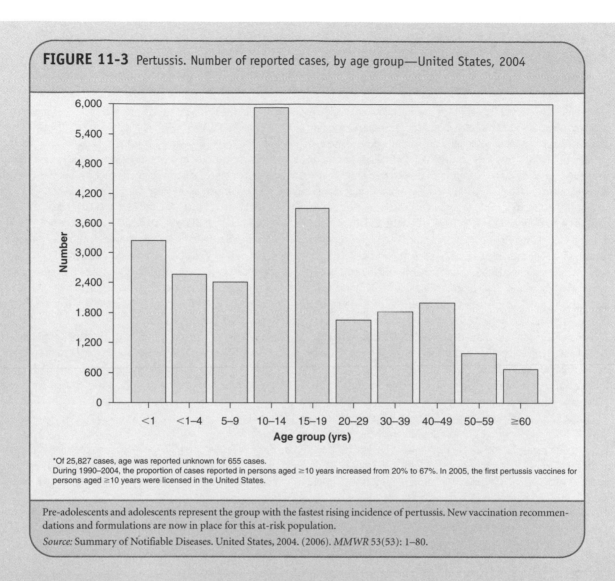

FIGURE 11-3 Pertussis. Number of reported cases, by age group—United States, 2004

*Of 25,827 cases, age was reported unknown for 655 cases.
During 1990–2004, the proportion of cases reported in persons aged ≥10 years increased from 20% to 67%. In 2005, the first pertussis vaccines for persons aged ≥10 years were licensed in the United States.

Pre-adolescents and adolescents represent the group with the fastest rising incidence of pertussis. New vaccination recommendations and formulations are now in place for this at-risk population.

Source: Summary of Notifiable Diseases. United States, 2004. (2006). *MMWR* 53(53): 1–80.

What about the nonrespondents—the 43% of households that did not return the survey? This is important to consider. It may be that they had no symptoms or had already been vaccinated, thus they did not feel it important to participate. Perhaps they were not able to read or understand the survey. Perhaps they had already been hospitalized or died of pertussis. Irrespective of the reasons, they are important to take into account when analyzing any dataset. Nonresponse is a significant source of bias and, unfortunately, there is not much we can do about it. The information is missing and thus the information it could provide is similarly so. In this case, the primary problem in an immediate sense was that those households could not be evaluated or treated. In the long term, though, there were other consequences. The survey queried respondents about their perceptions of vaccinations; having this information on the community would have enabled better development of social marketing tools to improve vaccination rates in the future.

measurement; or because information is "guessed" incorrectly. Major categories of why misclassification occurs include:

- Inaccurate or incomplete recall of prior exposure or symptoms by participants
- Inaccurate reporting of disease or exposure information (intentionally or unintentionally)
- Systematic error due to subconscious or conscious gathering of selective data by interview and field staff; may occur while asking questions as well as during data abstraction, data entry, or analysis/interpretation
- Inaccurate measurement of exposure or disease-related parameters
- Inaccurate diagnosis of disease

Some of these will be systematic, or differential, in nature, whereas others will be nondifferential, more like noise, such as inaccurate measurement.

How Can We Study Misclassification?

Misclassification is a serious concern in epidemiologic studies. As mentioned in the text, when there are only two cells on each axis—exposed/nonexposed or diseased/nondiseased—one wrong turn lands the counts squarely in the opposite domain. The exposure and disease status can all of a sudden land one in an opposite direction from the truth, and wrong conclusions can quickly result.

In an outbreak investigation, this is of particular concern. One way misclassification can be easily demonstrated is to imagine the situation that Harris and colleagues evaluated.[3] In looking at antimicrobial resistance—that is, bacteria that are resistant to antibiotic treatment—case-control approaches are frequently taken. Cases can be identified in the hospital, because they have undergone laboratory testing to identify the specific resistance patterns. Hospital-based controls may be identified in two key ways: random samples taken from individuals who have antibiotic-sensitive (nonresistant) cultures, and those who are admitted to the hospital at risk of having resistant strains but who have not (yet) been cultured. There are potential limitations of each approach: In the former, there is the risk of selection bias, because patients with less severe disease would not be included in the study. (This could occur because they did not require laboratory assessment initially; this is also known as a severity of illness bias) In the latter, there is the problem of what the authors dub *control group misclassification bias*. In this case, some of the controls, by virtue of not having been tested, may actually be cases that have not been shown to be cases. Should this occur, the bias would be towards the null (that is, odds ratio [OR] = 1.0) because the cases and controls would appear more similar than they in fact were.

Harris et al.[3] conducted a study to assess the degree of misclassification that could occur in these two different control-selection approaches. They compared results from two case-controls studies performed with each of the control group types, in a hospital-based study of imipenem-resistant *Pseudomonas aeruginosa*, a gram-negative bacillus that is often the cause of pneumonia.[4] They found that although there was a degree of control group misclassification bias, and the estimates derived from use of the healthier controls could have been biased towards the null. The effect of the severity of illness selection bias was worse. The controls who had a culture conducted as a requirement for control section were sicker individuals, thus introducing a selection bias that was worse than the potential misclassification, in the opinion of the authors.

Deciding on an appropriate control group is always difficult. This study provides guidance on the relative strengths and limitations of different types of control groups. As you develop your own studies, taking into account methodological studies such as this one in the evaluation of an appropriate control group is very helpful. Unfortunately, as seen here, sometimes one has to live with a little bias to avoid a lot of it.

Misclassification and Surveillance: What Happens When There Is Confusion in a Case Definition?

Syphilis is a difficult disease to correctly stage, thus rendering surveillance—a critical part of disease control—challenging. Stages of syphilis are as follows:[4–6]

- *Primary syphilis:* This stage usually begins 3 weeks after infection, but ranges from 10 to 90 days after infection. It is usually accompanied by a painless ulcer called a chancre at the point of infection.
- *Secondary syphilis:* Several weeks or months later the patient may have one or more systemic manifestations of disease, including a generalized rash that is also on the soles of their feet and palms of their hands, hair loss, and swollen lymph nodes. Symptoms of secondary syphilis tend to spontaneously resolve within weeks to a year.
- *Latent syphilis:* The period of latency is only detectable serologically, and then staged based on duration of disease. Early latent is the first year of the latent phase; late latent occurs thereafter. There is a third category, unknown duration, for situations with missing information. The duration is established through a combination of laboratory testing data and recall of symptoms.
- *Tertiary syphilis:* During late latent syphilis, the patient can develop tertiary syphilis (though not all do), which is characterized by central nervous system involvement, cardiovascular effects, disabling systemic lesions, and finally death.

With use of antibiotics, complications from syphilis have decreased dramatically—just one injection of benzathine penicillin G generally cures primary, secondary, and early latent infections; three weekly doses cure late latent. But tracking syphilis can be difficult, which makes it difficult, in turn, to fully have faith in surveillance estimates as we will discuss in Chapter 12.

Peterman and colleagues took a systematic look at local health department records to assess the degree of misclassification of syphilis.[6] What they found reflected the challenges involved in classifying the latent stages. Out of 973 records assessed, primary, secondary, and late latent showed excellent or very good agreement with the case definitions described above, with 94.0%, 95.4%, and 80.2% agreement, respectively. Agreement for early latent (48.4%) and unknown duration (49.7%) were not nearly as good, with misclassification having taken place more than half the time each. Some locations changed substantially with restaging, indicating the value of systematic evaluation and the risk of misclassification. As a result of this study, the authors recommend consideration of a new classification scheme that would evaluate the latent stage not on duration, which is not always attainable, but on whether the person has a high or low indicator in the blood (nontreponemal titer).

What were some of the barriers to accurate classification of disease? To identify these, and propose means of reducing misclassification, the authors conducted a comprehensive evaluation using both quantitative and qualitative methods:

- Not all of the health departments used systematic forms to help classify disease; those that used the forms had less misclassification than those that did not.
- Not all of the health departments were using the Centers for Disease Control and Prevention (CDC) case definitions.
- There were individual differences between staff members based on misunderstanding or individual interpretations of the case definitions. These interpretations differed from person to person and from patient to patient..
- Not all personnel at a given site agreed on definitions; for example, clinicians and disease investigation specialists did not always agree.
- Sometimes partner notification personnel, feeling that a case should be traced despite the late latent stage, would document early latent status, to facilitate contact tracing and partner notification.

Most of these issues could be addressed with increased training and education. In addition, refinement of the operationalization of the latent stage case definition was suggested as a means to improve consistency in diagnosis. Improved surveillance of syphilis will allow better tracking of the disease, as well as comparison between when cases are being identified and when they are being treated (as those emerge from use of latent case data).

In differential misclassification, we have situations in which the errors are systematic in direction only. For example, imagine you are conducting a community-based study of varicella titers to gauge the duration of the response to the chickenpox vaccine among college students. The study is conducted at the student-health center, where there is one STD screening room. Every time a person goes into the STD screening room, they have a blood test taken in the correct type of blood collection tube. All other patients, however, have it taken in an incorrect tube that actually alters the processing of the specimen and consistently makes the titer appear lower than it actually is. In this situation, we have a systematic difference in the way the data are being collected. Whether the titer was collected in the correct tube or the incorrect tube is consistently associated with the STD status of the student. STD screening room—correct tube; all other rooms—incorrect tube. Now, it may be that this will not affect your findings. However, if the predictor of interest is whether the student had signs or symptoms of STDs then we will have misclassification, where the outcome of interest (titer) is misclassified based on the exposure (STD status).

The problem with this type of situation is that it is impossible to know; in general (though this example would have hopefully been identified by supervisory staff), that such a problem is occurring and leading to misclassification. Often it is impossible to detect. Therefore, bias can lead to differential misclassification, but other things can as well. With differential misclassification, it is generally impossible to determine the direction of the inaccuracy or bias: Your estimate may bias towards the null or away from the null—and you will not be able to tell.

Now take this situation again, only this time there is one nurse who just plain confuses the tubes. Whether the person is there for a cholesterol checkup or an STD screening or a broken leg, this one nurse uses the wrong tube for the study. Here, some study participants will inevitably be counted as low titer when they should in fact be high, and vice versa, but this is not occurring systematically. And, most importantly, it is not associated in any way with the way in which the predictor or confounders of interest were collected. Here we have just random "noise" or variability entering into our equation. When this is the case, in general, the "noise" makes it harder to see if there is a difference between the exposure and the disease of interest; this attenuates the relationships and in almost all cases biases towards the null (i.e., OR or relative risk [RR] = 1.0). In the case of nondifferential misclassification, we may have difficulty finding an association if one does exist.

Sometimes it is hard to see the difference between the multiple words and categories we have to describe differential misclassification and nondifferential misclassification and biases. One easy way is this:

1. Misclassification is generally the result of bias.
   a. Information bias, which is whether one correctly classifies information once they are in the study. This relates to internal validity: was the study done correctly and without bias?
   b. Selection bias, which is whether a representative sample makes it into your study. This relates to external validity, also known as generalizability.
2. These categories of bias relate to misclassification of exposure or disease, which is differential—that is, it is systematic. They occur when the item is being misclassified.
3. Misclassification can also be the result of random phenomena, which creates "noise." This is called nondifferential misclassification. This type of misclassification can occur at any time, with either exposure or disease. This problem is easier to fix because increased knowledge about the exposure and disease axes, supervision, and quality assurance activities can often identify the problem and fix it. Nonsystematic error is thus not a bias, and yields problems on a smaller scale.

4. Finally, we have missing data. Missing information makes it very hard to know what we are doing altogether. This generally leads to misclassification if the data are estimated, imputed, or otherwise placed in our analysis in the absence of certainty about the exposure or disease category. If eliminated from the analysis, bias results from that elimination if the data were systematically missing; now the whole cases are systematically excluded, which may give us false impressions of the information we have.

Bias and misclassification are the primary bane to researchers' goals. It affects everything from how the study is designed, implemented, data are collected, managed, analyzed, and interpreted. Obtaining inaccurate information, which is systematically out of sync with the reality of the participants, or that fails to study the correct subjects, invalidates the reason for the study: to learn about a relationship between an exposure and an outcome. As a student of infectious disease epidemiology, your job is two-fold:

1. Learn how to identify bias in the studies you read. If you can do this, you will better understand the interpretation of the study (and whether you believe the author is correct), and their implications on public health practice. The more you read and critically analyze all you read for bias in design, analysis, and interpretation, the better your own research skills will be.

2. Learn how to avoid bias in the studies you conduct, as well as to quantify and rigorously explore the biases that are present in your data.

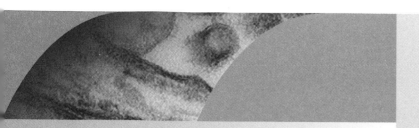

Discussion Questions

3. Write a table listing the most salient biases for each study design type we have covered thus far: the randomized controlled trial, the cohort study, the case-control study, the cross-sectional, the ecologic study, the outbreak investigation, and the case series/case report. For each, write one way to reduce bias through study design methods.

1. Go to your favorite peer-reviewed journal and find one article. Identify at least one type of selection bias, information bias, and potential source of misclassification. How could you assess if these are present? Did the authors do anything to assess if they were present? How could the authors have designed the study differently in order to avoid these problems?

2. In Chapter 10, there was a question regarding a large concurrent cohort study evaluating the association between drinking alcohol and likelihood of contracting an STD over the course of a year. [Note: these numbers are hypothetical.] After data collection is complete, your 2×2 table looked like this:

	STD	No STD	
Alcohol	295	2116	2411
No alcohol	160	3929	4,089
	455	6045	6,500

Both alcohol use and STDs are sensitive issues to some. What if there were misclassification of exposure and outcome in the following ways:

   a. 20% of people who had had an STD stated they did not; what would the RR be?

   b. 40% of people who had drank alcohol stated they did not; what would the RR be?

   c. 30% of people who had had an STD stated they did not drink alcohol when they did; what would the RR be?

REFERENCES

1. Sackett DL. Bias in analytic research. *J Chron Dis.* 1979;32:51–63.

2. Delgado-Rodriguez M, Llorca J. Bias. *J Epidemiol Comm Health.* 2004; 58:635–641.

3. Harris A, Carmeli Y, Samore MH, et al. Impact of severity of illness bias and control group misclassification bias in case-control studies of antimicrobial-resistant organisms. *Infect Control Hosp Epidemiol.* 2005;26:342–345.

4. Heymann DL. *Control of Communicable Diseases.* 18th ed. Washington, DC: American Public Health Association.

5. Nelson, K. Infectious Disease Epidemiology. Gaithersburg, Aspen Publishers, Inc; 2001.

6. Peterman TA, Kahn RH, Ciesielski CA, et al. Misclassification of the Stages of Syphilis: Implications for Surveillance. Sex Transm Dis 2005;32 (144–9).

7. Centers for Disease Control and Prevention. Pneumocystis pneumonia—Los Angeles. *MMWR.* 1981;30:250–252.

8. Babbie E. *Survey Research Methods.* 2nd ed. Belmont, CA: Wadsworth; 1990.

9. Alreck P, Settle R. *The Survey Research Handbook.* New York, NY: McGraw-Hill Professional Publishing; 1995.

10. Catania J, Binson D, Van der Straten A, et al. Effects of interviewer gender, interviewer choice, and item wording on responses to questions concerning sexual behaviour. *Public Opin Q.* 1996;60:345–375.

11. Catania J, Binson D, Van der Straten A, et al. Methodological research on sexual behavior in the AIDS era. *Ann Rev Sex Res.* 1995;6:77–125.

12. Fink A. *The Complete Survey Kit.* Thousand Oaks, CA: Sage Publications; 1995.

13. Fowler FJ. *Improving Survey Questions: Design and Evaluation.* Thousand Oaks, CA: Sage Publications; 1995.

14. Fowler FJ. *Survey Research Methods.* 3rd ed. Thousand Oaks, CA: Sage Publications; 2000.

15. Kissinger P, Rice J, Farley T, et al. Application of computer-assisted interviews to sexual behavior research. *Am J Epidemiol.* 1999;149:950–954.

16. Fenton KA, Johnson AM, McManus S, et al. Measuring sexual behaviour: methodological challenges in survey research. *Sex Transm Inf.* 2001; 77:84–92.

17. Kurth A, Martin A, Golden MR. A comparison between audio computer-assisted self-interviews and clinician interviews for obtaining the sexual history. *Sex Trans Dis.* 2004;31:719–726.

18. Strassberg D, Lowe K. Volunteer bias in sexuality research. *Arch Sex Behav.* 1995;24:369–382.

19. Paget W, Zwahlen M, Eichmann, AR, et al. Voluntary confidential HIV testing of STD patients in Switzerland, 1990–5: HIV test refusers cause different biases on HIV prevalences in heterosexuals and homo/bisexuals. *Genitourinary Med.* 1997;73:444–447.

20. Metzger D, Koblin B, Turner C, et al. Randomized controlled trial of audio computer-assisted self-interviewing: utility and acceptability in longitudinal studies. *Am J Epidemiol.* 2000;152:99–106.

21. Centers for Disease Control and Prevention. Pertussis—United States, 1997–2000. *MMWR.* 2002;51:73–76.

22. Centers for Disease Control and Prevention. Pertussis outbreak in an Amish community—Kent County, Delaware, September 2004–February 2005. *MMWR.* 2006;55(30):817–821.

23. Ward JI, Cherry JD, Chang S-J, et al. Efficacy of an acellular pertussis vaccine among adolescents and adults. *New Engl J Med.* 2005;353(15): 1555–1563.

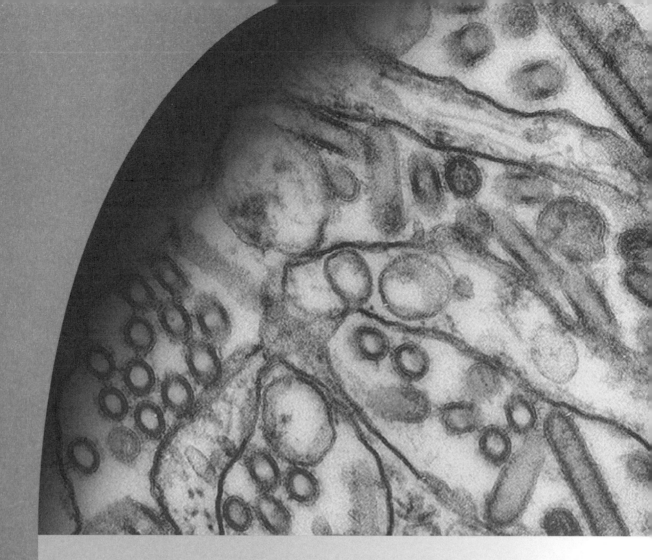

PART II

Special Applications

Surveillance of Infectious Disease

METHODS IN PRACTICE

Think back to Chapter 4 when we discussed outbreaks. Recall that one has to assess whether there actually *is* an outbreak before conducting an outbreak investigation. Is the occurrence of disease more than would ordinarily be expected for that time, area, or type of person? At that point, I did not mention the difficulty underlying that particular step: What data are collected that can answer these questions? How were these data collected? Who keeps this important information? How does one use that information to answer the crucial question preceding the outbreak investigation? Since so much of infectious disease epidemiology is understanding the prevalence and incidence of disease—and answering these critical questions—we need to be able to keep track in an ongoing fashion of the diseases that affect us. How can we do this?

Surveillance is the answer in most cases. Surveillance is a common concept, one with which most readers are already fairly familiar. Infectious disease surveillance is the most accessible of surveillance systems, one of the oldest to be sure, and one of the most readily intuitive as well. With communicable diseases, keeping count of the distribution of disease is obviously essential—few would disagree. Who is most vulnerable to disease, where the disease is spreading and at what rate, the manifestation of the disease, the rate of death, chronic illness, cure, and so forth. However, the details involved with setting up a comprehensive system that is able to do this is another story. In all forms of research we see how crucial methods are in the collection, management, analysis, and dissemination of data; surveillance is no different. Methods matter here as well, because we often need to characterize disease among a large target population. With surveillance, by and large we are not only looking for disease within a select group of participants or clinic attendees, we now must characterize it in large geographical regions such as states, countries, or even the globe. The search for evidence of disease can include coordination not only of personnel but of countries and governments at times. Yet only through a systematic, ongoing search for disease can we ascertain case counts, assess the effects of control measures, and monitor for emerging or re-emerging diseases. Only through this ongoing mechanism can we answer our question when confronted with various diseases, "Is this a true outbreak?"

The definition of surveillance is worth considering in some detail. The Centers for Disease Control and Prevention's (CDC) definition is a well-written one that has persisted (with modifications, truncations, and expansions—yet true to this central definition), and it provides a clear understanding of what surveillance is as well as how it works. It is a directive as well as a definition:

Public health surveillance is the ongoing, systematic collection, analysis, interpretation, and dissemination of data regarding a health-related event for use in public health action to reduce morbidity and mortality and to improve health.[1]

Let us dissect this a bit.

Public health surveillance has these facets that define it and direct us regarding how to implement systems. Note the following words and phrases in the definition:

Ongoing: Public health surveillance must be ongoing in nature in order to inform us about the state of disease under investigation by any particular system. Intermittent, sporadic, or casual systems will not be able to provide answers to the background rates of disease, because they would not contain sufficient information to allow comparison among places, time periods, or groups of people. Thus, any surveillance system must be ongoing.

Systematic: A surveillance system must be systematic. Just as our methods matter in other types of studies, so, too, do they in surveillance. There must be a systematic method that is universally applied in order to make a solid surveillance system. For example, imagine a surveillance system evaluating chlamydia that in some cities always required laboratory confirmation to define the disease, in others required clinical presentation, and in still others required self-report of clients. How would these data be compared? They would not be at all comparable. Imagine now that in one city chlamydia information is collected on nice, neat case report forms, and in another they are called in, and in still another they are just collected from nursing notes. How would these be compared? It would be extremely difficult and hardly systematic. Systematic means that a system—the same method—is applied to each and every potential case in each and every situation. If forms are used to collect data that include laboratory data, this same method is followed for all cases. Although this by no means should be taken to imply that data gathering is always perfect simply because there is a system (unfortunately that is not the case); it means that a specific and articulated system is in place to direct the method by which data are sought, collected, documented, recorded, analyzed, and disseminated. In order to be a surveillance system, there can be nothing anecdotal or haphazard about the means by which the information is retrieved. Note that the systematic nature of this applies to the *collection, analysis, interpretation, and dissemination* phases, not just one phase.

Health-related event: Many different types of surveillance systems are possible; the ones that we are concerned with here are those covering health-related events and, in particular, infectious disease events. The same concept can apply in a variety of settings, however. Surveillance of other events has a great deal in common with surveillance of infectious diseases.

Use in *public health action to reduce morbidity and mortality and to improve health:* The objective of surveillance is clearly put here: The data derived from surveillance should not gather dust, never being used, or simply be used for research that does not effect improvement of the health of the community. Surveillance data should be used to take public health action that does three things: reduces morbidity (sickness), reduces mortality (death), and improves health. Information gained through surveillance should be constantly fed back into the community to create an ongoing feedback loop of information knowledge→public health action→improved healthcare delivery→reduced rates of sickness and death, and improved health. Note that this feedback construct is similar to that of the evaluation construct that we will discuss in Chapter 13.

It is important to look at the characteristics of a surveillance system, in order to understand what such systems do, what features make them better or worse, and how methods are a part of surveillance activities.

INTRODUCTION TO INFECTIOUS DISEASE SURVEILLANCE

Counting occurrences of disease was one of the oldest forms of public health activity (see Appendix 2). As good histories of medicine describe, counting was one of the first public health activities ever. A novel idea at the time, the idea of counting became recognized as an increasingly important step towards quantifying the presence of disease in a community while also prompting prevention and control activities. Even before it was clear how different diseases were spread (e.g., Droplet transmission? Vector borne? Humours?) people realized that counting disease cases is a necessary step towards being able to control disease. As you will see in Appendix 2, some of the first steps towards the development of epidemiology as a science were that of counting death from disease). What do we do? Define the disease, try to figure out its cause, identify the mode of transmission, control the outbreak, and—hopefully—prevent future cases of it. As more infectious diseases emerged or were recognized, more diseases came to be under surveillance, where they could be mapped, counted, characterized, and, eventually, controlled and prevented.

Surveillance is somewhat like outbreak investigations, but on a meta scale. With surveillance, we count the occurrence of disease and its trends over a longer duration, and not just in one time-space cluster but overall. Here, knowledge is power. Characterizing individual cases or even individual outbreaks is not enough to understand, control, or prevent disease over lengths of time. Ongoing surveillance was early on recognized as necessary in order to understand disease over time as well as changes in the disease or its predictors and etiologies.

Imagine an investigation surrounding an *E. coli* outbreak at one birthday party. If you looked at the first few cases at this one party, how would you know if there was an outbreak?

Which Diseases Need to be Reported?

In the United States, the CDC regulates which diseases are notifiable on the national level. The World Health Organization (WHO) regulates which diseases are notifiable on the global level (Figure 12-1). Global coordination allows immediate response to threats to public health that cross international borders. Surveillance of HIV/AIDS is a good example of how many facets of a disease may be reported: from risk factors (behavioral surveillance) to death from AIDS (Figure 12-2).

FIGURE 12-1 Infectious diseases designated as notifiable at the national level— United States, 1997

Acquired immunodeficienty syndrome (AIDS)	Measles
Anthrax	Meningococcal disease
Botulism	Mumps
Brucellosis	Pertussis
Chancroid	Plague
Chlamydia trachomatis, genital infections	Poliomyelitis, paralytic
Cholera	Psittacosis
Coccidiodomycosis	Rabies, animal
Cryptosporidiosis	Rabies, human
Diptheria	Rocky Mountain spotted fever
Encephalitis, California serogroup	Rubella
Encephalitis, eastern equine	Rubella, congenital syndrome
Encephalitis, St. Louis	Salmonellosis
Encephalitis, western equine	Shigellosis
Escherichia coli 0157:H7	Streptococcal disease, invasive Group A
Gonorrhea	*Streptococcus pneumoniae,* drug-resistant
Haemophilus influenzae, invasive disease	invasive disease
Hansen disease (leprosy)	Steptococcal toxic-shock syndrome
Hantavirus pulmonary syndrome	Syphilis
Hemolytic uremic syndrome, post-diarrheal	Syphilis, congenital
Hepatitis A	Tetanus
Hepatitis B	Toxic-shock syndrome
Hepatitis, C/non-A, non-B	Trichinosis
HIV infection, pediatric	Tuberculosis
Legionellosis	Typhoid fever
Lyme disease	Yellow fever
Malaria	

In addition, some conditions are also reportable to WHO, as they have international implications as well as domestic (CDC 1997). These include cholera, associated coronavirus (SARS-CoV) disease, plague, yellow fever, West Nile virus, paralytic polio, and smallpox.

Source: CDC Case Definitions for Infectious Conditions Under Public Health Surveillance. *MMWR* 46 (RR-10): 1–64.

continued

Which diseases need to be reported?—continued

FIGURE 12-2 The multiple facets of surveillance for HIV/AIDS—from risk behavior to death

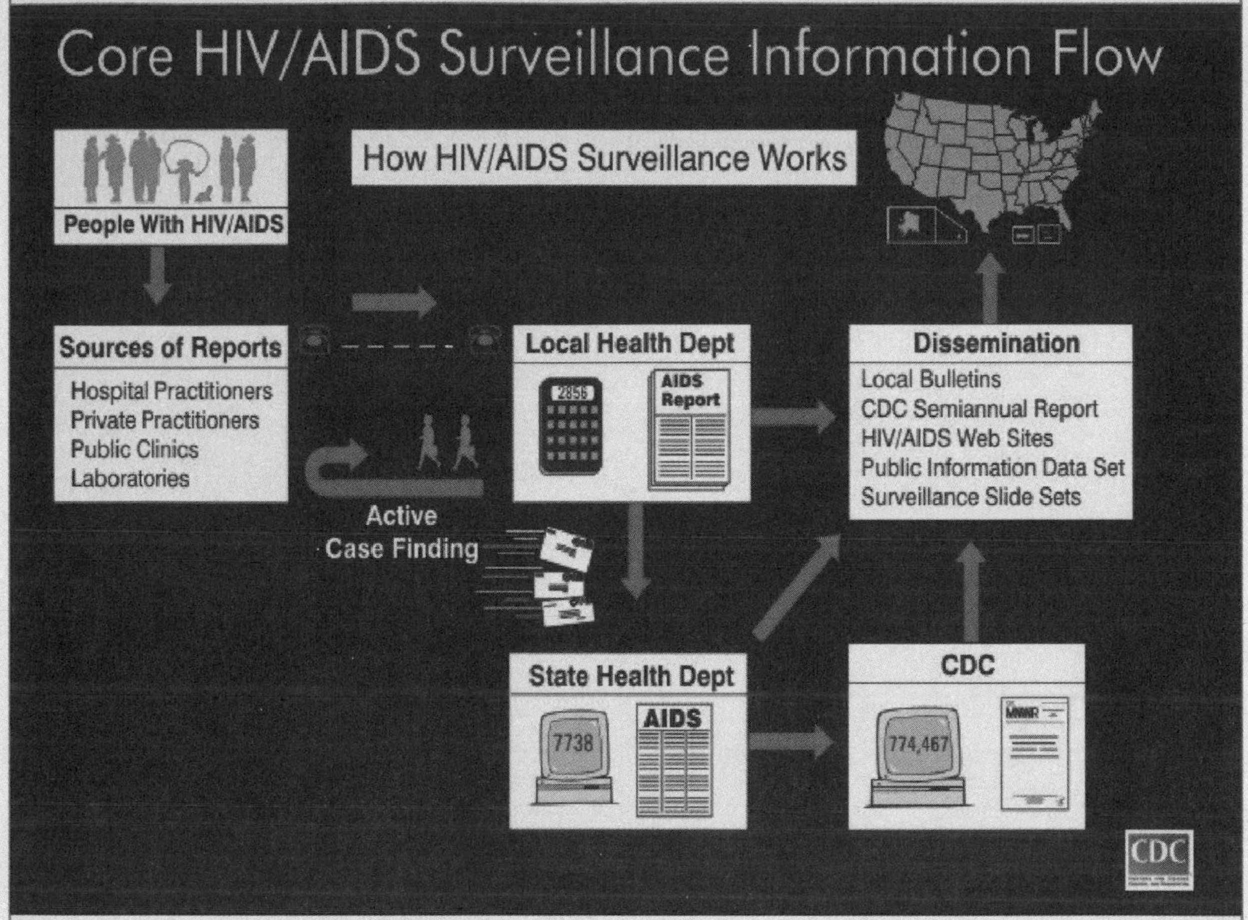

The data flow from diagnosis to submission of HIV/AIDS core surveillance data.
Source: CDC

But now, look at the outbreak in the context of the ongoing surveillance data. We know that one of the first steps in an outbreak investigation is to assess whether there is actually an epidemic. How can one know that there actually is an outbreak without ongoing trend or surveillance data? If you do not have baseline, prevalence, incidence, or mortality data on a specific disease, it is difficult to know if you have an epidemic. Maybe these cases are the only ones regionally—and while they are an outbreak locally, they represent a smaller number of cases in the region over the past year or the usually baseline. Surveillance data allow us to assess the "big picture".

To continue the parallel between outbreak investigations and surveillance, we see the need for case definitions in outbreak investigations: the person-place-time characteristics that define a case need to be clearly stated up front in order to ensure use of homogenous cases. Same, too, for surveillance systems. If we are measuring disease over decades with a primary purpose of comparing time periods, would it be worthwhile to track cases or deaths and put them on the same chart, if the definitions of what makes a case consistently change? No, of course not. That would not make sense—we would constantly be comparing apples with oranges and we would be unable to interpret our data. As much as we use case definitions in outbreak investigations, we must use them in surveillance as well. And we do, making surveillance an extremely useful tool for tracking, understanding, and preventing disease.

Surveillance can be applied to anything, from the behaviors necessary to contract a given illness, to acquisition of disease (incidence), to sickness or disease manifestations, to care services for, all the way to death from an illness. Although the counting that served as the foundation for surveillance systems originally surrounded primarily death, surveillance systems have evolved now to contain the whole pathway from health to death, making surveillance an even more useful tool. Take HIV/AIDS, for example. In the United States, we now conduct surveillance on behaviors that put individuals at risk for HIV acquisition (National HIV Behavioral Surveillance System), new HIV infections (HIV incidence surveillance), sickness from HIV disease and related care systems (morbidity monitoring project), core surveillance of AIDS, and death from AIDS (Figure 12-2). This entire pathway describes HIV/AIDS much more comprehensively than surveillance of death alone would, especially because we now have aggressive treatment regimens that forestall death from AIDS and prolong the duration from HIV acquisition to death. This evolution in disease surveillance provides us with rich information about the disease. It allows us to study all components along the acquisition to death pathway.

DISEASE REPORTING

Surveillance is generally divided into two types: passive and active. Passive surveillance relies primarily upon providers adhering to regulations that govern reporting requirements on the local, regional, state, or federal guidelines. It requires knowledge of the regulations, and requires that providers, such as providers' labs or other institutional personnel, identify an individual who has a reportable disease or condition. They are obliged to submit a full report to the local health department. Active surveillance is a more resource- and energy-intensive type of surveillance, which improves the yield over passive surveillance considerably. With active reporting, members (generally of the local health department in the locality under study) are sent out into the community in order to find new cases of the disease, actively pursuing case finding. They also do general training of the provider and laboratory staff in an effort to improve local passive reporting, thus increasing the yield of passive reporting as well.

Although specifics of how diseases are reported differ from locality to locality as well as between diseases, the surveillance path in the United States is fairly uniform. Those diseases that must be reported as per federal guidelines are ultimately reported to the CDC, which issues regulations guiding local surveillance activities. Systems differ more widely, however, in other countries with different rates of different diseases as well as varying infrastructure and resource settings. In the United States, surveillance paths generally involve mostly passive and some active identification of cases by local health departments. These are then managed to confirm cases as per required case definitions, using source documentation including laboratory reports, medical records, and so forth. Often there will be a deduplication process enlisted to ensure that multiple reports on the same person are not being submitted. This is an important step: Because reports may come from, say, laboratories, primary care physicians, and specialists—all on one person for one event—deduplication of reports ensures that there is an accurate count of cases. Otherwise, one case of, say, malaria could be reported as many times as the patient received care. Depending on the disease and the local and federal regulations, cases may be coded using a unique identifier or patient names. If a code is utilized, then its use must be managed by the local health departments, which will hold the one document linking name to code until they no longer need to do so. From that point, unlinked cases without names of those with reportable diseases that meet case definitions are then submitted to either the state health department or directly to the CDC. That agency tracks changes in the person-place-time characteristics of the disease—numerically, graphically, and conceptually—to develop profiles of the disease over time as well as to identify meaningful increases or decreases. Every surveillance system must have the following:

- The *case definition* for the disease under study. This case definition is the primary means by which people are included in or excluded from a surveillance system; its use is directly analogous to that of outbreak investigations. If there is not a solid case definition, then it is difficult to ensure that like cases are being compared over time points. This case definition must have specific diagnostic criteria within it, must balance sensitivity (How many sick people does the system pick up?) with specificity (If someone shows up sick, what is the probability that they truly are sick?). Note that these are different from clinical definitions: they are developed specifically to suit the needs of the surveillance system being developed. They may differ from clinical purposes or other research needs.

- The *population under surveillance* can be static or dynamic. It may be designed to be representative of all underlying people in the population or not, provided that whatever is chosen is clearly stated and articulated. Estimations of the presence of bias—that is, who is included and excluded from the surveillance system—should be available and quantifiable. If the system only assesses people receiving medical care, the data within this system will differ substantially from a system which is representative of the target population. Take deaths, for example. In the United States, death is more likely to be picked up by death certificates and, later, the National Death Index (NDI). If a surveillance system incorporates only hospital admissions, it will be composed of very different cases (those making it to the hospital, with resources, education, willingness to seek care, etc.) than if the NDI is used instead.
- *Confidentiality* must be assured by the system and all individuals who have access to the data. Whenever we deal with data, protection of that data is the highest priority. We can never be casual or flippant with the use of any type of surveillance data. In every surveillance system—as with data that come from a research study—each data point represents a person. If we do not take the utmost care of this data, then we are disclosing information that is not ours to share, or risking its disclosure. We are betraying the confidence that each of the persons in the system has given to us, the principal investigator, the city, or whatever governing body has ownership of the data. Surveillance data are generally covered by local, state, and/or federal regulations governing how confidentiality must be maintained. This includes handling of data by individuals, how data (electronic as well as paper or other media) are maintained, data transfer policies, and confidentiality training for all personnel coming into contact with the electronic or hardcopy data.

Outbreaks and Airplanes, Part I

As our world has become "smaller" with the advent of rapid air travel, infectious diseases that would, once upon a time, stay put in a given region (city, country, continent) are now readily transported from one place to another. Feeling well, we can board a jet and fly halfway across the world, where we emerge from the jetway, sick as a dog. Diseases, acquired in one part of the world by an unknowing carrier, are transported across oceans, transmitted to unwitting co-passengers on the plane, and ultimately shared with those at the destination point. It is the negative side of a great advance.

Fortunately, serious outbreaks seldom occur as a result of air travel. The common cold usually is transported, but the viruses responsible for the cold are so ubiquitous and not life threatening that it is generally not a problem. Several serious situations have arisen, however. There have been cases where individuals who were ill with infectious diseases were on planes and their presence on the plane ultimately led to full-blown outbreaks.[2-5] For example, in April 2006, there was an outbreak of mumps in Iowa, with as many as 515 possible cases.[5] The state health department identified two persons who had flown on commercial airlines at a time when they were potentially infectious. This information was communicated in the *Morbidity and Mortality Weekly Report (MMWR)* for that week, in an effort to make one more attempt (others methods of control were occurring simultaneously) to identify persons potentially exposed on the airlines to the two mumps cases. Active efforts using written and electronic dispatches[3] were immediately implemented in order to identify fellow passengers who could have been exposed; the *MMWR* published the specific flights the passengers were on in order to try to find potentially exposed persons.

A similar situation happened when a student, traveling from India back to the United States, was found to be infectious with measles.[6] Active engagement of the people exposed to the student on the plane, as well as their contacts, was undertaken. This effort successfully identified those at risk, and offered them postexposure prophylaxis in the form of immune globulin (if they had not been vaccinated against the measles previously and were susceptible). Three were found to be infectious and went into voluntary quarantine at their homes. This old-fashioned public health intervention was effective in preventing further cases from developing. Due to the energy applied to finding people who were exposed and their subsequent contacts, educating them, and providing them with care, a measles outbreak was stopped. These types of active involvement following exposures via air travel are essential. They are also a positive sign of our ability to evolve surveillance techniques to accommodate our changing infectious disease environment.

Outbreaks and Airplanes, Part II

In addition to the problem of transportation of pathogens via air travel, closed travel environments such as airplanes and cruise ships carry with them another concern: outbreaks en route, largely due to an inability to maintain the freshness of food and water. Sometimes, too, they are due to the source of the food, which may be from an area endemic for a specific disease. Norwalk and Norwalk-like viruses are common etiologies of outbreaks on cruise ships, causing gastroenteritis (and ruining many a vacation).[7]

An interesting case occurred in 1996 when there was an outbreak of cholera among passengers on a flight from Lima, Peru, to Los Angeles, California.[8] This was one of the biggest foodborne outbreaks on an airplane. In the early 1990s there was an epidemic of cholera in Latin America, with over 4,000 deaths (~400,000 cases).[8] A flight that began in Argentina, picked up food and passengers in Lima, and then moved on to Los Angeles included a seafood salad—uncooked—on the menu. Of the 336 passengers, 194 (58%) were located once in the United States and submitted specimens.[a] Over half (52%) of these were identified as having evidence of *Vibrio cholerae* infection; of these, three quarters (75%) reported symptoms. Ten were hospitalized; one man died. A case-control study was initiated to elucidate the source of cholera. Figure 12-3 displays a section of the actual data—just as we saw with our own example of an outbreak and analysis of food consumed in Chapter 4. Note that the seafood salad has an odds ratio (OR) of 11.6 (95% CI 3.3–44.5).[b] That the seafood salad would contain the offending organism makes sense. It may be that the water in which the fish

FIGURE 12-3 Food inventory for case and controls who ate selected food items on an airline flight from South America to Los Angeles, February 1992[8]

Food or drink	Cases number(%)	Controls number (%)	OR (95% CI)
(a) Items served between Buenos Aires and Lima			
Raw ham	14/19 (74)	23/50 (46)	3·3 (0·9–12·6)
Cooked ham	13/19 (68)	18/44 (41)	3·1 (0·9–11·6)
Melon	13/19 (68)	26/50 (52)	2·0 (0·6–7·2)
Drink without ice	5/17 (29)	8/46 (17)	2·0 (0·5–8·7)
Bottled water	7/19 (37)	13/50 (26)	1·7 (0·5–6·0)
Iced drink	8/19 (42)	25/48 (52)	0·7 (0·2–2·2)
(b) Items served between Lima and Los Angeles			
Seafood salad	26/30 (87)	27/75 (36)	11·6 (3·3–44·5)
Turkey sandwich	16/29 (55)	21/67 (31)	2·7 (1·0–7·4)
Ham and cheese sandwich	25/31 (81)	42/69 (61)	2·7 (0·9–8·5)
Bottled water	15/31 (48)	20/75 (27)	2·6 (1·0–6·8)
Chicken sandwich	16/31 (52)	22/68 (32)	2·2 (0·9–5·9)
Drink without ice	10/30 (33)	15/74 (20)	2·0 (0·7–5·7)
Cheese	15/31 (48)	30/79 (38)	1·5 (0·6–3·9)
Iced drink	19/30 (63)	43/74 (58)	1·3 (0·5–3·3)
Fresh fruit	5/23 (22)	16/66 (24)	0·9 (0·2–3·1)

This table shows the specific line items of the food inventory for each leg of the flight. A quick comparison of the case and control foods consumed reveals that 87% of the cases vs. 36% of the controls had eaten the seafood, with an OR of 11.6 (95% CI 3.3-44.5)—implicating the seafood salad.

Source: Eberhart-Phillips, Besser et al. 1996 with permission.

---

[a]The article does not indicate how many were identified but refused to provide specimens.
[b]After adjusting for other items eaten, an adjusted OR of 17.9 (95% CI 4.0 - 80.9) was found, strongly implicating the seafood salad and no other items independently contributing to illness.

continues

Outbreaks and Airplanes, Part II—continued

were caught was contaminated with cholera, other ingredients in the salad may have been washed with contaminated water or not washed at all, there could have been the usual food handling problems (e.g., staff not washing their hands), or the salad may have been contaminated en route somehow.

Important recommendations resulted from this outbreak.[8] Some are common preventive measures, whereas others are specific to air travel. If one is traveling to areas with suboptimal hygiene and sanitation, it is better to eat foods that are thoroughly cooked and hot when consumed (this is always true!), and commercial airlines should reconsider their policies in serving foods that are potential vehicles for contagions, either by their nature or their storage/serving process. These recommendations are especially relevant when the food comes from areas that are endemic for or experience epidemics of diseases such as cholera.

The authors rightly point out that this airline outbreak was noted primarily because of its size: smaller outbreaks almost certainly occur and may not be detected. Why was this detected? It was large, cases were fairly well localized in Los Angeles, the presentation was the same, and the appropriate laboratory diagnostics were conducted once in the hospital settings. Surveillance systems for cholera are in place, as it is reportable throughout the world. Were any of these features not in place, this outbreak may well have been overlooked.

Also, what about the 42% of people who were not contacted and/or did not provide specimens? This is an important methodological concern. One way we can address this is to conduct a sensitivity analysis, and calculate our measures of association imagining the outcomes of each of those missing data points at the extremes. For example, imagine if all of the people not located were exposed to the seafood salad and all were cases, such that location of the person was associated with their case and exposure status. We would miss crucial information about our association between the salad and the disease—leading us to the incorrect conclusion. What if they were all exposed and *not* cases? What if none was exposed? And so forth. Doing this creates bounds on what we see as our picture and refines our understanding of the impact of the missing data. If conducting a sensitivity analysis such as this indicates that in every circumstance the seafood was likely the culprit, then we are more confident in our interpretation. If, however, we find that it could have gone the other way, we have to be careful in extrapolating to the entire population of passengers on the plane in question. We can then only generalize our findings to those persons who were located and offered specimens for the outbreak investigation.

WHAT MAKES A GOOD SURVEILLANCE SYSTEM?

Nine basic characteristics have been identified to describe an optimal surveillance system.[1,7,9,10] These are general so that they may be applied to a variety of disease processes and diseases. Specifics for each disease under study, each region, or each target population are then incorporated so that the system is adapted appropriately for each system's specific needs:

1. *Simplicity:* Is the system simple, straightforward, and easy to conduct? Is the surveillance process clear and feasible from an implementation perspective? Are the case report forms readable and easy to complete? An overly complex system is less likely to be used or to collect accurate and optimal data.
2. *Flexibility:* Is the system flexible, such that it expands with the expanding knowledge base about the disease? If the system does not respond at all or responds too rigidly to growing information it will be difficult to keep it up to date and responsive to growing information. Particularly with infectious disease, there are likely to be significant changes in what we understand about disease and its impact on humans; given that, flexibility in the system is necessary.
3. *Data quality:* Is the information that is collected of high quality? Does it accurately and comprehensively reflect the reality of the disease under study? Haphazard data collection is necessarily of poor quality, and can render a surveillance system useless. If the system's data is not high quality, interpretations of the surveillance data will be incorrect and possibly of no use at all.
4. *Acceptability.* Is the system acceptable to the front-line providers and personnel who need to interface with it? If these key individuals are not engaged in the program and do not find it acceptable, they will be unlikely to report high-quality data or engage in the surveillance process. This is a problem for both active and passive surveillance

systems, but obviously especially so for passive systems. If the system is not acceptable to key stakeholders and users, the data are unlikely to be able to provide an accurate portrayal of the disease in the population.

5. *Sensitivity:* Of the true cases in the underlying population, how many of them does the system identify? If in a given region there are 150 cases of a disease, and 100 of them are detected by the surveillance system, then the sensitivity is 67%. The system should pick up the majority of cases—thus have a high sensitivity—and do so in a representative fashion. Sensitivity and specificity are measures used to describe screening programs, but the same measures are useful when evaluating surveillance systems as well. These are described briefly in Appendix 3.

6. *Predictive value positive:* Of the cases identified by the system as having the disease under study, how many of them meet the stated case definition for the program? If 200 cases are detected through passive and active reporting measures, and 57 of them meet the case definition, the predictive value positive is 28.5%. Also discussed in Appendix 3, this measure quantifies the probability that—given the system picks one up as a case—how likely is it to capture a case that is, in fact, a case?

7. *Representativeness:* Does the system identify a representative slice of persons with the disease in the underlying population? Or does it only identify certain types of people, certain socioeconomic strata, for example, or those who access care at particular locations? In order to be a good surveillance system, it must identify a representative sample of individuals with the disease in the base population, not just a select few, which could lead to selection bias.

8. *Timeliness:* Each disease has its own requirements for timeliness of reporting. Surveillance in general is a "real-time" activity; it is not intended to be something that takes many iterations or a long time to do. A lengthy reporting period and time to access surveillance data suggests a problem with the system. In order to have public health impact, up-to-date surveillance data must be readily available. Timeliness refers to how quickly data flow through the surveillance system, and how much time is required at each individual step of the process. Having a long gap between the time a case occurred and when it was reported to when the information was used would yield a less effective system.

9. *Stability:* Is the system stable? Is it expected to be durable over time or will it be replaced by some other system or forgotten as new issues come to the fore? With infectious diseases, we typically add diseases—very rarely do we remove them. If one looks at the list of reportable diseases in the United States and those in the world that are reportable to the WHO, one can see that even older diseases that are mostly eradicated still require reporting. This means that systems must be stable to continue to collect information about old diseases as well as new ones.

BENEFITS OF SURVEILLANCE ACTIVITIES

Although surveillance is critical for a variety of public health concerns—such as cancer, environmental hazards, injury, behavior, violence, and so much more—in no place is the use of surveillance data more intuitive than in infectious disease. Surveillance in this realm is hardly academic. SARS, avian flu, multiresistant tuberculosis, and so many more illnesses have developed or are on the rise just in the past decade. Without surveillance—active looking into the health status of populations—each of these could mushroom, turning into epidemics without our even knowing. For example, in the case of SARS, surveillance and resultant interventions stopped the spread. With avian flu, we have thus far been fortunate. Our global monitoring has led to interventions throughout the world to stop the spread of disease among poultry which, so far, has been associated with decreased risk among humans. Surveillance allows us to understand the natural history and the characteristics of the disease, including outbreaks, modes of transmission, persons at risk, control methods, the geographic location, socioeconomic relationships, and other demographics and characteristics associated with the disease. Surveillance allows one to generate hypotheses that can serve as the basis for later studies, or as a study in the system itself. Such surveillance systems can monitor feedback and improvements that take place in response to analyzing and interpreting the data.

BIAS IN SURVEILLANCE

Imagine conducting a multi-centered clinical trial, where there are multiple sites conducting the same study. You would usually have a protocol that details every imaginable specific of the study so that you can conduct it perfectly. Only instead of a rigorous, tight, and well-monitored protocol, this study has guidelines, a case definition, and suggestions about which way to go, but nothing more tangible than that. With surveillance, every imaginable type of bias that we learned about in the context of study design can happen—but worse, and without nearly the degree of control over data or design. These biases can take many shapes. For example,

New Strains of *Escherichia coli* and the Changing Needs of Surveillance

It used to be that one could order a juicy rare hamburger and eat it without hesitation. Same for licking the bowl and the mixers while mom made a cake, no matter the raw eggs, which can be a common source of salmonella. Times change, though. In recent years, juicy rare hamburgers that were not fully cooked have been associated with outbreaks of *Escherichia coli* O159:H7, a particularly dangerous strain of *E. coli*. This strain has been associated with severe and bloody diarrhea, abdominal pain, and, for approximately 2% to 8% of those infected, can progress to hemolytic uremic syndrome (HUS), a syndrome that includes blood abnormalities and renal failure.[7,11-15] The case fatality rate is high, ranging from 3% to 5%. Over 90% of HUS postdiarrheal cases are associated with this hemorrhagic strain of *E. coli*.[7] Children are gravely affected; HUS is the most common cause of acute renal failure in this population.

This pathogenic gram-negative bacterium was first identified in 1982, and has been the cause of multiple outbreaks, primarily associated with undercooked ground beef, though there have been other sources as well (e.g., raw milk).[7,11,12] (See Figures 12-4 and 12-5.) During an outbreak that extended over 3 months and 4 states in 1992–1993, there were more than 500 confirmed cases and 4 deaths.[7,11,12] A case-control study conducted in Washington State, California, Idaho, and Nevada identified the source as hamburger patties eaten at a particular chain of restaurants and secondary transmissions (contacts with those individuals infected from the original point source). It was due to the Washington State Department of Health, which conducted an initial case-control study, that additional states were pursued and additional cases found. Unfortunately, the specific culture medium[c] needed to screen for *E. coli* O157:H7 in stool samples with bloody diarrhea or other questionable cases is not usually available. Thus, this screening is not routine, and it was not performed in the states other than Washington. It is unfortunate that so many individuals had to be exposed and become ill before the outbreak was stopped and the source identified. This is one problem with surveillance systems: Even as new infections

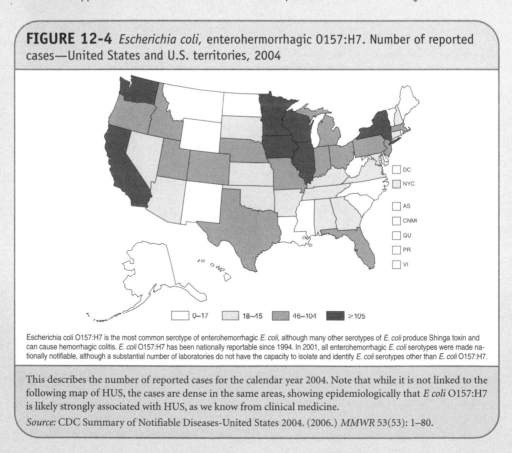

FIGURE 12-4 *Escherichia coli,* enterohermorrhagic O157:H7. Number of reported cases—United States and U.S. territories, 2004

Escherichia coli O157:H7 is the most common serotype of enterohemorrhagic *E. coli*, although many other serotypes of *E. coli* produce Shinga toxin and can cause hemorrhagic colitis. *E. coli* O157:H7 has been nationally reportable since 1994. In 2001, all enterohemorrhagic *E. coli* serotypes were made nationally notifiable, although a substantial number of laboratories do not have the capacity to isolate and identify *E. coli* serotypes other than *E. coli* O157:H7.

This describes the number of reported cases for the calendar year 2004. Note that while it is not linked to the following map of HUS, the cases are dense in the same areas, showing epidemiologically that *E coli* O157:H7 is likely strongly associated with HUS, as we know from clinical medicine.

Source: CDC Summary of Notifiable Diseases-United States 2004. (2006.) *MMWR* 53(53): 1–80.

---

[c]The specific culture medium required to identify this strain is called sorbitol MacConkey (SMAC).

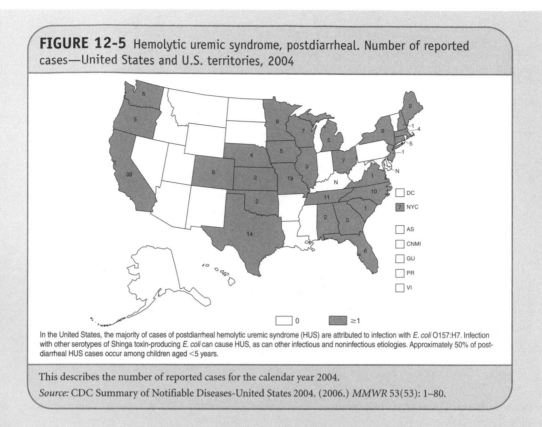

FIGURE 12-5 Hemolytic uremic syndrome, postdiarrheal. Number of reported cases—United States and U.S. territories, 2004

In the United States, the majority of cases of postdiarrheal hemolytic uremic syndrome (HUS) are attributed to infection with *E. coli* O157:H7. Infection with other serotypes of Shinga toxin-producing *E. coli* can cause HUS, as can other infectious and noninfectious etiologies. Approximately 50% of postdiarrheal HUS cases occur among children aged <5 years.

This describes the number of reported cases for the calendar year 2004.

Source: CDC Summary of Notifiable Diseases-United States 2004. (2006.) *MMWR* 53(53): 1–80.

become known and methods for diagnosing them are developed, it does not mean that they are automatically incorporated into clinical care; if not diagnosed appropriately, surveillance will obviously be suboptimal.

The postscript is that in 1994, this and similar strains of *E. coli* became notifiable in the United States under the name of enterohemorrhagic *E. coli* (EHEC), which includes other strains.[d] This resulted in better ability to diagnosis the disease, including the ability to send specimens to public health laboratories as needed. After a period of increase, cases have now decreased. Surveillance, together with improved regulation and enforcement, are helping to make a safer food supply. Still, the risk remains to some degree, and many local laws require that menus at restaurants disclose that there is a risk of consuming rare meat, raw eggs, and raw shellfish due to the risks of *E. coli* among other diseases.

---

[d]EHEC O157:H7; EHEC, serogroup non-0157; and EHEC, not serogrouped.

---

there can be self-reporting bias, such as people who experience food poisoning but are too embarrassed to disclose. There may be ascertainment bias, where information is sought on cases differentially from controls. Or misclassification, where information is missing making it look like someone who meets the case definition suddenly does not. Or selection bias, where there is not a representative distribution of cases that are identified when compared with the base population.

Like study design in general, it is only possible to see what you are doing, the people you are studying, and the results you are finding; it is never possible to see what you are not doing, the people you have not reached out to, or the results you happened not to have found. You only have what you have. Given this, you must be very diligent and consistent in assessing each surveillance system that you are reading about, evaluating, or creating, so that you know what biases are intrinsic to the data that result from that particular system. That way, estimations of the magnitude and direction of the bias may be made, in order to help identify what corrective measures must be taken. If it is not possible to eliminate or reduce the source of bias, then care can at the very least be taken that compensates for it and addresses the needs of those subgroups.

Changing Perceptions: What Used to Be a Disease Only of Travelers Becomes More Common Domestically

A great deal of being an epidemiologist, whatever your area of expertise may be, lies in embracing change. What holds true one day almost certainly will not the next. Akin to being a detective, epidemiologists must be able to think quickly on their feet and look to new—not old—paradigms. This is what makes epidemiology such an exciting field.

Infectious disease is particularly like this. A good example may be found in another strain of E. coli, called enterotoxin-producing E. coli serotype 0169:H41.[3,7,15] In the past, this strain was thought mostly to occur among travelers to developing countries, and it has a different presentation than the strain E. coli 157:H7. This so-called traveler's diarrhea is now the most common enterotoxigenic E. coli serotype in the United States. Sometimes it is difficult to identify the true etiology of an outbreak, with symptoms of many infectious agents being so similar. However, knowing the specific strain at work enables improved outbreak investigations. With laboratory identification, cases may be definitively linked to one another, and trace-back investigations can occur to identify the source and stop the contamination more effectively.

Cohort studies may be used in certain settings to assist in an outbreak investigation. Case-control studies tend to be utilized more often, because they do not have a requirement of exposure information before the outcome, which is often problematic. However, in occupational settings, this becomes more practical. For example, in order to identify the cause of a cluster of acute gastroenteritis at a company in Tennessee, a cohort study was undertaken.[15] Without it, the strain of E. coli, ultimately determined to be 0169:H41, might never have been discovered simply due to not thinking outside of the box.

In this situation, a company had a catered meal brought in to its employees; 5 days following the event, the local health department was notified about gastrointestinal disease among employees, and an outbreak investigation was initiated. Because it was an occupational setting, it was possible to assess all employees in the company, not just those who consumed the food. Data were ascertained on both exposure and outcome, and a case definition was developed. Cases were defined as employees having diarrhea, vomiting, or fever and cramps within one week of eating the meal (served on two specific dates). Stool specimens were collected to identify the pathogen in a laboratory that could measure enterotoxigenic E. coli as well as other strains. Of the 63 employees, 36 met the case definition (57.1%), and coleslaw was identified as the culprit (unadjusted RR 2.2, 95% CI 1.3–3.6, $p < 0.001$), with an attack rate of 79% among people consuming that dish. Two other foods were also associated significantly with being a case, but after adjusting for the effects of other illnesses, only the coleslaw was significantly associated (OR 4.4, 95% CI 1.1–17.0, $p < 0.05$).[e] Although a thorough examination of the catering company was performed, no confirmed source of the infection was identified. One employee who ate at the

FIGURE 12-6 Provisional cases of selected notifable diseases (50th week)

| | Shiga toxin-producing E. coli (STEC) | | | | |
| | | Previous 52 weeks | | | |
Reporting area	Current week	Med	Max	Cum 2006	Cum 2005
United States	94	53	297	3,026	3,156
New England	—	2	108	282	218
Connecticut	—	0	107	107	58
Maine	—	0	8	43	29
Massachusetts	—	0	9	82	85
New Hampshire	—	0	3	25	18
Rhode Island	—	0	2	8	7
Vermont	—	0	2	2	21
Mid. Atlantic	63	5	107	403	351
New Jersey	—	0	3	3	73
New York (Upstate)	—	0	103	10	133
New York City	—	0	4	35	17
Pennsylvania	48	2	25	197	128

This is an example of the weekly reports provided for all notifable diseases in the United States. This provides an ongoing count—by week, by previous year, by cumulative this and last years—of all diseases that are mandatory reporting. Counting is one of the critical advances made by our epidemiologic forefathers: without systematic counts of disease, it is impossible to know what public health measures are necessary, or, once implemented, effective.

Source: CDC Summary of Notifable Diseases-United States 2004. (2006.) MMWR 53(53): 1–80.

[e]Note that the relative risk (RR) was used in the unadjusted estimate of the association, as we would expect from a cohort study. This measure of association derives from the 2 × 2 table as RR = [a / (a + b) / c / (c + d)]. The adjusted estimate derives from a multivariable logistic regression, a maximum likelihood estimation; thus, even though it is a cohort study, the OR is used to describe the adjusted association.

event had been traveling abroad and also became sick, but given the short incubation period, the fact that that individual, too, became ill 5 days after the event (and not closer to the date of travel, which was 4 weeks prior) suggests that the employee was not the source. It is possible that the lack of refrigeration of the coleslaw was the culprit, but no specific source was ever found. The catering company had prepared more than 800 servings of coleslaw that were distributed to other places, and no other outbreaks were recognized, so there is the suggestion that the problem was at the local level and not with the catering company.

Notice in this example how the laboratory was a critical ingredient in the ability to identify the cause of the outbreak, and that without that step, it would have been easy to mistake the identity of the organism at work. Here we have a case where the symptoms were appropriately reported and followed up on, but had the specific diagnosis not been made, it would have been possible to think this was a different pathogen, simply because we do not expect to see this particular enterotoxigenic *E. coli* in the United States. This and similar studies help to remind us that we need to be on the lookout for strains once considered unlikely.[15]

Different Types of Surveillance

Surveillance is a magnificent part of the epidemiologist's toolkit that may be applied to nearly every condition, as well as stage of illness or health. We can monitor many things: injuries, consumption of vitamins, birth defects, infectious agents, cancers, care delivery—anything. Anything we can count with a systematic method we can conduct surveillance upon.

In the past, we would conduct surveillance on the most severe consequence of any disease or condition: death. This is a straightforward outcome to measure and is almost always the easiest counted of events. In resource-poor settings, counting deaths may be very difficult, but it is generally simpler than counting births, disease, hospitalizations, or behaviors. In the United States, we are fortunate to have the National Death Index, which captures the majority of deaths in the country. This amazing tool facilitates a great deal of surveillance; even if we can get nothing else, knowing if someone has died or not is a tremendous asset to surveillance and research in general.

There is also surveillance of morbidity (illness). This is the next most common form of surveillance. In some ways it is less informative than deaths, because the ability to be counted as ill depends in large part on whether one accesses care. If care is not accessed, a person will not be counted. Similarly, if someone accesses care but does not receive or have access to the appropriate diagnostic techniques, it is possible that they will again not be counted. A variety of estimates are available, and these can triangulate estimates of morbidity and make some helpful assumptions about the persons not counted and the true numbers being affected by a specific disease.

In infectious disease, one of the most exciting changes is a recent recognition of the need to conduct surveillance on antecedents to disease as well as disease and death. We can look at HIV/AIDS as a great example, as in Figure 12-7. At first we conducted surveillance on death from AIDS. Then we conducted surveillance on people with AIDS. Now that we have highly active antiretroviral treatment (HAART) and we have improved the number of people who can survive with HIV by delaying the onset of AIDS, we are conducting surveillance on HIV. Then it became possible, using a new technology, to assess the incidence of HIV, that is, new infections. It is now possible to quantify changes in IgG that accompany infection with HIV. This allows estimations to be made regarding the incidence of HIV, by virtue of how long someone, who has just tested HIV+, has been infected. This testing methodology is called Serologic Testing Algorithm for Recent HIV Seroconversions (STARHS), and it is a relatively new addition to the HIV/AIDS surveillance toolkit.[16] What is left? It would be helpful to understand what people in the population do that puts them at risk for HIV. Then we would have covered all the bases.

But how do we assess behavior? If we ask people who are already HIV+, we are not able to see the behavior of people *before* they are infected. Once infected, so many factors have changed—including the ability to accurately report on behavior prior to infection sometimes—so we need to find a way to assess behavior differently. Ideally, we would ascertain the general population's behavior; this would enable creation of improved outreach and prevention strategies. As we know, asking people what they

continues

Different Types of Surveillance—continued

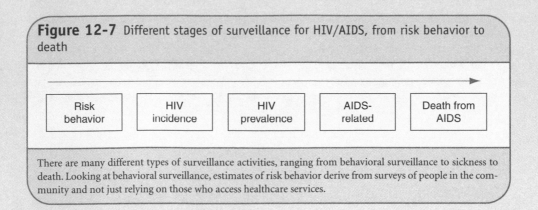

Figure 12-7 Different stages of surveillance for HIV/AIDS, from risk behavior to death

| Risk behavior | HIV incidence | HIV prevalence | AIDS-related | Death from AIDS |

There are many different types of surveillance activities, ranging from behavioral surveillance to sickness to death. Looking at behavioral surveillance, estimates of risk behavior derive from surveys of people in the community and not just relying on those who access healthcare services.

do is fraught with hazards and limitations; and yet, it really is the best option we have. With skilled creators of surveys and survey methodology, limitations of survey data may be limited to the extent possible, and reliable—and crucial—information may be gathered. This information can inform us about what people do that puts them at risk for disease, so that we can improve our prevention activities.

In the United States, this is being conducted in a novel fashion via the National HIV Behavioral Surveillance (NHBS) system. Originally conducted in just 17 studies with a handful conducting HIV testing in conjunction with the survey, this unique study is now conducted in 25 cities, all of which perform HIV testing. This novel surveillance approach is conducted in annual cycles: the first was in men who have sex with men (MSM), the second in injecting drug users (IDU), and the third in heterosexuals at high risk of HIV infection. Thus every 3 years, the cycle begins again. This allows coverage of these very distinct risk groups. The MSM cycle uses venue-based sampling, whereas the IDU cycle uses respondent-driven sampling.[i, 17-23] The heterosexual cycle is underway as of this writing, with a pilot cycle. The pilot cycle has half of the 25 sites conducting venue-based and the remainder respondent-driven sampling. Because it is unknown what the best design for this population will be, one of the research questions of this cycle is to identify the optimal sampling strategy to be used in the future. What is essential about both of these sampling methods is that they allow population-based estimates of the underlying population. This is different from a clinic- or organization-based sample. A comprehensive behavioral survey is then conducted with participants, and a rapid HIV test is offered.

Results from a subset of the first MSM cycle were surprising and highlight the utility of behavioral surveillance. One of the findings was that a quarter (25%) of the respondents were HIV+ (prevalence estimate); 46% of black MSM were positive, 21% of white, and 17% of Hispanic. The most alarming finding: almost half (48%) of these positive individuals did not know their status. Positive participants under 30 and nonwhite were most likely to not know their HIV status. Of those positive participants who did not know their status, 64% of them were black. These data alone convey the importance of identifying population-based estimates of risk and testing behavior, as well as positivity. Not only did this very high number of individuals have the opportunity to link into care as a result of the identification of their infection, their information was allowed to enter the other HIV/AIDS surveillance systems so that changes over time may be evaluated. Information from this important study continues to be collected and will most certainly inform our future approach to HIV surveillance and care for patients.

Figure 12-8 displays data from the aforementioned study.[21] Note that the prevalence ratio is correctly used, because this is a cross-sectional study.

---

[i]Venue-based sampling uses a time-space random sampling procedure, whereas respondent-driven sampling uses a snowball-like structure in which friends refer friends; data on the underlying social networks are then collected. Both allow population-based prevalence estimates of the underlying population.

continues

Different Types of Surveillance—continued

FIGURE 12-8 Prevalence of HIV testing during the preceding year among men who have sex with men, by selected characteristics—five NHBS cities June 2004 to April 2005[21]

Characteristic	Total previously tested	Last HIV test during preceeing year		Prevalence ratio	(95% CI[†])
		No.	(%)		
City					
Baltimore	404	260	64	1.00	Referent
Los Angeles	358	231	65	1.00	(0.90–1.11)
Miami	230	136	59	1.04	(0.92–1.17)
New York City	306	202	66	1.03	(0.92–1.14)
San Francisco	351	206	59	0.91	(0.81–1.02)
Age group (yrs)					
18–24	350	285	81	0.86	Referent
25–29	285	200	70	0.86	(0.79–0.94)
30–39	547	330	60	0.74	(0.68–0.81)
40–49	346	180	52	0.64	(0.57–0.72)
≥50	94	40	43	0.52	(0.41–0.66)
Race/Ethnicity					
White, non-Hispanic	589	345	59	1.00	Refernet
Black, non-Hispanic	391	254	65	1.11	(1.00–1.23)
Hispanic	422	289	68	1.17	(1.06–1.28)
Asian, Pacific Islander	85	55	65	1.10	(0.93–1.31)
Native American/ Alaska Native	7	6	86	1.46	(1.07–2.00)
Multiracial	79	52	66	1.12	(0.95–1.34)
Other	34	25	74	1.26	(0.36–1.13)
Education					
<High school	142	97	68	1.00	Referent
High school or equivalent	343	227	66	0.97	(0.85–1.11)
>High school	1,135	709	62	0.91	(0.81–1.03)
Sexual identity					
Homosexual	1,256	787	63	1.00	Referent
Bisexual	320	219	68	1.09	(1.00–1.19)
Health-insurance status					
Private physician or HMO[§]	954	616	65	1.00	Referent
Public	149	91	61	0.95	(0.83–1.08)
None	495	312	63	0.98	(0.90–1.06)
Health-care use					
Visited provider during preceding year					
No	317	156	49	1.00	Referent
Yes	1,305	879	67	1.37	(1.22–1.54)
Provider recommended HIV test[¶]					
No	809	476	59	1.00	Refernet
Yes	496	403	81	1.38	(1.29–1.48)
Most recent HIV test result[**]					
Negative	1,285	874	68	1.00	Referent
Unknown	95	72	76	0.90	(0.80–1.01)
Total	**1,622**	**1,035**	**64**	—	—

*National HIV Behavioral Surveillance
[†]Confidence interval
[§]Health maintenance organization
[¶]Among those who visited a health-care provider during the preceeding year
[**]Results of last HIV test before participation in NHBS

Data from the National HIV Behavioral Surveillance system, indicating the very high prevalence of MSM who are HIV+ and also who do not know their HIV status.

CHANGING CASE DEFINITIONS

Since the identification of the first five cases of *Pneumocystis carinii* pneumonia in men that ushered in the era of HIV/AIDS in 1981, there have been two major case definitions in use for adults and adolescents in the United States:[f] that from 1987, and a revision in 1993.[g, 25,26] Changing case definitions used for surveillance requires more than just making sure there is consensus about the new definition. Attention also needs to be paid to the impact the change will have on case counts and surveillance, past and future. In 1993, the CDC issued a change to the case definition for AIDS for adults and adolescents. This allowed inclusion of people who had absolute CD4 counts less than 200/μL or a CD4 percentage less than 14, and those with invasive cervical cancer, pulmonary TB, or recurrent pneumonia. The most salient change is that regarding CD4 counts. This marker of immune status is a key diagnostic tool in the care of HIV+ persons, providing an understanding of the stage of the disease. As CD4 counts decrease, the immune system is increasingly compromised. Many people were ill enough to be experiencing symptoms at and below this CD4 cutoff, but not ill enough to be considered as having AIDS.[h] This change in guidelines recognized the increased incidence of invasive cervical cancer among HIV+ women (as well as recognizing the different HIV-related manifestations between men and women, and HIV infection in women in general), and the role of TB and recurrent pneumonia.

What happened when the change was made? The impact may be seen in Figure 12-9.

Comparing the 1993 first quarter and the same time period for the previous year, a 21% increase in cases was seen; 89% of those were due to the immunosupression criterion alone. Approximately 75% more AIDS cases were expected to be reported in the total of 1993 as a result of the new case definition, and that may be seen clearly in Figure 12-10. In addition to the absolute number of cases added, there was the issue of diagnostic times. By changing the definition and adding

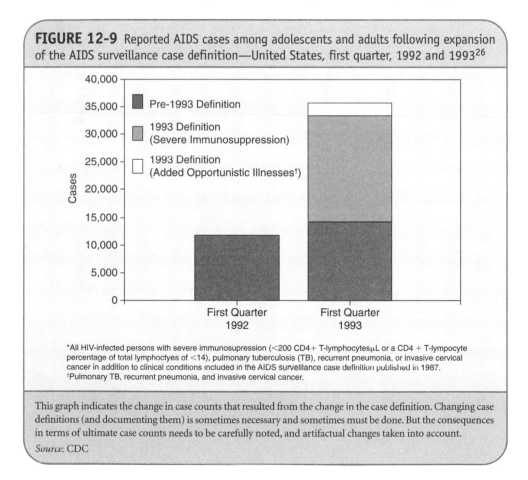

FIGURE 12-9 Reported AIDS cases among adolescents and adults following expansion of the AIDS surveillance case definition—United States, first quarter, 1992 and 1993[26]

*All HIV-infected persons with severe immunosupression (<200 CD4+ T-lymphocytesμL or a CD4 + T-lympocyte percentage of total lymphoctyes of <14), pulmonary tuberculosis (TB), recurrent pneumonia, or invasive cervical cancer in addition to clinical conditions included in the AIDS surveillance case definition published in 1987.
†Pulmonary TB, recurrent pneumonia, and invasive cervical cancer.

This graph indicates the change in case counts that resulted from the change in the case definition. Changing case definitions (and documenting them) is sometimes necessary and sometimes must be done. But the consequences in terms of ultimate case counts needs to be carefully noted, and artifactual changes taken into account.
Source: CDC

---

[f] The pediatric case definition currently in use is from 1994.[24]
[g] This does not include working case definitions that helped to identify early cases, however.

[h] For many, this also impacted availability of support from government agencies and employers.

the laboratory criterion alone, there was an increase in the median interval between date of diagnosis and date of report of AIDS; this increase went from 3 to 5 months for those with pre-1993 case definition, and 3 to 9 months for those with the new condition compared with 3 to 5 months for those with the older definition from 1993. Notice how in Figure 12-10 (and every AIDS surveillance slide since 1993) there is a clear delineation of the change in guidelines, to prevent a reader from thinking there was an increase in cases not due to the surveillance guideline changes.[22] This is an important thing to note; although over time case definitions may change, keeping track and communicating those changes is essential.

Surveillance is an excellent merging of several cornerstone epidemiologic methodologic issues:

- The importance of case definitions and clear operationalization of exposure and disease. Surveillance systems necessitate a clear definition of who will be included in the system as diseased or exposed, and how information on these individuals will be ascertained. This is true for all the study designs we work with, from randomized trials to outbreak investigations to case-control studies.
- The method by which data are collected is critical, and informs us how the system's data may be applied. This is important from the type of data collection forms as well as the way the system itself is operated.

- The use of similar surveillance techniques around the world allows us to understand disease in a way that includes time and space (when, where). The methods that drive surveillance must be uniform enough to compare findings—or the systems will be useless.
- The measures used to describe surveillance data are the same as those used in epidemiologic studies.
- Multidisciplinary approaches to development and implementation of surveillance systems enhances their validity, reliability, and applicability. Without the input of a variety of disciplines—as well as the end users of the system—surveillance techniques are unlikely to succeed.
- Ethical components of surveillance must be considered, just as they do in research and evaluation studies. Methods of reporting and maintenance of absolute confidentiality of data are essential. In addition, understanding the continuum of care for each case is important, such that reporting to the surveillance system does not prevent care delivery to the patient.

Many public health students will find themselves working in surveillance activities, many at departments of health in the United States and abroad. Surveillance is one of the most exciting and important public health activities, one which works not only to study but to control and eventually prevent the spread of infectious disease.

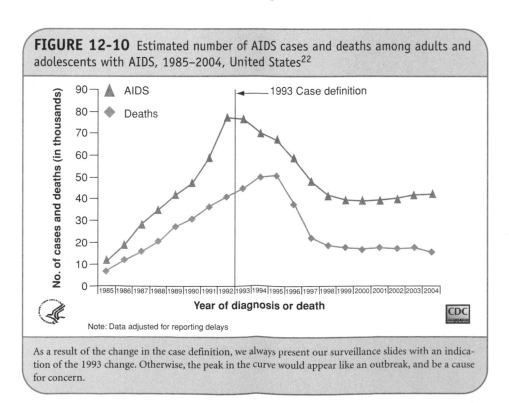

FIGURE 12-10 Estimated number of AIDS cases and deaths among adults and adolescents with AIDS, 1985–2004, United States[22]

Note: Data adjusted for reporting delays

As a result of the change in the case definition, we always present our surveillance slides with an indication of the 1993 change. Otherwise, the peak in the curve would appear like an outbreak, and be a cause for concern.

Surveillance Following a Natural Disaster in the United States: Hurricanes Katrina and Rita, 2005

On August 29, 2005, the gulf coast of the United States was hit by Hurricane Katrina. This historic storm ravaged Louisiana, Mississippi, Alabama, and Georgia, with over 1,000 dead in Louisiana and over 200 in the remaining states, in addition to severe property damage throughout the region. It is not possible to properly describe the damage in words; the many images shared across the media or better yet, by those who visited the region (or visit even now) are necessary to chronicle the depth of the wounds to the environment and its people. Insult was added to injury when, on September 24, 2005, Hurricane Rita hit the south again.

Through a confluence of events—Category 5 winds in the Gulf of Mexico, storm surge conditions, and weakening of the levee system that holds back the waters—New Orleans experienced substantial and life-altering flooding of over 80% of the city. The damage to person and property caused by Hurricane Katrina and the water was extensive, and brought with it infectious disease—and the fear of it. In the absence of surveillance systems, how would we be able to observe if there were a change in disease incidence? It would be impossible. Surveillance systems allow us to observe changes—for the better, for the worse—in disease patterns. Surveillance following this natural disaster was implemented in a number of ways. Infectious diseases, such as cholera that are common in areas without access to clean water or that have flooding, were of particular concern. Other diseases carried by vectors that harness the stagnant waters for reproductive purposes, such as mosquitoes (that can carry malaria, dengue fever, encephalitis, among many others) were a significant worry. This was in addition to concerns of other health needs: access to care, mental health, exposure to environmental dangers, injuries, and more.

On the infectious disease front, there were several approaches taken. In addition to the usual Internet Reportable Disease Database, to which Louisiana usually reports, there were other innovative surveillance methods implemented, and diseases of concern kept under keen watch.[27] Here are some examples of the surveillance that went on following Hurricanes Katrina and Rita:

- Toxigenic *Vibrio cholerae* 01, the bacterium that causes cholera and is generally very rare in the Unite States, was of particular concern with the rising waters. Two cases were identified in persons in Louisiana, following the second hurricane event. The infected individuals had been exposed to floodwaters as well as eating seafood, a common mode of transmission of the disease. Routine surveillance of cholera allowed these cases to be reported to the surveillance system and counted. Although there were other suspected cases, diagnostic studies did not reveal toxigenic *V. cholerae* 01 or 0139 in them. Figure 12-11 shows the number of cases by year and source of infection of *V. cholerae* 01. This is a good example of where surveillance revealed less to worry

FIGURE 12-11 Number of toxigenic *Vibrio cholerae* 01 cases, by year and source of infection—United States, 1996–2005*[27]

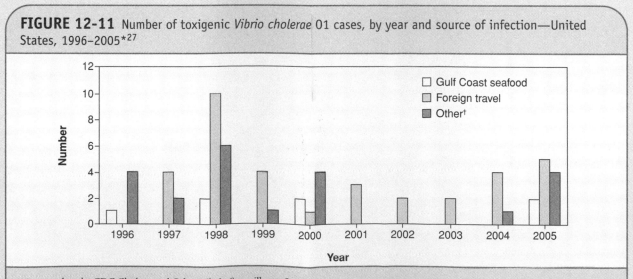

*Reported to the CDC Cholera and Other Vibrio Surveillance System.
†Not associated with either foreign travel or consumption of Gulf Coast seafood. Thirteen of these 22 cases were associated with consumption of seafood from areas other than the Gulf Coast, and nine exposures were undetermined. Thirteen of the cases occurred in the states outside of the Gulf Coast, eight occurred in U.S. territories (seven in Guam and one in the Mariana Islands), and one case occurred in Louisiana.

Surveillance Following a Natural Disaster in the United States: Hurricanes Katrina and Rita, 2005—continued

about than expected. Without a surveillance system, however, and systematic screening for diseases with catastrophic potential among humans, it would not be possible to measure the effect of the natural disaster on this outcome.

- With one of the largest evacuations in the history of New Orleans underway, nearly 50,000 persons sought shelter and refuge in evacuation centers in Louisiana. In addition to routine reporting via the Internet Reportable Disease Database, the need for active surveillance of communicable disease within the evacuation centers was noted. By September 8, 2005, surveillance was activated at the centers using syndromic surveillance. This surveillance system counted the number of times care was sought at each evacuation center of the following symptoms:[27]
  - fever (>100.4°F [>38°C])
  - watery diarrhea (three or more watery bowel movements per day)
  - vomiting
  - bloody diarrhea
  - influenza-like illness or other severe respiratory infection
  - rash
  - scabies, lice, or other infestation
  - conjunctivitis
  - other potentially communicable diseases
  - injury (e.g., self-inflicted injury, intentional injury, unintentional injury, dehydration, or heat related injury)
  - mental health disorders (e.g., preexisting psychiatric disorder, new psychiatric disorder since hurricane, or alcohol/substance abuse or withdrawal)
  - chronic medical conditions (e.g., diabetes mellitus, high blood pressure and other cardiovascular disease, and asthma or chronic obstructive pulmonary disorder)

Why were these symptoms selected? These are general symptoms and syndromes that can indicate the presence of an infectious, communicable disease. Nearly 3,000 (2,975) surveillance forms reporting on 39,217 patient encounters during its 49 days of operations were submitted to the system; Figure 12-12 shows a graph of the reports, while Table 12-1 displays the average daily incidence of disease at the evacuation centers.

Epidemiologists reviewed the data to look for clusters of potential diseases of concern; potential clusters were followed up either by telephone or in person, by the Louisiana Office of Public Health. This is an excellent example of how a low-tech (no diagnostic capacity, limited on-site personnel, high stress situation) approach to surveillance can be effective. It appeared that the majority of the clusters were, in fact, due to overreporting. However, without this innovative system, it would have been impossible to track or stem potential outbreaks. For this type of system, it is better to have a more sensitive system with a low yield, so that problems can be stopped before they become unstoppable.

- Another surveillance system was instituted to assess injuries and illnesses at acute care facilities and hospitals between September 25, 2005 and October 15, 2005. [27] This system was paper based, and providers and staff completed case report forms (CRFs) that were entered into a database and analyzed every 24 hours for trends or indications of increases in injuries or diseases. In this system, there were 17,446 CRFs submitted; 8,997 (51.6%) for illness, 4,579 (26.2%) for injury, and 3,870 (22.2%) for non-acute (e.g., medication refill and follow-up visits) or undetermined reasons; 178 CRFs reported both an injury and an illness (1.0%). Note that while on the surface this system and the one at the evacuation centers *seem* similar they really are not: this one only captures persons that accessed care in an acute care facility or hospital while the other was only located in the evacuation centers. These are largely mutually exclusive systems (unless a sick person at a center was referred to a hospital, for example). In addition, the hospital-based system collected information on injuries as well as syndromic surveillance. Both systems work in tandem to keep track of potential signs of outbreaks that need attention. And these ancillary, situation-specific systems work together with the usual infectious disease surveillance, such as that described for the *V. cholerae*. Tables 12-2 and 12-3 display the data from this surveillance system. Note that the columns break the results into categories (also known as stratifying) of relief worker, resident, or unknown. This assists us in seeing if there may be particular categories of people at risk, as well as taking into account the risks that individuals are facing.

continues

Surveillance Following a Natural Disaster in the United States: Hurricanes Katrina and Rita, 2005—continued

FIGURE 12-12 Number and percentage of persons under surveillance in hurricane evacuation centers (ECs), by date —Louisiana, September–October 2005[27]

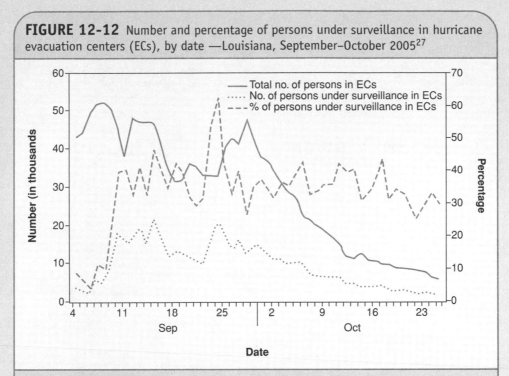

Note that this graph shows on one Y-axis the number in thousands and the percentage on the right Y-axis. The date is along the X-axis.

TABLE 12-1 Average daily incidence* of communicable disease signs and syndromes among persons in hurricane evacuation centers (ECs), by selected conditions—Louisiana, September–October 2005[27]

	Average daily incidence	Range	Largest reported cluster (no. of cases)
Fever only (>100.4°F[>38°C])	0.5	(0–1.9)	10
Bloody diarrhea	0.1	(0–0.7)	6
Watery diarrhea with or without vomiting	1.8	(0–4.0)	22
Vomiting only (one episode or more)	1.3	(0–6.0)	13
Influenza-like illness	4.7	(0–8.8)	47
Rash	2.7	(0–13.8)	35
Scabies, lice, or other infestation	0.6	(0–3.8)	60
Wound infection	1.6	(0–8.5)	34
Conjunctivitis	0.4	(0–1.8)	10

This table provides information on selected signs and syndromes tracked under this surveillance system. The case definitions used refer to the symptoms—for example, the definition of fever is >100.4° F—instead of diagnostic certainty or laboratory-based diagnosis.

*Per 1,000 persons

continues

Surveillance Following a Natural Disaster in the United States: Hurricanes Katrina and Rita, 2005—continued

TABLE 12-2 Number and percentage of persons with selected illnesses after Hurrican Rita, by residency status—New Orleans, Louisiana area, September 25–October 15, 2005[27]

Illness	Relief worker No.	(%)	Resident No.	(%)	Unknown status No.	(%)	Total No.	(%)
Infectious-disease-related								
Skin or wound infection	62	(8.8)	361	(9.9)	459	(9.9)	882	(9.8)
Acute respiratory infection	179	(25.5)	538	(14.8)	587	(12.6)	1,304	(14.5)
Diarrhea	18	(2.6)	92	(2.5)	123	(2.6)	233	(2.6)
Other infectious disease	28	(4.0)	219	(6.0)	223	(4.8)	470	(5.2)
Noninfectious-disease-related								
Rash	59	(8.4)	170	(4.7)	290	(6.2)	519	(5.8)
Heat-related	28	(4.0)	86	(2.4)	118	(2.5)	232	(2.6)
Nondiarrheal gastrointestinal	24	(3.4)	200	(5.5)	253	(5.4)	477	(5.3)
Renal	11	(1.6)	49	(1.3)	104	(2.2)	164	(1.8)
Other classifiable illness*	76	(10.8)	758	(20.8)	1,030	(22.1)	1,864	(20.7)
Other illness†	217	(30.9)	1,166	(32.0)	1,469	(31.6)	2,852	(31.7)
Total	**702**	**(100.0)**	**3,639**	**(100.0)**	**4,656**	**(100.0)**	**8,997**	**(100.0)**

*Includes diabetes, cardiovascular conditions, obstetric/gynecologic conditions, and dental problems.
†Includes other nonclassifiable illness.

TABLE 12-3 Number and percentage of persons with selected injuries and exposures after Hurrican Rita, by residency status—New Orleans, Louisiana area, September 25–October 15, 2005[27]

Illness	Relief worker No.	(%)	Resident No.	(%)	Unknown status No.	(%)	Total No.	(%)
Injury								
Fall	64	(12.0)	449	(25.0)	479	(21.3)	992	(21.7)
Bite/Sting	52	(9.8)	114	(6.3)	173	(7.7)	339	(7.4)
Motor-vehicle crash	20	(3.8)	161	(9.0)	235	(10.5)	416	(9.1)
Intentional injury	11	(2.1)	32	(1.8)	46	(2.0)	89	(1.9)
Other intentional injury*	334	(62.7)	934	(51.9)	1,143	(50.8)	2,411	(52.7)
Undetermined etiology	44	(8.3)	96	(5.3)	158	(7.0)	298	(6.5)
Toxic exposure/Poisoning								
Carbon monoxide poisoning	1	(0.2)	1	(0.1)	3	(0.1)	5	(0.1)
Other toxic exposure	7	(1.3)	11	(0.6)	11	(0.5)	29	(0.6)
Total	**533**	**(100.0)**	**1,798**	**(100.0)**	**2,248**	**(100.0)**	**4,579**	**(100.0)**

Note that surveillance can be used for many things in addition to infectious disease. This table displays injuries and exposures, tracked in the same way and with the same system as the hospital and acute care surveillance that tracked infectious diseases.

*Includes cuts, blunt trauma, burns, and environmental exposures.

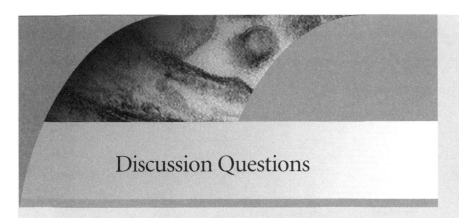

Discussion Questions

1. You have been asked to develop a new surveillance system to address the risk of a new strain of an STD, found only through laboratory diagnosis. How will you accomplish this?

2. What are the key defining characteristics of a good surveillance system?

3. Using existing literature, pick one disease in which you are interested. How is surveillance conducted for that disease? Is it reportable to the CDC? WHO? Why or why not?

4. Do you think that existing surveillance systems for avian flu are sufficient? If not, how would you propose improving them?

REFERENCES

1. Centers for Disease Control and Prevention. Updated guidelines for evaluating public health surveillance systems recommendations from the Guidelines Working Group. *MMWR.* 2001;50(RR-13):1–51.

2. DeHart RL. Health issues of air travel. *Ann Rev Public Health.* 2003;24:133–151.

3. Centers for Disease Control and Prevention. Summary of notifiable diseases—United States, 2004. *MMWR.* 2004;53(53):1–80.

4. Brownstein JS, Wolfe CJ, Mandl KD. Empirical evidence for the effect of airline travel on inter-regional influenza spread in the United States. *PLoS Med.* 2006;3(10):e401.

5. Centers for Disease Control and Prevention. Exposure to mumps during air travel—United States, April 2006. *MMWR.* 2006;55(14):401–402.

6. Centers for Disease Control and Prevention. Postexposure prophylaxis, isolation, and quarantine to control an import-associated measles outbreak—Iowa, 2004. *MMWR.* 2004;53:969.

7. Heymann DL. *Control of Communicable Diseases.* 18th ed. Washington, DC: American Public Health Association.

8. Eberhart-Phillips J, Besser R, Tormey MP. An outbreak of cholera from food served on an international aircraft. *Epidemol Infect.* 1996;116:9–13.

9. World Bank. World Bank surveillance kit. Available at: www.worldbank.org. Accessed January 1, 2003.

10. Aschengrau A, Seague GR. *Essentials of Epidemiology in Public Health.* Boston: Jones and Bartlett; 2003.

11. Centers for Disease Control and Prevention. Preliminary report: foodborne outbreak of *Escherichia coli* O157:H7 infections from hamburgers—western United States, 1993. *MMWR.* 1993;42:85–86.

12. Centers for Disease Control and Prevention. Update: multistate outbreak of *Escherichia coli* O157:H7 infections from hamburgers—western United States, 1992–1993. *MMWR.* 1993;42(14):258–263.

13. Cunin P, et al. An epidemic of bloody diarrhea: *Escherichia coli* O157 emerging in Cameroon? *Emerg Inf Dis.* 1999;5(2).

14. Walford D, Noah N. Emerging infectious diseases—United Kingdom. *Emerg Infect Dis.* 1999;5(2):189–194.

15. Devasia RA, Jones TF, Ward J. Endemically acquired foodborne outbreak of enterotoxin-producing *Escherichia coli* serotype O169:H41. *Am J Med.* 2006;119:168.e7–168.e10.

16. Parekh B, Pau C, Kennedy MS, et al. Assessment of antibody assays for identifying and distinguishing recent from long-term HIV type 1 infection. *AIDS Res Human Retroviruses.* 2001;17:137–146.

17. Heckathorn D. Respondent-driven sampling: a new approach to the study of hidden populations. *Soc Problems.* 1997;44:174–199.

18. Heckathorn D. Respondent-driven sampling II: deriving valid population estimates from chain-referral samples of hidden populations. *Soc Problems.* 2002;49:11–34.

19. Sackett D. Why randomized controlled trials fail but needn't: 1. Failure to gain "coal-face" commitment and to use the uncertainty principle. *Can Med Assoc J.* 2000;162:1311–1314.

20. Salganik M, Heckathorn D. Sampling and estimation in hidden populations using respondent-driven sampling. *Sociolog Methodol.* 2004;34:193–239.

21. Centers for Disease Control and Prevention. HIV prevalence, unrecognized infection, and HIV testing among men who have sex with men—five U.S. cities, June 2004–April 2005. *MMWR.* 2005;54(24):597–601.

22. Centers for Disease Control and Prevention. HIV/AIDS surveillance report, 2004. *MMWR.* Available at: http://www.cdc.gov/hiv/stats/hasrlink.htm. Accessed January 1, 2005.

23. Reynolds SJ, Risbud AR, Shepherd ME, et al. High rates of syphilis among STI patients are contributing to the spread of HIV-1 in India. *Sex Transm Inf.* 2006;82:121–126.

24. Centers for Disease Control and Prevention. 1994 revised classification system for human immunodeficiency virus infection in children less than 13 years of age. *MMWR.* 1994;43(RR-12).

25. Centers for Disease Control and Prevention. 1993 revised classification system for HIV infection and expanded surveillance case definition for AIDS among adolescents and adults. *MMWR.* 1992;14.

26. Centers for Disease Control and Prevention. Impact of the expanded AIDS surveillance case definition on AIDS case reporting—United States, first quarter, 1993. *MMWR.* 1993;42:308–310.

27. Centers for Disease Control and Prevention. Public health response to hurricanes Katrina and Rita—Louisiana, 2005. MMWR 2006;55:1-64.

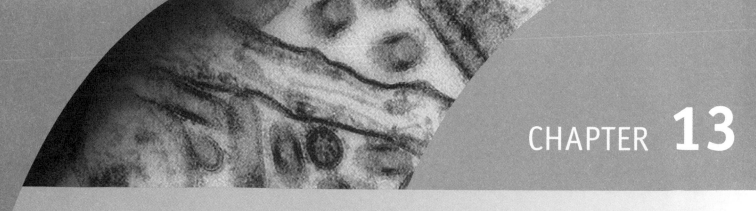

CHAPTER 13

Program Evaluation in the Infectious Disease Setting

What is the difference between research and evaluation? Some feel the two are synonymous: many researchers conduct evaluation, and many evaluators conduct research. Some even feel the difference is more a matter of jargon than of practice or theory. Both take similar steps toward the exploration of the research question at hand. One difference, however, is that evaluation typically is done in the field, looking at programs whose primary purpose is not to answer research questions but rather to serve some function. On the other hand, research generally creates and studies exposures, interventions, predictors, or other independent variables, whether they are intentional or otherwise. Evaluation assesses similar types of exposures, but they are usually within a context of what is already there programmatically. The evaluation paradigm is such that evaluation findings may be incorporated into an overall program design, and used to improve it. Evaluation results suggest changes that may be made to a program, and those changes—once made—are similarly evaluated; this allows for a feedback loop by which the evaluation improves the program.

Several examples may help distinguish research from evaluation—as well as illustrate their areas of overlap.

- Imagine you have an ancillary service program that provides intensive case management to persons with chronic hepatitis. The program will benefit from a comprehensive and prospective evaluation, allowing sponsors, staff, and clients to see if the ancillary services "work." The exposure, or "intervention," is the program, but this program's offerings are quite extensive, ranging from bus token dissemination to intensive case management to medical case management. To prospectively research each intervention being utilized would be complicated, although useful. Still, the program has only minimal funding for evaluation or research, and cannot afford the research faculty and staff to conduct studies. But assessing the program in an overall sense, evaluating it, is possible and is, in fact, mandated by the program's funding sponsors. Once the program specifics are operationalized (that is, defined in a way for this study), and what it means to the evaluators for the program to "work" is operationalized, then the program may be evaluated. The information that results from an evaluation of the program may not be generalizable to other programs, but will be critical to the operations of this one.

- Imagine you have a mobile van providing methadone, needle exchange, and counseling to heroin addicts. The program is not doing anything particularly innovative, yet still needs to document each and every service provided to the community and, where available, outcomes associated with the program. For example, the program director and the funding agencies would like to know precisely how many methadone doses were given, needles exchanged, and counseling sessions provided. They would like to know the number of new and existing clients, the number who stay off heroin and on methadone, and the number who stop using substances altogether.

- Imagine a free vaccination registry, which automates all vaccination information for children 0 to 12 years of age. The registry collects and maintains all information about each child's vaccine records, so that the parent does not need to worry in case of loss of records. The program also sends reminders to parents when vaccinations are due. The program has been running smoothly for over 10 years, and has recently received funding to support a mobile van that not only tracks vaccinations and serves as a clearinghouse for vaccination education, but also provides vaccines free of charge to all children under 12 years old, irrespective of insurance. This well-established organization wants to evaluate the effectiveness of the expanded program in getting new users of its registry, encouraging improved timeliness in vaccinations among children who were previously getting vaccinations, and engaging children in the program who were not previously getting any vaccinations. This particular program is well funded and benefits from having a staff of two evaluators and four evaluation field staff. They opt to have one evaluator and two field staff work exclusively on evaluation studies—that is, keeping track of services delivered, new and continuing users, timeliness of vaccinations, and counts of new, previously unvaccinated clients. The other half of the evaluation team is assigned to the research component of the program, and begins developing an observational, prospective study design. Following receipt of institutional review board (IRB) and other relevant approvals at the participating programs, parents of children born at hospitals in the local catchment area will be asked to participate in a study of factors that might improve participation in the vaccination program. Following provision of informed consent, parents will be randomly assigned to one of three arms of the study: 1) standard of care (handouts and information regarding vaccination and free vaccine program and registry) plus referrals to pediatricians in the area; 2) standard of care plus one reminder phone call one week prior to the vaccination due date; 3) standard of care plus one reminder postcard received one week prior to the vaccination due

date. The goal of the study is to identify cost-effective and feasible methods for improving vaccination rates. The researchers also adapt existing validated survey instruments to assess parent satisfaction with the program. This is developed and a telephone survey is conducted, drawing on a random sample of participants in the program.

Within these examples of program contexts, certainly research can be and is frequently conducted. As you saw in the last example, research and evaluation were performed alongside one another. In general, however, evaluation is more commonly conducted, because it builds upon the underlying program without needing to alter it or develop new programs. In the last example, you can see that the evaluation team was studying what the vaccination program was doing and creating as far as outcomes, while the research team had to develop something new—the experimental study, the satisfaction survey—in order to address its research questions.

Program evaluation is designed to answer the question of what the program is doing (process evaluation) and whether it works (outcomes evaluation). In addition, there are other types of program evaluations to address certain specific informational needs. These include

- Cost analyses to determine the ability of the program to attain its goals relative to the program's cost.
- Time studies to determine the time savings a program may be able to convey.
- Quality improvement evaluation to assess whether the program meets objective measures of quality care
- Satisfaction studies to assess levels of satisfaction with the program

Evaluation is usually required by funding agents to monitor the progress of the program in attaining its goals. This assists programs in justifying monies that have been allocated as well as future monies that are being requested. It also is used to inform the evolution of the organization in a constant feedback loop. Evaluation is central to the operations of many community-based, academic, and foundation organizations interfacing with topics of infectious disease, both in the United States and abroad. Many evaluation tools are based on epidemiologic methods, yet evaluation is seldom presented to programs in epidemiology. Through exploration of evaluation methods, the goal of this chapter is to provide a foundation that will allow you to have several basic program evaluation tools at hand when entering the workforce or moving ahead to more advanced evaluation studies.

DIFFERENCES BETWEEN RESEARCH AND EVALUATION

One key differentiating factor between research and evaluation is that evaluation is often conducted after the fact rather than designed in advance (*a priori*). When data collection procedures can be developed up front for evaluation purposes, and they sometimes are, the resulting data can be very good. But when they cannot, the data sources generally pertain to the needs of the programs to manage themselves rather than to ask specific research questions; the data can range from unusable to excellent, depending on the data sources available, and the care with which each datapoint was collected and entered. Each dataset has its own reason for being. This has several implications:

- Data may not have been collected using instrumentation designed specifically for the research questions at hand; it may have been developed for a program-specific purpose.

- Power and sample size were not considered, because the research question came after the program's initiation; thus the sample size may not yield adequate power.

- Individuals staffing the program may not be skilled at or fully comprehend the need for program evaluation; they may perceive any instrumentation as "paperwork," or that the evaluators are "grading" them, and they may be resistant to the evaluation efforts underway.

- Evaluation usually has an element of a feedback loop. Unlike a research study in which the intent is, and must be, to retain fidelity to the intervention and original instrumentation, evaluation is more fluid and flexible. The operationalization of the variables, the instrumentation, or any part of the study may change based upon results identified during the preceding parts of the study at hand. In this way, the evaluation findings contribute in an ongoing fashion to the program being evaluated. This is in contrast to researchers, who are often obliged to await the results of the entire study in order to contribute to public health or the research question being investigated.

- The research questions and null and alternative hypotheses in a typical research study are designed to produce information that is generalizable to other populations, settings, or situations. This is in contrast to evaluation, which is generally intended to inform the specific program that is being evaluated. Whereas researchers function autonomously within a structure of external sponsorship, evaluators generally function in response to the sponsor's research agenda. The essential goal of evaluation is to improve a specific program, whereas that of a research study is to learn about a phenomenon and generalize its findings to a larger target population. This feedback loop intrinsic to evaluation allows it to identify areas for improvement, take action towards improvement, evaluate the changes, and then begin again. If an evaluation is not providing information to improve the program, then the study may not be viewed as particularly worthwhile and does not meet the definition of evaluation.

- Although publishing findings from a research study are generally an expected and hoped-for outcome of a research undertaking, evaluation does not have this same expectation. Findings from evaluation studies may be published in peer-reviewed literature or as monographs, newsletters, and other informative documents, but sharing information beyond the sponsor and the program itself is usually not a priority because it takes too long to find out "answers" from the study. Evaluation needs to be accessible and in real-time; waiting too long for information hampers the feedback loop, and prevents the evaluation findings from being used to improve the program. Evaluation is designed to have a real-time element to it, allowing changes and improvements to the program to be made based on the evaluation findings.

- Although research interventions usually require that the intervention stay the same throughout the study period to ensure that all participants receive identical treatment, evaluation usually does not. The recognition that programs change over time and also that the evaluation itself will often influence the program to change is a critical difference between these designs. As evaluation methodologies become more complex and refined, the evaluator can actually develop means to study the changing intervention. This may be quite complicated at times, and requires expertise to address the methodological challenges intrinsic in a changing intervention. The static—and clean—randomized trial paradigm is not part of evaluation. Measuring the intervention may be made more difficult with changing interventions offered to changing groups of people with changing settings. For those "bored" with the clarity of experimental studies, program evaluation offers a wealth of challenges and delights.

- Research studies are developed with careful attention paid to the protection of patients, the safety, health, and rights of participants, as well as protection of the integrity of the study itself. Evaluation studies are developed with equal attention paid to the safety, health, and rights of participants. However, in some respects the study's internal validity is less important relative to ensuring the knowledge gained from the study is readily incorporated into the program itself. To this end, sometimes individuals who staff community-based or other programs needing evaluation have doubts about both research and evaluation studies, perhaps confusing the two somewhat. For example, take a clinical trials environment—it definitely has more research than evaluation. Sometimes information from the trial is not analyzed on a real-time basis, to preserve the integrity of the trial and the study; some may believe that the analysis did not illuminate the results quickly enough to be useful to those that were in the study or the target population, or did not get analyzed quickly enough to be useful in improving the program on a real-time basis. The trial might be highly valid but for a staff member in the field, may be perceived as taking to long to be immediately meaningful.

- Research is always planned up front, even when the data are collected prior to the development of the research study design. This allows data collection mechanisms to be created and refined prior to implementation, and generally lends itself to a higher quality of data designed to answer the specific research questions. Although this sometimes happens in evaluation studies, more often the evaluator is called to assess a program that has already begun. Thus the data collection procedures, databases, training, and all the elements of the study, which eventually determine the quality of that study, are in place. This can be a tremendous problem when the program's data collection procedures are less than optimal. However, in cases where they have not yet been initiated, the evaluator can play a tremendous role in developing them, to the benefit of the data. In cases where the evaluator is invited into the program after the program—or even the data collection—has begun, the evaluator can then contribute to the refinement of the data collection tools and processes as well as analysis and interpretation.
- Putting studies of any type—research or evaluation—into action in the field can be treacherous, just as field medicine can be. There are unknowns, staffing issues, implementation difficulties, and real-life practicalities that interfere with the clean execution of a study. Of the two, research is cleaner than evaluation. Lines of command in a research study are more direct as far as goals,

objectives, and protocols go; those of an evaluation study are less so. Evaluation studies dive into the core of programs, evaluating the very structures and people who operate them. Not being designed specifically to assess programs, and relying heavily on existing data sources, evaluation studies are frequently more confusing and far less linear than their research counterparts. Evaluation is thus attractive to researchers with a sense of daring about the work they are doing; they often have a level of tolerance for the messier aspects of field research than those who prefer the more controlled research environments.

Table 13-1 summarizes the differences between evaluation and research.

There are many similarities between research and evaluation, however. This lends itself to a situation in which many times researchers use their evaluation skills, and evaluators use their research skills as they work together.

- Both designs require *a priori* research questions, null and alternative hypotheses in order to be properly conducted. Due to the difficulties in ascertaining funding and starting programs in the field, many community-based or other types of service delivery programs are initiated without having an evaluation plan in place, even though this is far from ideal. But when the evaluation begins, development of these fundamental tools takes place. In this way, the underlying research questions and hypotheses guide the study's design development, implementation, analysis, and ultimate dissemination—as in a research study—even when the data or processes under study cannot be altered or created afresh as in a research study. So in this sense, the research questions, null, alternative hypotheses are developed but after—not before—the program begins.
- Traditional quantitative and qualitative methodology, data collection, and analytic and presentation techniques are appropriate for both designs. Although evaluation may not always utilize techniques as sophisticated as research will, they are all available to the evaluator and are the techniques used to answer the questions at hand.
- Professional and ethical treatment of participants is mandatory no matter what type of study is being conducted. Just because the evaluator may take a more passive role than the researcher, or may come in after the fact, this never implies that ensuring participant safety is not a priority. If the evaluator becomes aware of any infringement—or potential for infringement—on the

TABLE 13-1 Differences Between Evaluation and Research

Evaluation	Research
Data collection for program management or other purposes	Data collection specifically for research design
No sample size considerations, as intervention is applied to persons receiving program services; power calculations are necessary in the case of negative findings to assess if sufficient power exists to see a difference if there were one.	Sample size and power calculations required prior to study's initiation.
Staff collecting data may no be trained specifically on data collection mechanisms; they may not see the utility of program evaluation and may view it as "paperwork" or being "graded" instead of assessing their work and improving the program.	Research staff usually extensively trained on data collection needs; generally they understand the need for meticulous data collection activity.
Program and intervention changes possible over time; feedback loop paradigm.	More difficult to make changes over time, less flexible in terms of intervention and program alterations.
Informs program leadership to effect change; sometimes findings to local or regional community.	Generalizable to a wider audience, including the scientific community.
Publication of findings possible, but lower priority than communication of findings to staff, local collaborators, and other persons operating within similar program contexts.	Publication of findings essential; need to communicate findings to scientific community to lend information to scientific—not just local—feedback loop.
Analysis in real-time, with real-time feedback.	Analysis generally waits for stopping rules or until study is completed.
Can assess program before it starts, but more often, evaluate existing program, with all tools already developed.	Develop evaluation procedures and study designs a priori.
Sometimes difficulty in fitting evaluator into chain of command; staff already in place makes it difficult to establish clear lines of authority.	Clear lines of authority for study and data related procedures.

participant's health or rights, then this must be reported and the infringements stopped. For example, if the evaluator comes into a program setting and begins analyzing data that are being collected on a routine basis for the program's operation without proper consent, the evaluator must halt the evaluation study and immediately seek counsel for the appropriate source regarding how to proceed. Even if the data collection was not under the evaluator's purview, to use inappropriately gained information is unethical. It is the responsibility of the evaluator to rectify the situation just as much as it would be for a researcher to halt a study that was enrolling subjects without having their informed consent. Guarding the rights of participants, clients, and patients—no matter what the context—is always critical. It is incumbent upon all staff involved with any evaluation or research to guard the rights of those generous

individuals giving their time and selves to the evaluation study.

Table 13-2 summarizes the similarities between evaluation and research.

TABLE 13-2 Similarities Between Evaluation and Research

Evaluation and research both...
... require *a priori* research questions, null and alternative hypotheses
... can use traditional quantitative and qualitative methodology, data collection, analytic, and presentation techniques
... demand professional and ethical treatment of participants

TYPES OF EVALUATION

There are several broad categories of program evaluation, each of which may use different techniques of conduct and analysis. These techniques may include epidemiologic methods, qualitative and formative research, or specialized tools. As funding sponsors increasingly require program evaluation, methods have become more sophisticated, allowing for more breadth in the methods selected. These categories are listed below, and summarized in Table 13-3.

- *Process evaluation:* The primary goal of process evaluation is to describe which services are being provided, and to whom. Process evaluation can range from the very simple to the very sophisticated. For example, a program might count the number of condoms given out at a drop-in center for homeless youth and also handle a complex instrument detailing attendees at an HIV 101 workshop and the specific lessons they received. Process evaluation is the nitty-gritty of how the program is running and what is being done with its funding. Within this basic framework, several specific study designs can be conducted
  - ○ *Cost analyses:* This type of study evaluates the costs of the program, sometimes including an assessment of costs relative to benefits, outputs, and expenditures.

TABLE 13-3 Summary of Types of Evaluation

Type	Description
Process evaluation	Counting the services the program delivers, processes used by the program
Cost analyses	Assessment of costs of program, sometimes in relation to benefits and outcomes
Satisfaction studies	Evaluation of user or provider satisfaction with a program or its services
Quality improvement studies	Evaluates services being delivered against a benchmark or a minimum standard
Quality improvement	Assesses whether program meets specific minimum standards
Outcomes evaluation	Assesses outcomes associated with the program

Cost analyses may range from the simple calculation of money spent on the program and money expected to be saved from the program's existence (cost-threshold analysis) all the way to sophisticated modeling of cost-effectiveness.

- ○ *Satisfaction studies:* This type of study evaluates the satisfaction of individuals participating in the program, from the providers to the consumers to community stakeholders. These studies are essential and assist program personnel in ensuring that the service they provide is appropriate for those for whom it is intended, and meeting the stated program goals. In cases where program satisfaction is lower than expected or required, the program can take active steps towards improving service delivery. This is another example where immediate changes are implemented based on results of the evaluation. If there is low satisfaction with the services the program is delivering, then changes can be made to improve satisfaction right away.
- ○ *Quality improvement studies:* This type of study evaluates the services being delivered against benchmarks or standards developed from either other studies or specific and agreed-upon guidelines. Quality improvement studies are generally formal, systematized, and institutionalized to allow the program to be assessed in objective and measurable terms. This type of evaluation is especially prevalent in clinical care and case management–type settings, where care must be up to at least a minimum standard.
- *Outcomes evaluation:* Outcomes evaluation offers the highest degree of overlap with our epidemiologic toolkit. The purpose of outcomes evaluation is to see whether the program is successful in achieving its stated goal. As in our research designs, in this type of evaluation we ensure that we have research questions, null and alternative hypotheses to guide our study's implementation. Outcomes evaluation can be conducted on the aggregate level as well as on the individual level. The design approaches for outcomes evaluation are infinite. Any research design that can be used to test a null hypothesis can be used to assess an intervention and related outcomes. For example, randomized controlled trials can be used to compare partner notification strategies for HIV and syphilis. Observational studies can be used to compare different modes of testing for strep throat. Ecologic studies may be used to assess aggregate changes in diet and the incidence of a potentially related disease. Cohort studies can be used to evaluate associations between program arms and longer-term outcomes. It is

important to remember that the same strengths and limitations attend use of these designs in the evaluation setting as well as the research, however. The most rigorous scientific methods, the randomized trial, can be used in evaluation and will be more rigorous than will an ecologic study, just as in a more traditional research paradigm. But creative use of the epidemiologic toolkit in the evaluation setting is an important advance in the field of evaluation. When we do not have the luxury of advance planning or a perfect research setting, evaluation can lead to important findings and help shape real-life programs in a significant way.

- *Outcomes-based quality improvement:* Outcomes-based quality improvement studies represent an intersection of study that is somewhere between process and outcomes evaluation. In quality improvement activities, there is a systematic study of services delivered (process evaluation), but in conjunction with specific outcomes (outcomes evaluation). Generally, the focus of these studies is on ensuring that a minimum set of standards is met. For example, in a hospital nursery, there is likely a standard regarding provision of hepatitis B vaccination prior to hospital discharge. One activity might be to assess how many children were discharged prior to being offered the vaccine. The outcome here is whether the program (the nursery) meets the recommendation for clinical services, so in this sense, it is an outcomes evaluation. Still, the real data being collected are the process data, that is, the number of children vaccinated prior to hospital discharge. A good example of what might be an outcomes evaluation might be the number of children vaccinated prior to hospital discharge who, when given information about where to get the second and third vaccinations in the series, actually return for their shots. A longer-term outcome might be to assess the number of vaccinated children who acquire hepatitis B (though clearly this is another research question altogether, going beyond the scope of a standard evaluation).

DEVELOPING EVALUATION STUDIES

What can be evaluated? Anything—and therein lies the beauty of evaluation. What evaluation lacks in the strict methodology of a randomized controlled design, for example, it makes up for in its ability to respond to a variety of needs and program types. These then may be adapted for infectious disease settings. Programs that address specific disease processes are easily developed to evaluate the unique needs of the clients, outcomes, or overall framework. Examples of types of programs that can be evaluated include:

- Ancillary service delivery programs
  - Direct service utilization, such as case management services
  - Indirect service utilization, such as financial support in the form of bus tokens to a clinic
- Policies
  - City policy requiring directly observed treatment (DOT) for persons with tuberculosis
  - School district policy regarding sex education in schools
  - Clinic policy to require all staff to have a PPD test annually
  - Surveillance systems and reportability of diseases in jurisdiction
- Community-based programs
  - Condom distribution programs
  - Education in juvenile detention centers regarding hand washing to reduce transmission of viruses during flu season
  - Social marketing campaigns to reduce exposure to mosquitoes through encouraging environmental change, following a West Nile Virus outbreak
  - Training programs for peer educators in working with transgender persons at risk for HIV and hepatitis related to silicone injection needle use
- Clinical programs
  - Specific infectious disease–related diagnostic procedures
  - Outbreak investigations, in the field, in hospital, or clinic settings
  - Administrative systems, such as information technology (IT), electronic health records, and electronic clinical decision support
  - Infrastructure development

These are just examples. Any program that can be developed to do anything or serve any population can and should be evaluated in an ongoing fashion.

EVALUATION FRAMEWORKS

There are many evaluation frameworks that can be used to build evaluation studies. Many organizations have their own models for evaluation, as well as unique goals and objectives, although the underlying constructs remain similar from organization to organization. The Centers for Disease Control and Prevention (Available at: http://www.cdc.gov/eval/framework.htm) presents a particularly useful framework that is circular in nature, reflecting the nonlinear, iterative, and feedback loop qualities of evaluation (see Figure 13-1).

Within this framework, there are six key steps in program evaluation, which are bound by four standards to guide the study. Irrespective of the conceptual framework you opt to follow in your own practice of evaluation, these are important topics that should be integrated into your everyday work.

The six key steps are as follows

1. *Engage stakeholders prior to starting the evaluation:* Stakeholders are individuals that either use the services, provide the services, or implement or disseminate ultimate evaluation findings, or even those who are negative about the program. Working with the community in which the program operates to identify stakeholders and then engaging them actively benefits the evaluation in several ways:
   ○ The stakeholders are included in the process such that they are aware and, hopefully, supportive of the evaluation.
   ○ As key informants, they may be able to provide information about the program that would otherwise be unavailable.
   ○ They can assist the evaluator in addressing community needs better by making the evaluator aware of community and stakeholder concerns.

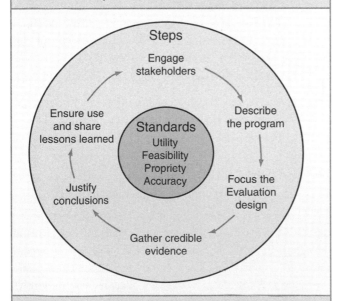

FIGURE 13-1 CDC Framework for Program Evaluation (MMWR, 1999, Framework for Program Evaluation in Public Health; available at: http://www.cdc.gov/eval/framework. htm)

The four standards underscore each and every step of the evaluation framework, and also help to identify the appropriate type of evaluation.

Working with stakeholders should never be a perfunctory exercise. People are readily able to tell whether their input is being sought genuinely or they are just being "used" as a community advisory board, but not actually listened to. More value can come from listening to stakeholders than almost any other activity, thus it should be taken seriously.

2. *Describe the program:* This step should use any and all available methods, from formative/qualitative to quantitative. The evaluator should become well acquainted with the entire program being assessed, through observations, interviews, comprehensive review of standard operating procedures, and more. One primary barrier to effective evaluation is the failure of the evaluator to really get to know the program being evaluated. When the evaluation is a world apart from the day-to-day program realities, the evaluator is likely not evaluating the actual program but rather a set of program ideals. This approach generally will not result in program improvement. One of the most important first steps of any evaluation is to thoroughly get to know the program in its most naked state. Often, this will not "match" the program's stated goals or design—or aspirations. This is what makes it so important to evaluate what the program really is, what the program is really doing: If you evaluate the program on paper and not the truth, the evaluation will never be able to improve the program or contribute to its growth.

3. *Focus the evaluation design:* After learning about the program, the evaluator identifies research questions, null and alternative hypotheses, and data sources, and then can identify the optimal study design. This may range from process all the way to outcomes evaluation, using techniques ranging from traditional to novel. As with research, the research questions guide the study and should remain in focus for the duration of the study, from design and implementation to analysis and dissemination. In evaluation studies, there is often a need to refine the research questions and design in tandem with evaluation findings along the way, making the evaluation design somewhat iterative in nature.

4. *Gather credible evidence:* As in any study, quality data sources are imperative. In evaluation, as you have seen, data sources are often developed and maintained for purposes besides evaluation. For example, a database may be used by the clinic for billing purposes, and ICD-9 diagnostic coding may be used. Documentation of diagnoses for billing purposes generally differs from

that used for clinical purposes, which differ again from study purposes, so this difference must be taken into account when the design is put forth. In evaluation, one must often use whatever data are available, but the inherent limitations in each data source need to be acknowledged. If quality data sources are not available, the evaluator may have to investigate the feasibility of developing new ones specific to the research questions under study.

5. *Justify conclusions:* Quality data analysis is the one element of evaluation that is in the complete control of the evaluator and not subject to the problems that emerge from studying existing programs and data. A deliberate and well-executed analysis, with a clear understanding of the limitations of the data sources, is what makes an evaluation worthwhile. In tandem with the in-depth understanding of the program and stakeholders, the data may be interpreted and appropriate recommendations made. Interpretation follows from quality data analysis: the evaluator is responsible for ensuring that correct and sufficiently rapid conclusions are extracted from that analysis, and then communicated to the program and relevant stakeholders. Conclusions need to be data-driven at all times, well-supported, and justified. Documentation for every element of the research (both qualitative and quantitative) should be quality assured and maintained to allow for future support of conclusions and recommendations.

6. *Ensure use and share lessons learned:* Going back to the differences between research and evaluation, the evaluation study must improve the program it is evaluating. It is not sufficient to find out about the program and not report upon it. Evaluation findings must be fed back into the program and then the cycle must begin again. This ensures that the findings are used, shared, and improve the program. After this has been accomplished, the evaluators may wish to share their findings with a larger audience and make them more generalizable, if applicable.

Figure 13-2 compares the research and evaluation frameworks. Where the research paradigm is generally fairly linear and unidirectional—moving from question to data collection to analysis and interpretation, followed by communication to community, scientific literature, and public health action, the evaluation paradigm is generally circular. Note below how feedback and findings move from every step of the research flow to informing and improving the services delivered. This

impacts the research questions and design, as the program is continually changing. This is one thing that makes evaluation studies challenging—and exciting.

1. *Utility:* Information must be useful in order for it to have impact. Will the information gained by the evaluation be "academic" or will it help modify and improve the program? In order to have utility, it must meet the needs of the stakeholders, paying particularly close attention to the program staff. Discussion with the program leaders and working with them to gain support of the design selected is essential.

2. *Feasibility:* Is the proposed evaluation design realistic? Is it reasonably priced? Does it maximize existing resources? Is it possible to conduct given the context of the actual program's needs? Like most things, even the best ideas may not be all they seem if they are not feasible and realistic. One reason why becoming acquainted with the program being evaluated is so central is that without knowledge of the actual program, determining feasibility of the evaluation is not possible. Before embarking on any study, be sure that it is realistic.

3. *Propriety:* Like research studies, evaluation studies must be ethical, protecting the rights of all persons affected by the evaluation. This includes those individuals who are contributing just their data, even if they are not aware that the evaluation is being conducted. Use of an institutional review board (IRB) may be required depending on the evaluation design and the institutional regulations. At no time should an evaluator do anything that would be unethical or alter the ethical treatment of program participants, staff, or community members. In addition, the evaluation must be culturally competent in all of its facets, ensuring that the unique cultural elements of the program and its clients are acknowledged and represented in the evaluation.

4. *Accuracy:* Here, too, there is no difference between research and evaluation. Accurate, high quality study design, data collection, data analysis, interpretation, and dissemination are mandatory. Just because evaluation may allow the investigators less direct control of the study or data sources does not imply that there can be lapses in the degree of accuracy of the study. In fact, with the limitations inherent in evaluation, the evaluator must be more meticulous and must better understand the limitations of the data sources in order to maintain an ethical as well as informative evaluation. There may be no compromise about this at any time.

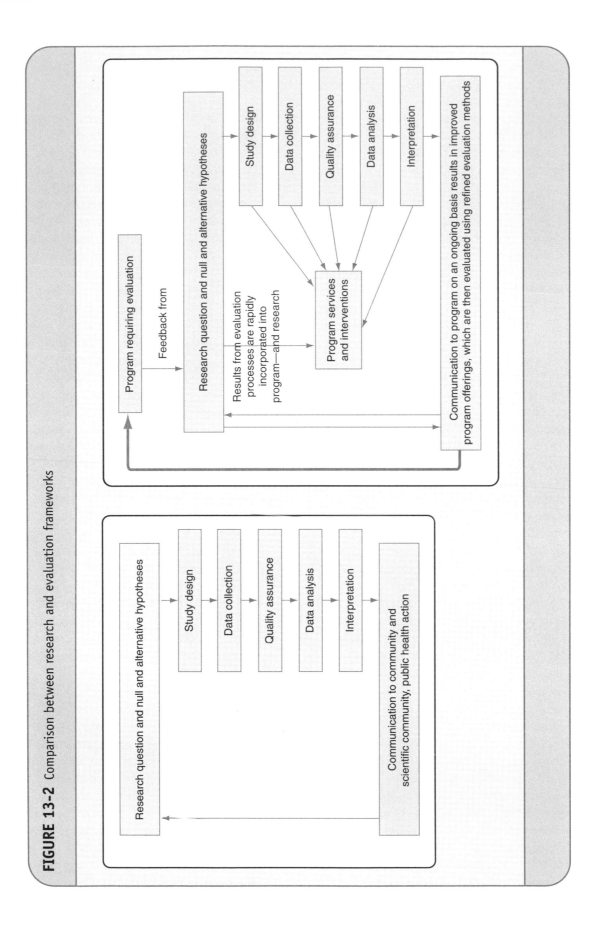

FIGURE 13-2 Comparison between research and evaluation frameworks

THINKING THROUGH EVALUATION IN THE INFECTIOUS DISEASE SETTING

The following is an example of an evaluation study to provide a sense of the unique study designs utilized in evaluation of programs surrounding infectious disease. This is a hypothetical program that provides HIV prevention services to adolescent males at high risk for HIV infection, as well as linkage into adolescent-specific HIV primary care. The program has been operating for 5 years and is growing rapidly; they have just been awarded a new 4-year grant to provide services specifically to at-risk and HIV-infected adolescent males. The program wishes to evaluate the program that will pay for client services, to see how well they work and to keep a close eye on the program so they may improve it in "real time." What does the evaluator do?

First, the evaluator spends two full weeks with the program. This phase is not casual: The evaluator observes the central office, the outreach van, and the clinical services, and then asks detailed questions to learn all about the program. He looks at the original program records and related documents, extending back to the program's birth. This way, he is fully aware of the history, the needs, the mission, and the day-to-day issues facing staff and clients.

The evaluator needs to decide what the key predictors and outcomes of interest are to the evaluation. For the purpose of this example, this is somewhat abbreviated; this list could be considerably longer. He wants to conduct primarily process evaluation, with a small outcomes evaluation. He develops a logic model for the evaluation, to keep straight the variables he is working with. A logic model is similar to a research question matrix, although it is generally used for evaluation purposes. It assists evaluators, funders, and program managers in articulating what services they are providing and the outcomes that are expected to result from this. There are several logic model templates, of which the United Way Logic Model format shown in Table 13-4 (Available at: http://national.unitedway.org/outcomes) is one.

Definitions

It is important to define for your logic model—just as with eligibility criteria and case definitions—operationalizing specifically what each outcome means. For example:

- *Adherence with antiretroviral treatment regimen:* Missing fewer than 10% of prescribed doses over the past week
- *Engagement in care:* Having at least two initial visits with clinical partner
- *New clients:* Clients who have not received services at the mobile van ever or in the past 12 months

- *Retention in care:* Having one visit every 3 months over 1 year
- *Safer sex behavior:* Increased abstinence or use of condoms during sex during the past 3 months, based on response to the question, "The last time you had sex, did you or your partner wear a condom?" If the client responded yes to the question, ask "Have you had vaginal or anal sex with a man or a woman in the last 3 months?"

After describing the program using the logic model, the evaluator needs to think through the objectives of the program, as well as define specifically which variables on which to collect data. One method of assessing objectives for the project is called the SMART acronym, to help remember how to develop "smart" goals and objectives. This stands for goals and objectives of the project that are specific, measurable, appropriate, realistic, and time-based (see Table 13-5). Use of this paradigm can be helpful when assessing the program and developing an evaluation strategy. First one can see whether the program's goals and objectives meet the SMART criteria. This will help the evaluator understand the underlying program in measurable terms. (If the program does not have its programming sufficiently articulated to be able to present SMART goals and objectives, the evaluator may have to work with the staff on basic program issues prior to beginning an evaluation.) Then evaluation questions can be developed that will assist in understanding whether these goals and objectives are actually being met.

It is often useful to create a list of process variables—services that the program offers—and of the outcomes of interest. This list can be an excellent tool for the evaluator while he ensures that all of the program's services—educational tools, condoms, peer-education visits, clinical documentation, and so on—are documented and recorded. Sometimes the process evaluation is the hardest part of the process. It can be difficult to even keep track of the services that the program provides. Moving from the logic model to a process variables list is very helpful. The same can be done for the outcomes of interest.

Deciding where to obtain data for predictors and outcomes can be tricky. In this hypothetical example, the program maintained process data on all of its services already, so the new services under the grant, for adolescent males, could be readily incorporated into the evaluation analyses. Outcome data were more difficult, however. In the case of this example, outcome data were not available. The program kept pre- and post-test quiz data after their group-level HIV 101 activities, but never did any data collection on their outreach program; the clinical linkage part was new. The evaluator had a big job ahead: develop data collection methods consistent with the program's goals, objectives, staffing patterns, and availability

TABLE 13-4 Logic Model for Program Evaluation

Inputs	Activities	Outputs	Outcomes
Inputs are the resources dedicated to or consumed by program: • Dollars from grant • Donations to this non-profit • Staff time and expertise • Peer educators • Condoms • Outreach brochures • Mobile van and personnel • Adolescent-specific HIV primary care clinic • 24 hour on-call providers, including mental health staff	**Activities** are services the program provides; how the program will use the inputs it has to achieve its goals: • Innovative outreach program using vans to go outside of schools, with consent of school system • Culturally-competent print media and condoms, developed by peer educators, and assessed by target population • Linkage agreement with adolescent-specific HIV primary care clinic	**Outputs** are the products of the program's activities and services, in a tangible, day-to-day sense: • Mobile outreach • Peer education • Adolescent males aged 13 to 24 given condoms, brochures, and outreach • Peer education contacts • HIV tests (including pre- and post-test counseling) • Number of new HIV+ clients identified • Referrals made to clinical partner • Number of clients engaged in care • Number of clients retained in care	**Outcomes** are benefits or changes in participants during or after involvement in program activities. These may be divided into program- and client-levels. Based on the nature of this example, client-level outcomes are provided. These are generally broken down into initial, intermediate, and long-term outcomes, and quantified where possible: **Initial:** • Expose at least 100 adolescents per month to culturally-appropriate HIV 101 materials. • Provide condom packets to at least 100 new adolescent males per month. • Screen at least 50 adolescent males for HIV each month. • Identify at least one HIV+ males aged 13 to 24 years identified per quarter and link into adolescent-specific HIV care. **Intermediate:** • Increased safer sex behavior among adolescent males, based on survey data. • For HIV+, adherence with recommended treatments and retention in care **Long-term:** • Improvements in condom use and drug use behavior. • Reduced HIV (and other STD) risk • Improvements in health care utilization demonstrated by engagement and retention in care (for HIV+). • Improvements in adherence to antiretroviral regimens

TABLE 13-5 SMART Charactistics of Goals and Objectives

Characteristic	Questions to guide the development of goals and objectives
Specific	• Are objectives stated as changes in particular behaviors? • Is the amount of change expected made explicit? • Can the changes be achieved through one intervention?
Measurable	• Can the objective be measured in such a way that the success of the intervention can be determined? • Can these numbers or facts be presented in a report? • Are there data to compare these dates with? (e.g., from a baseline or a control group)
Appropriate	• Are these objectives culturally and educationally appropriate? • How will this program be accepted by the community? • Does the intervention fill a gap in current services?
Realistic	• Are the goals and objectives attainable given the level of risk and the anticipated difficulty changing the risk behavior(s)? • Can the providing agency implement the proposed intervention? • Are the resources available to achieve the stated objectives?
Time-based	• Can these objectives be accomplished within the available time frame? • Can we reasonably expect to detect changes within this time frame?

Source: Evaluating CDEC HIV Prevention Programs—Volume 2: Supplemental Handbook

that could collect data on some difficult outcomes, namely, abstinence, condom usage, adherence to antiretroviral treatment regimen, referrals, linkage, and retention in care.

Here is where research and evaluation studies dovetail: now the evaluator has a chance to be creative, in order to ascertain outcome data that he needs. He might opt for a one-time, anonymous cross-sectional survey of clients receiving outreach services. He could also conduct a prospective design, which would evaluate clients repeatedly over time, either the HIV+ or the high-risk seronegatives. He could conduct a case-control study, using as cases those that seroconverted during a given time period, and controls as a random sample of age-matched males receiving outreach services or HIV screening. If the proper design to attain information on the necessary outcomes is elusive, returning to the steps outlined in Chapter 6 can help. Clearly identifying the research questions, null and alternative hypotheses, independent and dependent variables, potential confounders, and effect modifiers is a good first step. A clear look at the resources available at the program to conduct the study, as well as training needs and staff, if there is a need, is necessary as well. In this case, data collection for outcome information is its own research study. Nevertheless, the information obtained should be cycled back to the program as it becomes available.

Ongoing supervision, quality management and assurance, data analysis, and interpretation of information are the final steps before dissemination of information. (Though information will be provided to the program on an ongoing basis as well.) Analysis of and reporting on even process data for this program will be very useful in attaining future funding; knowledge of outcomes and their association with the program will help the directors know whether their interventions are having the intended public health effects. If so, the information may well be useful to disseminate to a wider audience. Other agencies—and adolescent males at risk for HIV—can then benefit from this organization's findings.

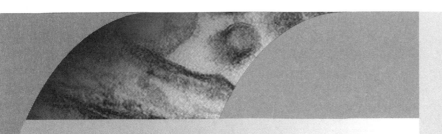

Discussion Questions

1. You are the evaluator asked to develop an evaluation of a screening program for a hospital-based program to reduce the number of syphilis-infected pregnant women. Create a logic model to describe your program.

2. Imagine there is a program providing directly observed therapy (DOT) for tuberculosis patients. What are six process measures and three outcomes that could be developed for this program? Propose four existing data sources that could be used for process indicators and outcomes (two for each), and two new sources for each that you would need to develop.

RESOURCES LIST

There are abundant informative textbooks, monographs, and guidelines to assist in program evaluation, many of them related to infectious disease. If you are interested in learning more about evaluation research, consult some of the resources below. This resources list is just a beginning.

The American Journal of Evaluation: http://aje.sagepub.com

A practical guide to evaluation and evaluation terms for Ryan White CARE Act Grantees, Report #4, September 1999.

The CDC Evaluation Working Group has listed multiple evaluation resources and references: www.cdc.gov/eval/index.htm

Centers for Disease Control and Prevention. Evaluating CDC HIV prevention programs. Volume 2: Supplemental handbook, 1999a. Available at: www.cdc.gov

Centers for Disease Control and Prevention. Framework for program evaluation in public health. *MMWR.* 1999b;48:1–40. Available at: http://www.cdc.gov/eval/framework.htm

Evaluation guidance handbook: Strategies for implementing the evaluation guidance for CDC-funded HIV prevention programs; March 2002.

Fitzpatrick JL, Sanders JR, Worthen BR. Program Evaluation: Alternative Approaches and Practical Guidelines, 3rd Edition. Boston, Allyn & Bacon. 2003.

Medical Outcomes Trust Instruments: http://www.outcomes-trust.org

Outcomes evaluation technical assistance guide: Primary medical care outcomes. HIV/AIDS Bureau, Division of Service Systems; 1999.

Outcomes evaluation technical assistance guide. Case management outcomes: Titles I and II of the Ryan White CARE Act, 2001. Available at: http://www.hab.hrsa.gov

Outcomes evaluation technical assistance guide. Getting started: Titles I and II of the Ryan White CARE Act, 2001. Available at: http://www.hab.hrsa.gov

Patton MQ. Qualitative Research & Evaluation Methods, 3rd Edition. Thousand Oaks, Sage Publications; 2001.

United Way of America. *Measuring program outcomes: A practical approach.* Alexandria, Virginia: Author; 1996.

United Way's Outcome Measurement Resource Network: http://national.unitedway.org/outcomes

U.S. Department of Health and Human Services. Centers for Disease Control and Prevention. Office of the Director, Office of Strategy and Innovation. *Introduction to program evaluation for public health programs: A self-study guide.* Atlanta, GA: Centers for Disease Control and Prevention; 2005.

W.K. Kellogg Foundation. *Evaluation handbook.* Battle Creek, MI: W.K. Kellogg Foundation; 1998. Available at: http://wkkf.org/Publications/evalhdbk

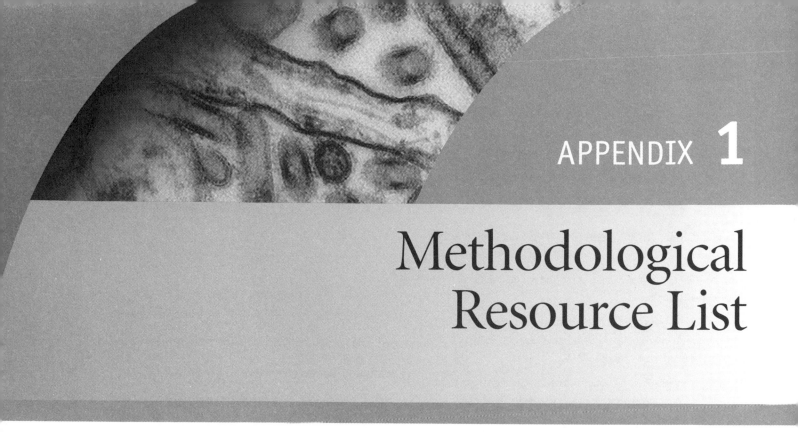

Methodological Resource List

General methodological reference list:

The methods discussion covered in this textbook draw on a wealth of literature written in the field, applying it to infectious disease epidemiology. While the specific examples are cited in each chapter as you have seen, the depth of the methods material has been synthesized from many sources as listed below. Each of these has its own unique approach to this field and material. I strongly suggest reading as many of these texts and articles as you can, to gain understanding of epidemiology, infectious disease, evaluation, and research in general. Of course, this list is just a few of my favorites: you will find your own favorites, and help this list grow. As I have taken the essentials—the basics—and applied them to one field, once you gain further knowledge of the epidemiologic toolkit, you will be able to have a deeper approach, and apply it to other arenas of study. This book is only an introduction. Don't stop here! Read and practice what you learn as much as you can. This is only a beginning, so harness your interest and allow it to take you further into this exciting profession.

Alcamo IE. *AIDS: The Biologic Basis,* 3rd Edition. Sudbury, MA: Jones and Bartlett Publishers. 2003.

Alreck P, Settle R. *The Survey Research Handbook.* Columbus, OH: McGraw-Hill Professional Publishing. 1995.

Aschengrau A, Seage GR, III. *Essentials of Epidemiology in Public Health.* Sudbury, MA: Jones and Bartlett Publishers. 2003.

Babbie E. *Survey Research Methods,* 2nd Edition. Boston, MA: Wadsworth Publishing Company. 1990.

Buck C, Llopis A, Najera E, Terris M. The Challenge of Epidemiology: issues and selected readings. *Scientific Publication No. 505.* Washington, D.C., Pan American Health Organization. 1988.

British Medical Journal (BMJ): "How to read a paper" series of articles. These articles summarize specific types of papers, statistics, and study methodology. The website is: http://bmj.bmjjournals.com

Catania J, Binson D, Canchola J. Effects of interviewer gender, interviewer choice, and item wording on responses to questions concerning sexual behaviour. *Public Opin Q,* 1996;60 (345–75).

Catania J, Binson D, Van der Straten A. Methodological research on sexual behavior in the AIDS era. *Annual Review of Sex Research.* 1995; 6 (77–125).

Choi BCK. Bias, overview. In: Gail MH, Benichou J, eds. *Encyclopedia of epidemiologic methods.* Chichester, U.K.: Wiley, 2000:74–82.

Daniel WW. *Biostatistics: A Foundation for Analysis in the Health Sciences.* New Jersey, Wiley; 2004.

Defoe D. *A Journal of the Plague Year.* New York, Modern Library. 2001.

Delgado-Rodrigues, Llorca J. Bias. *J Epidemiol Community Health.* 2004;635–41.

DeMets DL, Furberg CD, Friedman LM. *Fundamentals of Clinical Trials.* New York, Springer; 1999.

DeMets DL, Furberg CD, Friedman LM. Data Monitoring in Clinical Trials: A Case Studies Approach. New York, Springer; 2005.

Ellenberg JH. Selection bias in observational and experimental studies. *Stat Med.* 1994;13:557–67.

Fan HY, Conner RF, Villarreal LP. AIDS: Science and Society, 4th Edition. Sudbury, MA: Jones and Bartlett Publishers. 2004.

Fink A. *The Complete Survey Kit.* Thousand Oaks, CA: Sage Publications. 1995.

Fitzpatrick JL, Sanders JR, Worthen BR. Program Evaluation: Alternative Approaches and Practical Guidelines, 3rd Edition. Boston, MA: Allyn & Bacon. 2003.

Fleming D, Wasserheit J. From epidemiological synergy to public health policy and practice: the contribution of other sexually transmitted diseases to sexual transmission of HIV infection. *Sex Transm Infect.* 1999; 75:3–17.

Fowler FJ. Improving Survey Questions: Design and Evaluation. Applied Social Research Methods Series. Vol. 38. Thousand Oaks, CA: Sage Publications. 1995.

Fowler FJ. *Survey Research Methods,* 3rd Edition. Thousand Oaks, CA: Sage Publications. 1995.

Fenton KA, Johnson AM, McManus S, Erens B. Measuring sexual behaviour: methodological challenges in survey research *Sex. Transm. Inf.* 2001;77;84–92.

Frerichs R. History, maps and the internet: UCLA's John Snow site. *SoC Bulletin.* 2001;34:3–7.

Friis RH, Sellers TA. *Epidemiology for Public Health Practice,* 3rd Edition. Sudbury, MA: Jones and Bartlett Publishers. 2004.

Garrett L. *The Coming Plague: Newly Emerging Diseases in a World Out of Balance.* New York: Penguin. 1995.

Garrett L. *Betrayal of Trust: The Collapse of Global Public Health.* New York: Hyperion. 2001.

Giesecke J. Modern infectious disease epidemiology. London, U.K.: Arnold Publishers. 2002.

Glesby MJ, Hoover DR. Survivor treatment selection bias in observational studies: examples from the AIDS literature. *Ann Intern Med* 1996;124:999–1005.

Gordis L. (2004.) *Epidemiology,* 3rd Edition. Philadelphia, PA: Elsevier Saunders.

Grosskurth H, Gray R, Hayes R, et al. Control of sexually transmitted diseases for HIV-1 prevention: understanding the implications of the Mwanza and Rakai trials. *Lancet.* 2000;355:1981–7.

Heckathorn D. Respondent-Driven Sampling: A New Approach to the Study of Hidden Populations. *Social Problems.* 1997;44:174–99.

Heymann, DL. Control of Communicable Diseases, 18th edition. Washington, D.C., American Public Health Association. 2004.

Kleinbaum DG, Kupper LL, Morgenstern H. *Epidemiologic research.* Belmont, CA, Lifetime Learning Publications. 1982.

Kleinbaum DG, Morgenstern H, Kupper LL. Selection bias in epidemiologic studies. *Am J Epidemiol.* 1981;113:452–63.

Kleinbaum DJ, Kupper LL, Muller KE, Nizam A. Applied Regression Analysis and Multivariable Methods. Boston, MA: Duxbury Press. 1997.

Lachin JM. Statistical Considerations in the Intent-to-Treat Principle. *Controlled Clinical Trials.* 2000;21:167–89.

Last JM. *A Dictionary of Epidemiology.* New York, Oxford University Press. 2000.

Lillienfeld DE, Stolley PD. Foundations of Epidemiology, 3rd Edititon. New York, Oxford University Press. 1994.

Montori VM. Guyatt GH. Intention-to-treat principle. *CMAJ Canadian Medical Association Journal.* 2001;165:1339–41.

Nelson, K. *Infectious Disease Epidemiology.* Gaithersburg, PA: Aspen Publishers, Inc. 2001.

Neyman J. Statistics: servant of all sciences. *Science.* 1955;122: 401–6.

Orroth KK , Korenromp, EL, White RG, et al. Comparison of STD prevalences in the Mwanza, Rakai, and Masaka trial populations: the role of selection bias and diagnostic errors. *Sexually Transmitted Infections.* 2003;79:98–105.

Patton MQ. *Qualitative Research & Evaluation Methods,* 3rd Edition. Thousand Oaks, CA: Sage Publications. 2001.

Reingold AE. Outbreak investigations—a perspective. *Emerg Inf Dis.* 1998; 4:21–27.

Riegelman RK. *Studying a Study and Testing a Test: How to Read the Medical Evidence.* Philadephia, PA: Lippincott Williams & Wilkins. 2004.

Rothman K, Greenland S. Modern epidemiology. 2nd ed. Boston, MA: Lippicontt-Raven. 1998.

Rosen G. A History of Public Health. Baltimore, MD: Johns Hopkins University Press. 2003.

Sackett DL. Bias in analytic research. *J Chron Dis* 1979;32: 51–63.

Sackett DL. Why randomized controlled trials fail but needn't: 1. Failure to gain "coal-face" commitment and to use the uncertainty principle. *CMAJ.* 2000;162:1311–4.

Schlesselman JJ. *Case-Control Studies: Design, Conduct, Analysis.* New York: Oxford University Press. 1992.

Selvin S. *Statistical Analysis of Epidemiologic Data* (Monographs in Epidemiology and Biostatistics, V. 35). New York, Oxford University Press.

Simon R. Length biased sampling in etiologic studies. *Am J Epidemiol.* 1980;111:444–52.

Smith GD. Commentary: Behind the Broad Street pump: aetiology, epidemiology and prevention of cholera in mid-19th century Britain. *International Journal of Epidemiology.* 2002;31: 920–32.

Snow J. *Snow on Cholera.* Cambridge, Harvard University Press. 1965.

Steineck G, Ahlbom A. A definition of bias founded on the concept of the study base. *Epidemiology.* 1992;3:477–82.

Stratton IM, Neil A. How to ensure your paper is rejected by the statistical reviewer. *Diabetic Med.* 2004; 22:371:3.

Szklo M, Nieto J. Epidemiology: Beyond the Basics, 2nd edition. Sudbury, MA: Jones and Bartlett Publishers. 2006.

Tashakkori A, Teddlie CB. Handbook of Mixed Methods Social and Behavioral Research. Thousand Oaks, CA: Sage Publications. 2002.

Taubenberger J. 1918 influenza: the mother of all pandemics. *Emerg Inf Dis,* 2006; 12:15–22.

Tufte E. (1997). Visual & Statistical Thinking: Displays of Evidence for Decision Making. Cheshire, CT: Graphics Press. 1997.

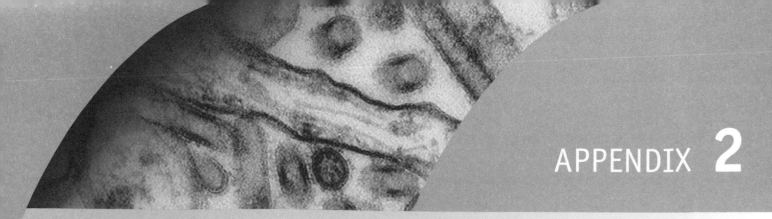

Essential Moments in Infectious Disease History

So much of our current clinical and epidemiologic approaches have been shaped by infectious disease in history, that it is worth considering key public health influences in a nutshell. These are covered extensively in other infectious disease textbooks and history of medicine texts. But a brief primer of essential moments to remember is provided here for your quick reference. What do you think will be next on the timeline?

Hippocrates (~400 bc)

First proposes a relation of disease to environment

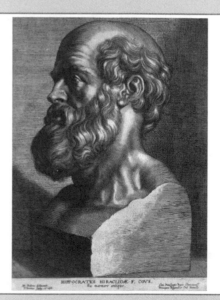

Hippocrates, engraving by Peter Paul Rubens, 1638

Source: Courtesy of the National Library of Medicine

Black Death (1300s)

Pandemic of plague in Europe, believed to be bubonic plague caused by Yersinia pestis and spread by fleas, killing over 20 million people.

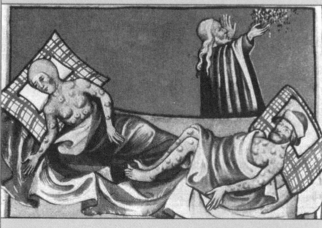

Illustration of bubonic plague in the Bible (1411)

Source: Courtesy of the National Library of Medicine

Frascatoro (late 1400s, early 1500s)

Writes On Contagion, contagious diseases and their treatment. This is one of the earliest known works to postulate a cohesive theory of infectious diseases, presenting the notion that diseases can be spread person to person via tiny, unseeable particles or seeds ("seminaria").

Arrival of Spanish in the Americas, Bringing With Them Smallpox (early 1500s)

Introduction of smallpox into Aztecs without immunity to disease decimates over half of the population.

John Graunt (1662)

Natural and Political Observations Made upon the Bills of Mortality, one of first to record data regarding births and deaths, and note that there were patterns—determinants of distribution of disease.

Anton van Leeuwenhoek born, who later invents the microscope (1632)

For the first time, microbes become visible.

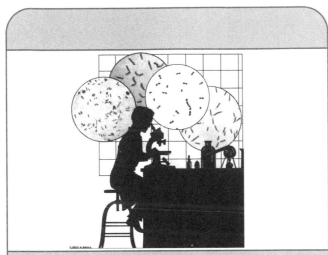

Source: CDC/Minnesota Department of Health, R.N. Barr Library; Librarians Melissa Rethlefsen and Marie Jones

Edward Jenner (late 1700s)

Grandfather of modern-day vaccination. Experimented with administration of cowpox exposure to prevent contraction of smallpox, following observation that dairymaids (who were constantly exposed to cowpox) seldom were infected with smallpox.

John Snow (mid-1800s)

Used epidemiologic methods to identify source of cholera infected water in London.

William Farr (1839)

Complier of Statistical Abstracts for the General Registry Office in Great Britain. Identified need for and developed new way of coding disease, the godfather of today's clinical coding schemes.

Ignaz Semmelweis (1840s)

Identified importance of hand washing in the clinic, and reduced post-partal mortality due to puerperal fever ("childbed fever"), a bacterial infection leading to sepsis and, often, death, following delivery of infants. After his death, took many years—and many more deaths—for his studies and recommendations regarding hand washing to be implemented.

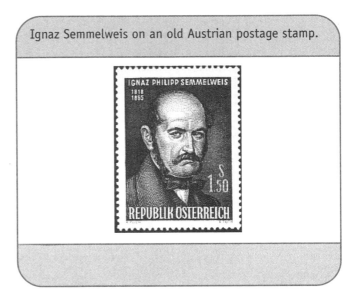

Ignaz Semmelweis on an old Austrian postage stamp.

Robert Koch (late 1800s)

Landmark thinking in infectious disease epidemiology. Robert Koch causally linked disease with specific causal microorganisms, and developed postulates (Koch's Postulates) that remain useful today in determining the relation between exposure to a microorganism and disease—or even more broadly applied to other health conditions. These are (summarized)

- The microorganism must be found in all cases of the disease.
- The microorganism must be isolated and grown in a pure culture medium.
- If introduced into a susceptible animal, this pure culture must cause the same disease.
- This microorganism must be observed in and recovered from this newly infected animal.

Spanish Influenza Pandemic (1918)

Killing over 20 million people around the globe, the virus is responsible for more deaths than World War I, which it is partly responsible for halting.

Alexander Fleming and Colleagues Identify Penicillin (1940s)

Landmark treatment identified from growth of mold. Effective against syphilis pneumococcal, gonorrhea, and countless other bacteria. A major advance in public health in the 20th century. Later in the 20th century, we witness strains of resistant bacteria, including newer generations of penicillin-like medications. In the 2000s, community-acquired methicillin (a latter generation penicillin cousin) resistant strains of S. aureus become increasingly prevalent. Vancomycin-resistant (a still latter generation penicillin cousin, only available drug to treat MRSA) strains of bacteria become reportable to the CDC in the United States.

Syphilis Brought Under Control (1940s)

In tandem with newly available penicillin, U.S. Surgeon General Thomas Parran recommends active notification and treatment for partners of syphilis infected persons. Despite availability of penicillin, Tuskegee experiment in Alabama denies treatment to black men with syphilis in an unethical study of catastrophic proportion. Increasing syphilis outbreaks continue, however, to this day.

Alexander Langmuir (1949)

Establishes epidemiology branch of what becomes CDC and, later, the Epidemic Intelligence Service (EIS).

Salk Polio Vaccine Successful (1955)

Jonas Salk invents polio vaccine, which is tested and found effective in humans, stemming a terrifying polio epidemic in the United States and elsewhere.

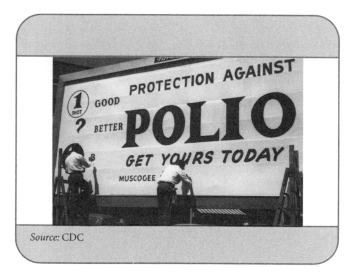

Source: CDC

Filoviruses Identified (1967)

Family of emerging viruses with high case fatality rates and ability to decimate populations rapidly is identified. This includes Marburg virus and multiple strains of Ebola virus.

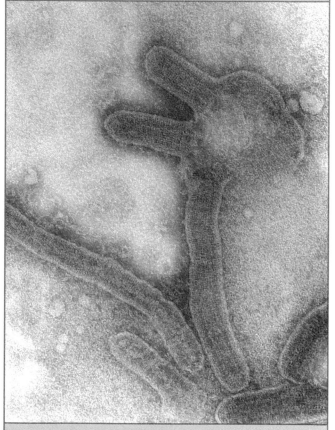

This negative stained transmission electron micrograph (TEM), captured by F.A. Murphy in 1968, depicts a number of Marburg virus virions, which had been grown in an environment of tissue culture cells. Marburg hemorrhagic fever is a rare, severe type of hemorrhagic fever, which affects both humans and non-human primates. Caused by a genetically unique zoonotic (that is, animal-borne) RNA virus of the filovirus family, its recognition led to the creation of this virus family. The four species of Ebola virus are the only other known members of the filovirus family.

Source: CDC/F. A. Murphy; Cynthia Goldsmith

Legionnaires' Disease Outbreak (1976)

Outbreak of new disease at Legionnaires' conference in Philadelphia

Toxic Shock Syndrome Case-Control Studies Initiated (1980)

Link between high absorbency tampons and life-threatening reaction to S. aureus bacteria

Smallpox Eradication Successful (1980)

WHO declares smallpox eradicated throughout the globe. Similar eradication campaigns underway for polio and measles; neither attained by 2007.

First Cases of PCP Pneumonia Disclosed in MMWR (1981)

Five cases of PCP pneumonia, generally found only in elderly or severely immunocompromised persons, found in healthy homosexual males. This is the first notice of what becomes the era of AIDS.

Identification of Virus that Causes AIDS (mid-1980s)

HTLV-III/LAV identified from blood of AIDS patients (1983–1985); in 1986, virus that causes AIDS called HIV.

Prions identified (1980s)

Family of neurological diseases including scrapie, kuru, Creutzfeldt-Jakob Disease, bovine spongiform encephalopathy, and new variant Creutzfeldt-Jakob Disease identified to be caused by an infectious protein. Previously not thought possible, the prion contains no nucleic acids at all. It is not susceptible to medications nor to usual extremes of heat (only autoclaving at >121° C). Prion-caused diseases have generally lengthy incubation periods, and are spread though tissue transplantation or consumption. An outbreak of "Mad Cow" disease took place in late 1980s/early 1990s, primarily derived from consumption of diseased cows from the United Kingdom.

Emergence of E. Coli 0157:H7 (1982)

Identification of extremely dangerous pathogen for humans, spread primarily through food sources, such as beef or plant products.

Bacterial Agent Linked to Ulcer Formation (1994)

Helicobacter pylori linked to gastrointestinal ulcer formation, leading to new avenues of treatment. Other potential links with coronary heart disease possible.

Human Papillomavirus Infection (strains HPV-16 and HPV-18) Associated with Cervical Cancer (1990s)

HPV infection associated with cervical cancer development, in addition to condylomata (genital warts). In 2007, a study suggests that oral and throat cancers may also be linked with HPV infection.

SARS (1996)

Severe Acute Respiratory Syndrome identified. Readily transmissible and with high case fatality rate, rapid global coordination reduced deaths despite potential for widespread epidemic.

Avian Influenza (1997)

First cases of new strain of influenza, dubbed Avian Flu for the animals most likely to carry it and share with humans. This H5/N1 virus is highly dangerous and increases in livestock-to-human cases have been seen by 2007, though person-to-person transmission remains either nonexistent to date, or extremely rare.

Which other moments in infectious disease history would you like to see on this brief listing? There are so many—which do you think should be added?

What moments do you think will come next?

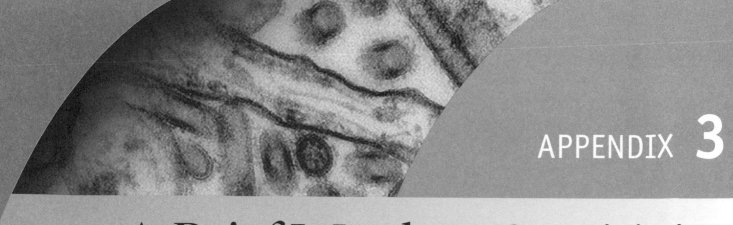

A Brief Word on Sensitivity and Specificity

Sensitivity and specificity are treated in nearly every introductory textbook. However, the concept is useful as a tool to characterize screening programs as well as surveillance systems. Thus the simple definitions and calculations are provided for you as a ready reference. For more information regarding screening programs, refer to the Resource List in Appendix 1 for textbooks that may be useful.

Using the 2 × 2 paradigm introduced in the text, we have only a slight modification. Instead of the rows being labeled exposed/non-exposed, they are now screen positive/screen negative. This refers to whether a person, who has been both screened as well as tested using the "gold standard", screened positive or negative. The columns are labeled disease/non-diseased as before, but referring now to the "gold standard", which is the best diagnostic tool in use.

	Gold standard positive	Gold standard negative	
Screen positive	a	b	a + b
Screen negative	c	d	c + d
	a + c	b + d	a + b + c + d = N

- Sensitivity of the screening program is described as a/(a + c). That is, of the people that are positive, what proportion are revealed as positive on the new screening tool? A high sensitivity suggests that there are fewer people given false negative results.
- Specificity of the screening program is described as d/(b + d). That is, of the people that are negative, what proportion are revealed as negative on the new screen-

ing tool? A high specificity suggests that there are fewer people given false positive results.
- Predictive value positive of the screening program is described as a/(a + b). That is, of the people that screen positive, how many really are positive? This is a measure of program yield. As the prevalence of the disorder under study increases within the population, the predictive value positive also increases.
- Predictive value negative of the screening program is described as d/(c + d). That is, of the people that screen negative, how many really are negative? This measure is affected by the number of false negatives in the program.

You can also look at the table like this:

	Gold standard positive	Gold standard negative	
Screen positive	Number who screened positive who were positive (true positives)	Number who screened positive who were negative (false positives)	Total screened positive
Screen negative	Number who screened negative who really were positive (false negatives)	Number who screened negative who were negative (true negatives)	Total screened negative
	Total with disease	Total with disease	Total participants

As applied to a surveillance system instead of a screening program, the idea of sensitivity can be used to see how many people are "caught" by the system, using various measures (e.g., case definitions, diagnostic studies) as the "gold standard".

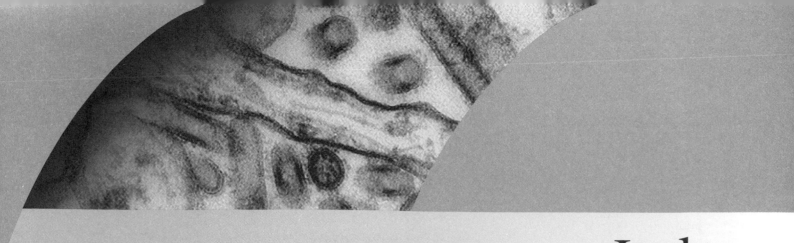

Index

Locators followed by *t, f,* or *n* denote tables, figures, and notes